The Caduceus Sword

The First Physicians' Strike

By

Adrian Philips, MD

This is entirely a work of fiction, and the events, settings, characters, insurance entities, medical societies, associations and organizations are fictitious and a product of the author's imagination. Furthermore, there is not, nor is there any intention to attempt to imply or portray, any similarity or resemblance to any existing person, living or dead, or any entity.

ISBN: 1-4107-6126-6 (e-book)
ISBN: 1-4107-6125-8 (Paperback)

Library of Congress Control Number: 2003093633

This book is printed on acid free paper.

Printed in the United States of America
Bloomington, IN

They are reproduced with the kind permission of Hunter Marine and the gracious assistance of Kit Keating

1stBooks - rev. 07/05/03

Dedication

To my Mother, who taught me to read
To my Father, who taught me to excel
And to my wife, who inspired me

Disclaimer

As is the case in any literary work, the author writes, at least in part, from his own personal life experiences. I am, in actual fact, a Board Certified surgeon in the private practice of medicine. This novel is broadly based on my observations in my practice, and written from the perspective of a dedicated physician, embattled and frustrated by the current dismal state of our national healthcare delivery system.

It is, however, a novel. It is entirely a work of fiction. None of the events described in this book ever occurred. The names, people, places, characters, events, societies, insurance entities, and all things are the product of the author's imagination and are fictitious. Any resemblance of events, places, things, or to actual persons, living or dead, is entirely and purely coincidental.

The Physician's Oath

I swear by Apollo Physician, by Asclepius, by Health, by Panacea, and by all the gods and goddesses, making them my witnesses, that I will carry out, according to my ability and judgment, this oath and this indenture...I will use treatment to help the sick according to my ability and judgment, but never with a view to injury and wrongdoing. Neither will I administer a poison to anybody when asked to do so, nor will I suggest such a course. Similarly, I will not give a woman a pessary to cause abortion. I will keep pure and holy both my life and my art...In whatsoever houses I enter, I will enter to help the sick, and I will abstain from all intentional wrongdoing and harm, especially from abusing the bodies of man or woman, bond or free. And whatsoever I shall see or hear in the course of my profession in my intercourse with men, if it be what should not be published abroad, I will never divulge, holding such things to be holy secrets. Now if I carry out this oath, and break it not, may I gain forever reputation among all men for my life and my art.

Attributed to
Hippocrates
460-377 B.C.

Translated by W.H.S. Jones (Loeb Classical Library)

Tampa Regional Medical Center
June 28
11:35PM

The Emergency Room was bedlam, total chaos. Patients filled every room and cubicle, with their family members overflowing into the corridors. Further congesting the packed hallways were ill patients laying on gurneys, their belongings in bright yellow plastic bags at their feet. The human stench was oppressive. Mixed with the pervasive, stale odor of urine and feces was the heavy, sickly sweet smell of human blood. Vomit streaked the floor where a drunk lay passed out, curled up in a corner. A nurse threw a towel over the putrid mess, glancing briefly at the prostrate form. Irate family members accosted personnel, each demanding immediate care for their loved ones. The staff rushed past, not having the time to explain triage in layman's terms.

Above the din of cries and moans, sharp commands and screams came from the trauma room where two MVA victims thrashed on bloody examination tables. The staff gravitated to the unfolding drama of their struggle, as X-ray technicians and support personnel rushed to assist in the Code Blue.

In the trauma room, the attending ER physician worked feverishly on one of the victims, a once pretty girl in her twenties. She had been ejected from a pick-up truck, and thrown onto the highway before slamming into a metal sign post. She was comatose, having suffered massive blunt head trauma. Dried blood caked her face and matted hair. A huge flap of scalp was torn away, revealing the white glistening surface of the skull. Black bruises on her flank indicated internal injuries, and the physician suspected she had fractured her spine horribly. He stabilized her neck, and ordered X-rays of the cervical spine, thoracic spine and lumbar spine. She had been intubated at the scene by the paramedics, and was already on a ventilator. He quickly evaluated her hemodynamic status, and turned to the other victim.

The driver of the truck was athletic and handsome, also in his twenties. He was screaming abuse and obscenities at the nurse as she tried to draw blood gases from his wrist. As he thrashed violently, the needle flew from her hand, skittering across the floor. The physician calmly scanned the man's twisting body and concluded that he had not suffered significant musculoskeletal trauma. His altered mental status concerned the doctor. This type of behavior could be the result of head injury, but judging from the unmistakable smell of alcohol on his breath, there were other factors to consider. The attending ordered the man restrained, and contemplated sedating him. His vital signs were strong, so he decided to watch him for a while, knowing that eventually the drunk would tire himself out. As he stood over the cursing man, he marveled how fate seemed to protect drunken drivers. Time and again, he had seen the victims of drunks die solitary gruesome deaths, separated from the comfort of their families, attended only by strangers like himself. Invariably, the drunks suffered minimal injury. Trauma experts had no theory to explain this phenomenon, but the doctor knew it to be fact, just as he knew that the full moon increased violent and bizarre human behavior. He recalled the medical school dictum: The First Lesson of Maturity - Life Isn't Fair. Nowhere is that rule more evident than in the ER, he thought as he strode toward his cluttered desk and telephone. He needed to discuss both cases with the neurosurgeon on call.

Outside the closed double doors of the ER, in the jammed reception area, another scene was being played out. Hundreds of people crowded the large waiting room, spilling out of the entrance into the ambulance driveway and blocking the transfer of patients as they arrived. Crying children sat on the filthy floors, aged infirm nursing home patients sat hunched over in wheelchairs where their attendants had abandoned them. Injured drunks and sick homeless lay curled asleep on the dirty gray linoleum, oblivious to the chaos around them.

Amid this pathetic throng of humanity, a pool of brilliant light illuminated an attractive news correspondent as she prepared to tape her story. The cameraman gently cleared an area for himself, as the light technician balanced his color and angles. The woman adjusted her Armani silk dress, and looked straight into the camera lens.

"This is Karin Sweetser, reporting live from the Emergency Room of Tampa Regional Medical Center, where the conditions are deteriorating rapidly. I am told that over seven hundred patients have been seen in the past eighteen hours, and it appears that there are at least another two or three hundred still waiting to be seen. This is more than twenty times the normal ER patient load, and clearly the system is stretched to the limit. The hospital spokeswoman has informed our local affiliate that the ER medical staff has been tripled and that patients are being diverted to the hospital's outpatient clinics, but you can see that even this measure has neither solved the backload nor improved the conditions within the Emergency Department."

She paused for drama. "I can feel the desperation of these patients as they wait interminably to be seen. Yet, tragically, this is a man-made crisis. This frantic scene is not the result of a terrorist attack or natural disaster or train derailment or plane crash or Ebola virus epidemic. This is the result of a hitherto unknown occurrence, a malignant and dangerous precedent in American healthcare. This is the third day of a city-wide physician strike. And as of now, there is no end in sight." She concluded the report as the waiting room swirled around her, the communal rage unaffected by the presence of the worldwide news coverage.

"This is Karin Sweetser, live from Tampa."

Chapter 1

Two months earlier.

Miami
April 25
11:05PM

His rage was intense, painful. For four nights and three days, Juan Gonzales, Jr. had been drinking and doing meth, sleeping fitfully on the damp couch in his aunt's living room. Their ramshackle two bedroom house was empty, save for him. Two years ago, Juan Gonzales, Sr., his father, had returned to his home in Coahuila, Mexico, to avoid several arrest warrants for auto theft. Nothing had ever been heard from him since his departure. Juan Gonzales Jr., known as Loco by fellow gang members, spoke proudly of his sire. He bragged of how mean his padron was, how he would return when the statute of limitations was run, that his father knew that Loco didn't need no help.

Loco's mother had never married Juan Gonzales, Sr. Loco was born at the county hospital, his birth weight low due to his mother's smoking and cocaine addiction. From the start he was an aberration, and he would do his best to make the worst of a bad situation. Loco spent his childhood in the care of his addict mother and her many boyfriends. He was valuable to her only because of the additional cash benefits she could demand with a dependent child. Eventually, her string of arrests for prostitution and drug possession landed her in jail, and Loco in the custody of the state. Subsequent hearings established that she was an unfit mother and the guardianship of Loco was given to her sister. He grew up with the sister, the both of them surviving on the money she made waitressing in bars. Many boyfriends came and went but the sister never liked one enough to keep him very long. Loco had been introduced to the gangs by one of these men, a tattooed felon with a small teardrop inked under his eye. Loco knew that it meant that he had killed a man in prison, that it signified mock regret for the taking of that life. Loco wanted to be bad, to be feared, to be dangerous. The gangs would do that all for him.

He found his way into Los Malvados, starting by holding weapons for his aunt's boyfriend. Children under the age of ten cannot be detained or arrested under Florida law for holding guns or drugs. They were perfect mules for the harder, older adolescents who used them to move automatic weapons and heroin, cocaine and speed across town and across county lines.

The ex-con gradually moved him up in the organization as he grew older and he became an initiated member on his thirteenth birthday. Four years later, the memory of that long night still sent a cold shiver down his spine.

But it was a much more powerful urge driving him to the limit of his sanity. The brutality and violence of his abbreviated childhood could not preclude the unavoidable development of passion and love. Juanita was the object of Loco's burning desire. She was rare and beautiful without question. Her smooth brown skin and green eyes teased him and drew him deeper, only to leave him lingering, aching. Her girlish body held pleasures that Loco wanted but did not yet fully understand. But Juanita was the property of rival gang.

He did not know that to her, he was only a stupid boy; easily fooled and useful to keep her lover jealous and interested as the novelty of her body wore off. Loco would provide her with drugs and money, knowing that she must love him, that soon she would leave the other and be his woman. The love and the ache in his chest, the gnawing emptiness in his belly when he thought of her in his bed drove him to the brink of insanity.

Tonight was worse than any before. Many nights he had waited for her to drive by or call him on his cell phone. He held the Motorola in one hand and drank the warm Corona with the other. He was coming down again, the cocaine high so sweet that it hurt to lose it. She had called hours ago, promising to be by at nine o'clock. It was almost eleven and her car still had not driven up.

Where the fuck is she? She knows I am waiting here with this dope, he thought bitterly. He cursed, pulling on the beer. He was holding a vial of crack and some powder. Two hundred dollars street value, to be given for free, for the elusive prayer of love, lust. He couldn't bring himself to believe what his homeboys told him. That she was a just a prick tease, that he would never get close enough to smell that pussy. They laughed at him, heightened his anger and shame.

Fuck them. Fuck her, he thought.

The cellular phone chirped, startling him. His heart sped as he answered.

"Loco? Baby, I can't make it tonight. Can you save the dope for me? Please? He knows about you and he is mad pissed. I can't come over no more." Her voice was slurred and thick from drugs.

"But why not? I can take care of you. You don't need him. I'll be your man, I will take care of you." He rambled, terrified by the fear of losing her before ever having her. The sure knowledge that this would mean an immediate, violent confrontation welled up in his throat, paralyzing him. He knew the reputation of his rival. He knew that to even speak of taking another man's woman is to invite death. Now neither man had any choice. The fatal dance had begun.

But she wasn't listening, didn't care. She never had any interest in him as anything other than a source of free cocaine. He was a punk, no power, no future. She was too stoned to lie anymore, and simply dropped the receiver of the pay phone and walked away.

Loco assumed that their conversation had been heard by her lover. He knew there was little time. He went quickly to his bedroom and pulled from a drawer his most prized possession, an Ingram MAC-11 machine pistol. There was beauty in its ugliness. The weapon had been designed as a sidearm for the US Military but was bypassed in the testing and selection process. The 9mm semi-automatic version of the weapon fired from an open bolt making it relatively inaccurate as a pistol, but it was completely legal, cheap and readily available. Loco had made a minor alteration in the bolt assembly that kept the sear from engaging, and transformed into a fully automatic weapon with a terrifying rate of fire and ease of control. He held it reverently, caressing the cold dull metal as he screwed on the cylindrical barrel extension. He had gotten the extension at a gun show for fifteen dollars, and it gave the gun an even more lethal appearance and better control. He tapped the heavy magazine as he had seen done in the movies, and slid it into the pistol grip.

He snorted four lines of cocaine mixed with speed for good luck. Then he turned off the lights in the living room, sat in the big yellow chair and watched the street.

Chapter 2

Miami
American Arena
11:36PM
April 25

It had been one of the wildest NBA games of the season. The Miami Heat had been eliminated in the Eastern Conference play-offs too many times by the Knicks in the past. They were determined to defeat them tonight, and there was bad blood between the two teams. The New York Knicks had been trash-talking in the press about how the Heat was even weaker now than in past years. The game had wide promotion and hype all over Florida, and had lived up to everyone's expectations. The contest was close from the start. The Heat were victorious with a three point shot in the last seconds of overtime.

John Strahan, Jorge Diaz and Mike Peterson had driven John's dad's BMW 750iL down from Tampa to see the game, under the provision that there would be no drinking on the trip. John's father David, a prominent CPA in town, had serious misgivings about the four hour trip at night, but his wife told him the boy was going to have to grow up sometime. John had never seen a live NBA game, and the Heat-Knicks game promised to be thrilling. So he gave John the keys to his new 750iL, thinking that if they did have an accident, the airbags and structure of the touring sedan would protect them from serious injury. Then he gave John a last stern admonition about drinking and driving and said good-bye, knowing that he would worry until they returned.

All three boys were seniors in high school and friends from the football team. They were good kids but still underage and unused to the effects of alcohol. Jorge and Mike had several beers at the game, enjoying the festive mood and happy to be away from home. No one here was likely to get word back to their parents that they were drinking in Miami, and by the time that they were back in Tampa, their family hopefully would be asleep. John, true to his word, was not drinking.

Their tickets had been given to John's dad by a physician client who could not attend due to a society meeting. For the boys, the night had been a taste of the high life. Outstanding seats, an outstanding basketball game, freedom and a couple of beers and now the drive home in an $80,000 European sedan.

"It don't get any better than this. Man, this leather smells good." Mike drawled from the back seat as they negotiated their way slowly out of the parking lot. Cars were lined up bumper to bumper and the going was slow. Mike was draped across the seats in the back, wishing he had pissed one last time before they left.

"Hey, John, I gotta take a leak, man." he concluded.

"You have to wait. We're in the parking lot."

"Shit, man, my bladder's about to bust."

"Hang on. We're almost on the road."

The line of cars slowly snaked out the lot and into the area around the enormous arena. Somewhere, blocks ahead of the boys, two drunken drivers had collided trying to merge lanes. The entire line of cars halted. After five minutes, horns began to start blowing. But no further motion of the line.

"I'm going to have to piss out the window." Mike pleaded.

"Wait till I can get to the next road and we will go down some sidestreet and you can piss in a fucking bush. You piss in the back of my dad's car and you'll be walking home." John found the next right turn and headed away from the jammed traffic.

They drove along the railroad tracks, still unable to find anywhere to stop. No suitable dark alley could be found to piss safely. The entertainment district gave way to deserted warehouses and tire recycling compounds between rows of tenement houses. After two turns and some long stretches of concrete brightly lit with the orange anti-crime lights, the boys were lost. No one said a word.

Finally they found themselves in a residential section. John slowed the car as they all looked out the tinted windows for a poorly lit bush, tree, or garbage can. Anywhere for Mike to relieve himself without commotion or discovery. They made a left onto Frio Street.

"Hey, John, stop. Back-up. There was an alley back there. It will work. It will work. Stop and let me pee." Mike was already opening the door.

"Wait up. I'll back up. Hang on for two more seconds." John backed the car past a cluster of metal garbage cans, and then pulled deep into the alley and shut off the lights.

Chapter 3

Frio Street
12:02AM
April 26

Loco had been watching the silver sedan drive by slowly, and had seen the three men inside. As he watched, the car drove into the alley next to his house, and the driver shut off his lights. By this time his fear and rage had risen to full pitch; his ability to reason lost to the fury and the drugs. When he heard the car door open, he knew they were the men who had come for him. He didn't know or care which man was Juanita's lover. They would all die. Or he would die. It didn't matter.

He released the safety on the MAC and sprinted out the back door and around the house. A wooden fence separated him from the alley where Mike leaned against a telephone pole and urinated. He rounded the end of the fence, spotted the car ten yards down the alley and stopped in the shadows. It was now or never.

He screamed incomprehensibly as he let the MAC fire on full automatic. A fireball of orange-yellow flame blossomed from the muzzle and he could hear the ripping of the rounds as they exited the short barrel. The empty cases flew past him on the right, the powder fragments burning his eyes and face. He saw movement in the car, someone trying to get the big BMW moving. But the car stalled with a jerk, and the engine died. For the first time he noticed the tall gringo standing to his right in the alley.

Mike had his back to the car when the shooting began and when he turned, the scene paralyzed him momentarily. He pissed all over himself. Loco seemed to turn in slow motion, bringing the weapon to bear on him. Mike thought how odd that he would die like this, pissing in an alley. He heard the first two rounds crack and felt a hammer slam into his left shoulder and spin him around. He looked up to see the wiry gunman looking down at his gun with puzzlement. A spent case had stovepiped in the ejection port, jamming the action. Loco had no idea how to fix it.

Mike responded instinctively, the result of years as a linebacker in varsity football. He rushed Loco, a low yell coming from deep in his chest. The distance was less than four yards between them and he felt no pain from his shoulder wound.

Loco heard the yell, and recoiled as Mike closed the distance between them. Realizing that his pistol was inoperable, he threw it in the face of the charging man. This split second action saved him, giving him the time to kick over a garbage can and duck around the fence. Then, he was gone.

Stunned and disoriented, Mike Peterson stood in the alley, watching the direction where Loco had disappeared. His shoulder throbbed, and he began to feel weak and nauseous. His heart pounding wildly and his mind numb, he turned and staggered to the bullet-ridden sedan. What he found within would stay with him for the rest of his life.

Strahan had been in the driver's seat, twisted around to see the source of the gunfire, when he was hit. Two bullets had struck him, one in the cheek and one in the side, after penetrating the seat. The bullet to the cheek had torn away the central part of the face and nose. Blood was everywhere, over the front seat, dash, and steering wheel. He had tried to exit the car, but was unable to release the shoulder belt. His body was collapsed half in and half out of the driver's door.

Jorge Diaz was not in much better shape. He had also been turning to the rear of the car when the shooting began. Loco had aimed for the rear window, and gotten great satisfaction as the bullets tracked an irregular pattern through the splintering glass. One of the projectiles, flattened and deformed by its passage through the glass-polymer laminate used in BMW automobiles, had impacted on the left aspect of his lower jaw. The shell fragment now was the size of a quarter as it passed from his left jaw, through the bone, through the tongue and then through the right central portion of the jaw. During this transit, it broke into two or three pieces and shredded the upper jaw and the central portion of his face.

The shock of the impact combined with the loss of blood and inability to speak turned Jorge into a zombie. He sat slumped in the passenger's seat, his head bobbing and blood and saliva dripping from the torn mass that had once been a handsome, young face. Mike looked closely at him, checked him quickly and then ran around the car to see to John. All the time, he yelled for help, for someone to call the police and request an ambulance. John was half out of the car, and Mike could see that he was not breathing or moving. Frantically he talked to him, cradling his head and begging him not to die. With tears in his eyes, screaming for help from the cautiously gathering group of locals, he ran back to Jorge and tended gently, as best he could, to his gravely injured friend. It was only when the paramedics came that anyone noticed that his shirt was soaked in blood.

Chapter 4

Bay Area Medical Society Meeting
Hillsborough Country Club
April 25
7:03PM

"I hate these medical society dinners," she whispered to her husband as the waitress passed with the coffee. There were three other couples at the table, physicians and their wives, chatting among themselves.

"Sorry sweetheart. It is just once a year and I promise you won't have to come to next year's meeting. This is my last term as Florida Medical Association delegate. Persevere, Britt. The food is great, isn't it? Have another Chardonnay." William Coltrane, MD, knew that the offer of wine would not placate his wife. But he had to try. The private practice of surgery, to be successful, required a great deal of socializing and politics. And his practice was successful. Hopefully, someday his lovely wife would accept that.

He had enjoyed the cocktail hour, when he could move around the reception and talk with his friends and colleagues. These meetings were one of the few times when doctors could talk freely with each other about patients, hospital issues, even other physicians. All other times, communication about patient care was limited to written notes in the patient record. One had to be very circumspect about what was written in the patient record. Often the truth was hidden between the lines. But during the cocktail hour, eased by the free flow of spirits, revelations were made, and secrets were divulged. In vino veritas.

But the cocktail hour was over, and they were seated with friends.

Coltrane looked around the club's main dining room, set elegantly with starched linen tablecloths and gold rimmed porcelain china place settings. He recognized all the faces, knew all the physicians and their reputations. From one of the head tables, Kathleen Brady, the Director of Physician Relations from Saint Mary's, smiled and nodded at them. Coltrane smiled back at her, remembering how she had navigated them through the process of opening his practice when he had arrived in Tampa years ago. The hospital had recruited nationally for a qualified hand surgeon, and Coltrane hadn't known why until he and Britt visited for an interview as he was finishing his training. Kathleen had told them that the only hand surgeon on staff was in his sixties, and consistently refused to take any ER call, or see indigent and Medicaid patients. The medical staff had finally forced him to participate in the ER call schedule, but when he was called at night or on the weekends, or at an inconvenient time, he would rarely respond. And if he did respond, he would tell the frustrated ER doctor that the injury was better treated by an orthopedic surgeon, or a plastic surgeon, or anyone but himself. She had made it very clear to Coltrane that if he was available, took ER call, and accepted all comers, he would establish himself in the medical community very rapidly.

Hard work for no pay was nothing new to Coltrane. He had spent the past eleven years as an indentured servant. Four years in medical school, where he got the privilege of paying tens of thousands of dollars to learn the art of medicine. Part of that training included performing countless hours of menial labor, grudgingly refered to as "scut work", for the nurses, residents, and attendings. Drawing blood, taking stool samples, running urine samples to the lab and checking lab reports. The tasks were unending. The medical student was the lowest form of life on a hospital floor, outranked even by the orderlies and nurses aides. Med students all got treated like shit. Then graduation, the swearing of the Hippocratic Oath, and a weekend of partying and tremendous relief, satisfaction.

The respite was painfully brief. Coltrane had gone directly into a General Surgery residency, five years of brutal hours, relentless stress and social deprivation. Three quarters of surgeons' marriages succumbed during this trial by fire. And the pay was below minimal wage. Coltrane had once calculated that he was being paid $2.47 an hour during his internship. After one year of surgical internship, he finished four more years of surgical residency, performing as surgeon or assistant in over four thousand major procedures. He was very well trained.

But in an era of rapidly advancing medical and surgical technology, new procedures and approaches, Coltrane had taken the difficult step of delaying private practice in order to pursue further specialty training. Arthroscopy, microsurgery and laser techniques were evolving, and he wanted to be skilled in their application. That meant two more years in fellowship, honing his art. Again at less than minimal wage. Again in a subservient position, with little true control of his life and time.

So working for free hadn't bothered Coltrane. At least now he was getting paid half the time, and now he had partial control of his life. And as time progressed, he earned the respect of the ER doctors and nurses, and the respect of the operating room nurses.

Initially, he had been sent only the worst possible patients, the worst possible cases. Patients that nobody wanted to have. Procedures that nobody wanted to do. Diseases that nobody wanted to treat. AIDS. TB. Hepatitis C. Modern day lepers. Drug addicts with abscesses where they had been injecting with filthy needles, homeless patients with tuberculosis who refused to take their medication, or were too insane to be regimented, hand fractures from bar fights, and countless unwanted, no pay patients. An established physician would not send one of his longtime patients to a new, unknown specialist. Even a well trained one. It took time to gain the trust and referrals of doctors. And many doctors already had referral patterns to another surgeon. Or maybe it was up to the office girls how and where to refer the patients. There were many obstacles to overcome.

Gradually, over the months and years, Coltrane had established a solid reputation as a skilled surgeon. More importantly, he was known for his integrity, and his honor. He was scrupulously honest with his patients, always placing their welfare above all other considerations. Coltrane was not altruistic; he had learned years ago that it is always better to do the right thing.

Graduation from medical school had been the proudest moment of his life. Each newly ordained physician recited the Hippocratic Oath, en masse, in unison. Each considered this significance in his or her own way. For Coltrane, he remembered two guiding principles.

Primum, non nocere.

Firstly, do no harm.

And secondly: Observe, and evaluate honestly. For him, the oath was sacred. His responsibility to his patients transcended religion, transcended secular law. Transcended self. His guiding principle was always the patient's best interest. Under no conditions had he ever violated that course, or would he. He could live by whatever that code brought him. It was simply karma that his ethical standards had made him the first choice among the hand and trauma surgeons in Tampa-St. Pete. As he looked around the ballroom, a feeling of pride and accomplishment washed over him.

"Bill, what's the current status of breast implants? Every new patient I see comes from the same attorney." Jack Farrara asked Coltrane. Jack was a brilliant internist who was seeing a record number of patients with complaints about their breast implants.

"Jack, as a general surgeon, I don't put implants in my patients. I refer all my breast cancer patients to a plastic surgeon who uses implants routinely, both for cosmetic and reconstructive indications. You can ask him for his opinion, but I know that the recent studies from the Mayo Clinic and Harvard show that there is no evidence of any causative link between silicone and the various autoimmune diseases that are the focus of the litigation. But it is a highly charged emotional issue, so I recommend implant removal to all my patients if they have serious concerns regarding the toxicity of silicone."

Jack agreed, but continued. "This attorney will send the woman to a quack in Miami where she gets a $25,000 work-up, including MRI, CT scans and blood tests for lupus and anti-silicone antibodies. I have seen the reports and the bills. Then the guy in Miami refuses to see her again. The patients all end up on our doorstep, confused. They have been told that they have silicone poisoning. It's outrageous."

Coltrane was about to mention that he had reported that particular doctor to the investigative branch of the Florida Medical Association, but was interrupted by an announcement from the podium.

"Ladies and gentlemen, it appears that I am the only candidate for President of the society this year. Dr. Fredricks had to withdraw due to other obligations," announced the incumbent president in his paternalistic tone. "As per the bylaws, nominations may come from the floor at this time, followed by voting this evening."

After a period of quiet murmuring subsided, silence fell on the group. The small faction of supporters of Dr. Fredricks were disappointed, however there was no recourse for them. Fredricks and the current president were similar in their age, views and standing in the community. Both had large internal medicine practices and held considerable sway in the community in terms of hospital committees and perhaps more significantly, in their referral and consultation patterns with the other specialists. They were crucial elements in the life-sustaining "food chain" of the private practice of medicine.

The silence continued.

Coltrane broke it. "I have been a member of this society for fifteen years now, and I have watched medicine change dramatically during that time. We all know the changes; I do not need to enumerate them for you. I wonder if I am the only member who feels that our society spends too much time and too much money in attempts at PR and the pursuit of political correctness; i.e. campaigns about the obvious perils of smoking, where to find a non-smoking restaurant, and our concerns about alcohol abuse and teenage pregnancies. These are all very important issues, don't mistake me; but they are national and cultural in scope, and we as a small local group of physicians have no chance or hope of making progress of any significance."

He was on a roll. The two glasses of Chardonnay certainly helped, but Coltrane was a man who didn't like public speaking, and had to be incensed to launch into such a tirade. Once started, however, he rambled effectively and passionately.

"My feeling is that this society should concentrate its efforts on improving the quality of patient care, firstly, and improving the quality of private practice, secondly. We need much greater input into hospital and insurance HMO, PPO, and managed care plans than we have now. We need power to determine treatments rather than asking the insurance bureaucrats what is available. We need adequate reimbursement for services, and the elimination of payer's red-tape and their tactics of intentional stalling. These trends will only continue unless we make a stand. The tail is wagging the dog, and we just allow it."

Coltrane sat.

"Nominate me," he whispered to Ferrara.

"I nominate Bill Coltrane for President." Ferrara voiced. Someone quickly seconded the nomination.

"Any further nominations?" the president asked. When none were forthcoming, he concluded the discussion sternly and ordered voting to take place.

The result was a landslide victory for Coltrane over the incumbent president. The opinions he had expressed mirrored much of the increasing frustration and impotence of the assembled doctors, and they wanted change as well. Somewhat surprised at the result of the election, Coltrane took the podium from his disgruntled predecessor. His acceptance speech was very brief, and was interrupted twice by the persistent distinctive ring of his cellphone, telling him he was being paged by his answering service. He concluded the meeting, thanked the assemblage for their vote of confidence. As he left the podium, he began scrolling through the alphanumeric messages, and searched for a quiet place to return his calls.

Chapter 5

Miami
April 26
1:13AM

While the paramedics worked feverishly on his two friends, Mike Peterson had the presence of mind to call home on the car's cellular phone. He quickly gave the details of the shootings to his sister when she answered, and told her to inform the Diaz and Strahan families as well. But before he could finish, the EMTs cut short his conversation. He was separated from the others and examined on the curb, then sent directly to the closest hospital.

It was a parent's most devastating nightmare. In Tampa, the situation was frantic, confused. The Peterson family had relayed the news of the shootings to the Strahans and the Diazes. Each family left a member at their homes to monitor the phone, and the parents assembled at Strahan's. The anguish was thick. All they knew was that all three boys had been shot in Miami, and that Mike had been able to talk on the phone. But why had someone taken the phone from him, and why didn't the other boys call? If they were at a hospital, then why didn't the hospital call? Were they all dead? Did the killers take the phone from Mike? Why would anyone shoot the boys? The mothers were too shocked to be in tears. The men were pacing, their frustration and anger rising.

"Have you called the car, David?" Diaz asked.

"I've called every two or three minutes since I heard, but the phone must be off or the car's ignition is off; the phone is inactive. I'll keep trying, but I don't want to tie up the phone," Strahan returned.

"You don't have call waiting?" Peterson asked irritably.

"My son is shot and you want to quiz me about my fucking phone services?" Strahan snapped.

"Screw this. I'm going to Miami." Peterson headed for his wife and the door.

"Please, please, let's not make this any worse. Why are you fighting? What has happened to our boys?" Mary Strahan started crying, and the room fell silent as the three mothers huddled together.

"Listen, I don't know what to do. I am going to call the Miami Police and see if any shootings have been reported." Strahan began to search numbly for the phone numbers of Miami Emergency Services.

Several phone calls later, he discovered that there had been a shooting near Port Boulevard that evening; and the three victims, all male, had been sent to different facilities. The names of the victims were unknown, but the disposition of one to Jackson Memorial Hospital and the other two to Bayside Community Hospital was verified by the police and the EMT service. Strahan made further calls and found that Mike Peterson had been taken to Jackson Memorial while the other boys were taken to the ER at Bayside.

"Why were they separated?" Peterson asked, calmer now and relieved that they were still alive.

"I don't know, but I am going to call the hospital and find out; then I suggest that we all go up to Miami." Strahan answered.

"Look, Mike is at a different hospital as John and Jorge. We are going to go in our car. I will keep in touch with you all by phone." Peterson gave Strahan his cell phone number, and hurriedly left with his wife to drive to Miami.

Strahan dialed the Bayside ER number. The triage nurse answered, and explained that both John and Jorge had facial trauma; gunshot wounds that penetrated the flesh and broke bones of the face. She described in carefully chosen layman's terms that the jaw bones were broken by the bullets and that a surgeon had been called to evaluate the boys. Their condition was stable and that the family could come and visit at any time. She then apologized and explained that she must get back to her patients.

Strahan immediately found William Coltrane's office number from his Rolodex. Coltrane and he had met at a charity benefit years ago and had been social acquaintances since, with Strahan helping with Coltrane's pension plan at times. It was Coltrane who had given Strahan his tickets for the game. Coltrane would know the best way to get the care that John and the boys would need.

Coltrane's answering service asked if the call was an emergency and if David was a patient. They would page the doctor.

Minutes later the phone rang, and a tired voice responded.

"Bill, this is David Strahan. I'm sorry to bother you this late, but John and two of his friends have been shot in Miami. I need your help. They're at Bayside Community Hospital and apparently have been shot in the face, both of them, in the jaw with broken bones. A surgeon is seeing them, but I don't know who. Can you see them; or can you tell me the name of a good plastic surgeon in Miami you recommend; or should they come down here?" Strahan rambled, anxious to form a plan of action, and leave for Miami.

Coltrane had been asleep, and was jolted quickly into awareness by the news. He often spoke to parents and relatives about their injured or sick loved ones, but rarely to friends in this manner. He listened to the details that Strahan provided.

"Based on the information that you have given me, I would have the boys transferred to Jackson Memorial Hospital as soon as possible. Now. *Tonight.* It may be that Bayside has good facilities for trauma, but I haven't heard of the hospital, so it is probably a community hospital with limited resources. The availability of specialty services may not be as good as at Jackson, and I can give you the names of several good surgeons there." Coltrane paused.

"Can you transfer him home to Tampa?" asked Strahan immediately.

"I would not bring him home yet. Once he has been stabilized at Bayside, request that he be transferred immediately to the Jackson Memorial Hospital in Miami, under the care of the Plastic Surgery Service. I'll call there when I get off the phone with you and arrange that the on call surgeon accepts your transfer. It should be no problem. They'll be able to take care of the immediate problems, and do any necessary surgery. If it is appropriate to bring him home, you can arrange that at a later date. I have no authority to act, since I am not the attending physician. You must do that yourself." Coltrane finished.

"That seems reasonable. I'm going to drive up now with Mary and the Diazes to Bayside and see how he is doing. Could you call and talk to the doctor in charge and find out what is going on? I have spoken to the nurse but you can get much more information, and understand it far better than I. I'll call you from Miami. Thanks for all your help. Hopefully, you will never have to know what this means to us." Strahan thanked Coltrane again and hung up. Grabbing his map of Miami, he headed out the door.

Coltrane found the phone number of Bayside through the operator, and called the ER. He asked to speak to the ER physician and was told that he was very busy with several patients. He then asked to speak with the nursing supervisor on call. She was likewise busy. His call was placed on hold and after several minutes, the administrative officer on call picked up the phone.

"Ralph Callahan here."

"Mr. Callahan, this is Dr. Coltrane in Tampa. I'm a trauma surgeon; I have been asked by the family of the Strahan boy to follow his status. I understand that both boys have gunshot wounds to the face. Can you give me some details about their condition please?

"Doctor, I would love to; but as you should know, since you are not the treating physician, I cannot release confidential patient information." Callahan responded coldly.

"Then perhaps you can answer questions about your facility? Do you have the new GE CAT scanner and MRI equipment?" Coltrane asked.

"Yes."

"Are you a Level I or II Trauma Center?"

"No."

"Do you have an anesthesiologist in house?"

"No, but one is on call and coming in right now. And we have called a plastic surgeon to evaluate the boys as well. I am quite sure that we have the situation completely under control. And now if you don't mind, it is late and I have a full day tomorrow." Callahan hung up.

Coltrane called the ER back several times, but was unable to get through to the ER physician. He left his home number and a message to call as soon as possible, then lay back in bed, wide awake.

Chapter 6

Miami
Bayside Community Hospital
April 26
4:50AM

When they arrived at Bayside Community Hospital, Strahan parked in the brightly lit driveway of the Emergency Room. As they got out of the car with the Diazes, an overweight security officer strode out and demanded that he move the car. Strahan bit back his rage and told the others to go inside as he reparked the car.

The hospital seemed brand new, and one could tell that the personnel were not fully accustomed to the new equipment and technology. No one was at the reception desk in the waiting area, and in the waiting room were the dregs of a long night; drunks gradually waking up, a victim of domestic assault sitting in the corner with filthy bare feet, trying to make amends with her attacker. Back from the bowels of the ER came the shrieks of an old woman, obviously drunk and obviously not appreciating the medical attention lavished upon her.

A nurse came through the swinging double doors, into the reception area. Strahan got a glimpse of the department before the doors shut. Disposable gowns and gloves and instruments littered the new tile floors, and several blood trails ran down the center of the aisle. People in white could be seen moving tensely; grim expressions on their faces. His stomach tightened and his pulse quickened.

"We are the parents of the boys involved in the shootings, Strahan and Diaz. Could we speak with the doctor?" Roberto Diaz asked softly.

"Yes, yes. Of course." The nurse pushed an intercom and spoke quickly into a phone, then was gone.

After a seemingly interminable wait, the nurse returned with the ER physician. Dr. Foster was in his late fifties; short, balding and disheveled. He snapped off his rubber gloves as he came through the door, and threw them in the direction of a wastebasket. His lids were heavy, and his eyes tired. Strahan became even more concerned by the physician's avoidance of eye contact during the nurse's introduction and while the doctor explained the boys' situation.

"Both boys were shot in the face by a high velocity projectile, ...er..., bullet, and John Straton was also hit in the right side of the abdomen as well.

I have stabilized them and we are waiting for a general surgeon and a plastic surgeon to further evaluate their injuries." Foster explained.

"It's Strahan, and I am his father, David Strahan. Am I to understand that the surgeons are not here yet? Weren't they called hours ago?" Strahan asked in disbelief.

"Yes, they were. I am sorry, but they're coming as fast as they can. It's not a concern; the boys are stable at this time. They are getting the best possible care. Please relax and I'll keep you posted on their progress. There is nothing that you can do to help at this time." With that, he turned to return to the ER.

"We want to see them. *NOW*!" Mary Strahan stated, slowly and forcefully.

Dr. Foster drew back from the intensity of the mother's fury. "I'm sorry, you can't see them just yet. We are in the middle of a procedure. When possible, I'll bring you all back."

"Then I want John and Jorge transferred at once to Jackson Memorial Hospital." Strahan looked to Diaz for agreement.

Diaz nodded concurrence. "Now."

Foster's face turned white, then red with anger and embarrassment. The request for transfer was a direct slap at his personal and professional ability, and implied that he and his staff lacked the training and talents to treat the patients in their care. In his arrogance, he refused to accept that there were others better trained, better equipped and better staffed to handle complex multiple trauma than he was. Without answering, he turned and strode back into the ER.

"What the fuck does that mean? Will he transfer them?" Strahan was becoming furious. A normally conservative professional, Strahan was raised in with a strong Protestant work ethic. He never cheated on his taxes, held the police in high esteem and paid respect to physicians by right of their extraordinary ability to aid the sick. But in the crucible of his child's severe injury, he was unable to control his mounting frustration and anger.

As Strahan paced and fumed, a tall slender man in a rumpled suit and tie emerged from a hospital corridor and approached the reception desk, speaking in low tones to the nurse behind the counter. Strahan overheard the conversation; the boys were the subject of the discussion. He walked over quickly.

"Are you the surgeon?" Strahan inquired hopefully.

"No, sorry. I am Ralph Callahan, Director of Hospital Community Relations. I'm the administrator on call this evening. I understand that you want the boys transferred to another hospital at this time?"

"Yes. We feel that they may get better support at a larger center." Strahan tried to be as tactful as he could.

"That is your choice, of course. Provided that the transfer is medically feasible. I will have our nurse coordinator help you with the arrangements." Callahan started to turn to speak to the nurse.

"What arrangements? What do you mean?" Strahan felt a heavy load descend upon him.

"Insurance pre-authorization for transfer. Acceptance of the patients by an attending physician at the facility you choose, Acceptance by the hospital administration, and so on. We can't just put the boys in a cab and send them off. Please be seated and I will have someone speak with you. You may want to get any insurance information you have organized. That will save time." He turned, spoke briefly with the nurse, and then strode out the glass doors to go home and back to sleep. He cursed the day he chose Hospital Administration over Hotel Administration. Patients' families were such a pain in the ass.

The nursing administrator on call was sympathetic. Strahan thought that there must really be a course in empathy in nursing school, just like there was a course in illegible handwriting in medical school. They talked about the need for more specialty services for the boys, and the supervisor agreed in theory. She asked for the name of John's family doctor. David said that neither John nor Jorge had seen a doctor for years except their team physician for the pre-season football exams. She inquired about their insurance plans, and David and Roberto gave her their wallet insurance cards. She explained that she would get the papers ready for the transfer, and be back with a progress report soon.

Time passed slowly. The vinyl seats stuck to their legs in the damp morning air, and the sullen looks from the white trash in the corner made them feel like a circus side-show. Why were people always so interested in the agony of others? Perhaps to diminish their own agony, Strahan thought. He returned the glare of the wiry, tattooed wife beater. Come on, *fuck with ME*, you little prick, Strahan thought as the man squinted at him. I'll give you a better dance than that little girl did.

He was awakened from his violent reverie by the supervisor's return.

"Mr. Diaz, your son will be transferred to JMH as soon as possible. He has been accepted by the Plastic Surgery Division there, and you can follow in a private car. I suspect his transfer will occur within the hour. Mr. Strahan, your insurance plan has refused to authorize transfer from this facility to JMH. They feel that this hospital has all the services that John needs, and transfer is unnecessary at this time." The nurse finished and looked hesitantly at Strahan.

"What do you mean?" Strahan was dumbstruck.

"Apparently you are in a HMO plan that does not allow unrestricted use of any hospital facility. This hospital is on the list of approved facilities, and by the terms of your coverage, you are required to use this facility," she explained. Strahan felt that she had recited this litany many times before.

"But we're not on a HMO plan. We have had the same coverage for years. It's not a HMO." Mary differed. She paid the bills regularly, noted the deductibles, and filed the contracts away in her computer's desk.

"This card and the 800 number I called gave me that information. You may give them a call and straighten it out if you like. Come with me to my office and we'll look into the problem. Mr. and Mrs. Diaz, you may go back and see Jorge before he is transferred." The supervisor started to turn and lead them into the administrative wing of the hospital, away from the ER and the boys.

Diaz looked apologetically at Strahan and touched his shoulder. "We will see to Jorge and take a cab to JMH. If I can help from there, please call me." Then he and his wife turned and hurried through the double doors.

Chapter 7

Bayside Community Hospital
April 26
5:50AM

The unraveling of the insurance situation was a nightmare. After dialing the 800 number on the back of the insurance card, and negotiating a slow and infuriating series of automated selections in English and Spanish, Strahan spoke with a weary operator in New Jersey. She only had access to limited information, but could tell him that they were indeed enrolled in a HMO product. He gave the phone to Mary. For several minutes, Mary argued to no avail with the representative. Mary was informed that the policy she purchased had been sold, along with thousands of other policies, to another insurance company. This was common practice in the insurance industry; not only with health, but also with life, home and car insurance products. The new guarantor of her policy had changed it into a HMO product, and had sent out information to that effect with the last renewal.

Mary asked to speak to the representative's supervisor. The woman responded by asking what her further questions were. Mary persisted in speaking to the supervisor, and was placed on hold. Then the line went dead. Mary cursed and slammed the phone down. She now began to recall that she had seen a two page letter and a list of local Tampa area hospitals enclosed with the last insurance bill. Since the list included their local hospital, she paid it no mind. Now, doubt crept into her mind. Was this her mistake? Would her failure to read the letter result in John being stranded here? Not getting the best care? Perhaps dying? She was overwhelmed with impending guilt, and broke into tears.

Strahan got back on the 800 line, but was repeatedly disconnected and finally gave up in frustration. He tried several times to have John transferred without the insurance pre-authorization, only to run into a wall of outright refusals and red tape. The hospitals would not even talk to him. He was told that transfer could only be arranged by physician to physician contact. When he became angry and screamed that they were talking about his son, the clerk just stated that it was a federal law; and hung up.

Strahan then tried to directly contact an ambulance company to arrange transfer, but was told that he would need payment pre-authorization from his insurance company first. He then went through the entire list of ambulances in the Yellow Pages to find one that would take MasterCard, but found that the minimum fee was $2900 and that his credit card had exceeded the available cash limit.

Finally, in frustration, he called Coltrane back.

Chapter 8

Tampa General Hospital
April 26
6:30AM

Coltrane was in the second floor nursing unit, finishing morning rounds when his cellphone messaged him. Seeing the Miami area code on the LCD display, he knew it was Strahan. He dialed the number. He hoped that it would be good news.

"Bill, I need your help. Jorge has been transferred to JMH, but John is still at Bayside, and I have been unable to move him. He's still in the ER. The doctors will not arrange transport, and the insurance company will not authorize transfer. I have nowhere to turn and I feel that he will die here if I can't get him out soon." Strahan pleaded.

Strahan was agitated and frustrated. He and Mary had been able to see John for a few brief moments earlier, and the visit had crushed their spirits. John had been heavily sedated, and had a large, clear plastic tube coming out of his side through which came volumes of bright red blood. His head was wrapped in dressings that were soaked in congealing blood and obscured his handsome face from the chin to just below the eyes. And the eyes were dull and lifeless. The effect had been crushing for Mary, and she sat in the corner, quietly weeping.

"David, can you patch me through to the general surgeon in charge?" Coltrane asked immediately.

Strahan arranged for the call to be routed to the ER with the help of the nursing supervisor.

"Dr. Meyer," an irritated voice responded.

"Dr. Meyer. This is Dr. Coltrane, a trauma surgeon in Tampa and a friend of the Strahan family. I'll be taking care of John when he's sent home. Can you tell me how he is doing?"

"Fairly well," the tired voice softened. "He has suffered a gunshot wound to the chest, through and through the right lower lobe of the lung. I've placed a chest tube and am doing a peritoneal lavage at this time. But I think that his chest wound has not communicated with the abdomen. His belly is benign. In addition, he has a gunshot wound to the midface which appears to be primarily a soft tissue injury. We're waiting for the plastic surgeon to evaluate that injury."

"He still has not been seen by a plastic surgeon, after five hours? Coltrane asked incredulously.

"Apparently the man on call has been in the OR at another hospital all night with a severe burn case, and we've had some trouble getting another surgeon. The ENT surgeon on call is an older guy who refuses to do facial plastic trauma. That's where we are now."

"What about the oral surgeon?" Coltrane demanded.

"They are not yet allowed admitting or operative privileges. This has been another problem that the medical staff has not yet resolved. You know, the usual turf wars that occur everywhere. You must have your share in Tampa as well."

"Dr. Meyer, this boy has been the victim of a random, drive-by shooting. He's not a criminal; he's a victim. He has insurance. Can you see what you can do to get the best available plastic, ENT or oral-maxillofacial surgeon to see him. Someone with experience in facial trauma. Midface wounds can be deceptive." Coltrane refrained from going into a lecture about the dangers of improperly treated facial trauma.

"Certainly. I'll do my best. The ER doc taking over the AM shift is Chas Nichols. He'll take good care of John, and I'll give him your number. I have 7:30 cases at Our Lady of Mercy. If I can help, please call." With that, Meyer hung-up.

"Shit," Coltrane cursed, and started the process of contacting David Strahan again. The nurse at the desk next to him smiled.

"Sorry," Coltrane grinned.

He finally got through to Strahan. "David, I spoke with the general surgeon who has seen John. He feels that the wounds are not life-threatening. John has a bullet wound to the lung, on the right side. The doctors have placed a plastic tube, a large but sterile plastic tube, to drain any blood or air out of his chest. The tube will stay for several days, and is not a serious concern. They are doing a peritoneal lavage, which is a procedure that injects fluid into the belly cavity to see if any organs have been injured. That is also a routine event. Dr. Meyer, the general surgeon, does not feel that the bullet injured any abdominal organ. That is very good news. What does concern me is that John has not yet been seen by a plastic surgeon. Meyer is going to try to call one, and if he has no luck, please call me within thirty minutes. Is the nursing supervisor that you spoke about nearby?"

"She is right here." Strahan looked over at her.

"Let me speak with her," Coltrane asked.

"Mrs. Davila," she took the phone from Strahan.

"Mrs. Davila, this is Dr. Coltrane in Tampa. Please bear with me; I'm not a member of your staff but I have an interest in the welfare of John Strahan. I am extremely concerned that his maxillofacial trauma has not been evaluated, and it is now seven hours after his admission. He needs an experienced max-face surgeon to evaluate his injury."

"A plastic surgeon has been called, and an ENT man as well. I will personally follow-up right now and see what is going on," she agreed, concerned.

"Thank you. Can you tell me who is the Chief of Plastic Surgery there?"

"Dr. Robert Westman. But he has already been called, and is in surgery at Miami General. You may not be able to reach him. May I have a number where I can reach you, Dr. Coltrane?" Mrs. Davila apologized.

He gave her his office number, and hung up. The nurse at the desk next to him had been half listening to the discussion. She glanced at him with a raised eyebrow.

"Not good," Coltrane shook his head slowly.

She nodded sympathetically.

Chapter 9

Bayside Community Hospital
April 26
7:18AM

Chas Nichols, MD arrived in the ER early, as usual. Nichols had just come off a weeklong rotation of the night shift, and his biorhythms were still slightly out of phase. He had been up since 4AM, reading journals and preparing for the 12 hour shift. Nichols loved the challenge of ER medicine, and thrived in the high stress environment. The imprinting of three years in the Marine Corps and two tours of duty in Vietnam, followed by seven grueling years of medical training had made him a highly organized and extremely methodical physician.

He was waiting in the staff lounge for the outgoing physician to brief him on the disposition and status of the current ER patients when the code was called. Over the hospital's public address system came the urgent *'Code Blue-Emergency Room'* announcement. Nichols jumped up and raced to assist.

The ER had been very quiet for thirty minutes before the code. All the technicians and nursing specialists who were in the ER earlier to stabilize John Strahan had returned to their stations throughout the hospital. The ER was empty when the nurse saw that John was not responding to stimulation any longer. He looked bluish, and she noted that the oxygen sensor had fallen off his fingertip. She listened to his lungs, and called the Code Blue immediately.

Nichols was the first physician at the bedside. He listened intently to the nurse's status report, and asked several quick questions about the nature and severity of the gunshot wounds. He then swiftly removed the blood encrusted bandages from John's face, and examined the wound. What he saw shocked and horrified him.

John's upper jaw had been badly fractured. The bone was reduced to three loose pieces, each free-floating in a red mash of blood and tissue. The palate and the fragments of bone had collapsed downward and backward to obstruct his airway. Earlier, John had been positioned flat on his back by the X-ray tech to facilitate taking his chest films. The technician had inadvertently left him in that position when he rushed to develop the X-rays. Flat on his back, and without reflexes, blood and secretions were forced down his throat and into his lungs. Unconscious, he was drowning in his own blood.

"Code Blue. Trauma Room 1. Find Foster. Get me the respiratory tech and Biomed tech STAT. Arterial blood gases STAT. Suction and ET tube." Nichols stood and yelled, his voice carrying throughout the department. He then turned to the nurse beside John's head and they began to work to clean the debris from his mouth, clearing his airway. They re-applied the oxygen sensor to John's finger, and Nichols cursed when he saw the readout. The level was dangerously low, indicating that he may have been oxygen starved for some time. The arterial blood gases were taken, and rushed to the lab for analysis.

Nichols took the suction tip and tried to clear the back of John's throat. He found and removed two loose teeth and a large fragment of bone with attached mucosa. Despite the powerful suction, he could not get ahead of the bleeding that his manipulation had stirred up. He opened John's mouth, and pulled the lower jaw forward in an attempt to establish an airway. He elevated the head of the gurney and suctioned again. None of these immediate responses helped.

The crash cart with the equipment to run and sustain a resuscitation attempt arrived and was opened. Nichols selected an 8.0mm ET tube and laryngoscope. He moved to the head of the gurney, pushing aside and ducking under the maze of tubes and wires connecting John to the monitors. He inserted his thumb into John's mouth, grabbed the lower jaw and pulled it upward. Clearing the debris from the throat with the suction, he tried to insert the clear plastic ET tube into the trachea. The first attempt failed, leaving the tube in the esophagus. The second attempt got the tube into the trachea, and the placement was verified by the nurse, using her stethoscope. Nichols then handed the black AMBU bag to the respiratory technician. She began the rhythmic, slow pumping of pure oxygen into John's lungs.

"ABGs pH 7.21, pCO2 65, pO2 59, Hematocrit 25.7," the lab technician read out loud to Nichols.

"*Damn. Damn. Damn.* He's severely acidotic and anoxic. Let's hook him up to the ventilator. Settings of 100% O2 and rate 24. One amp of Bicarb. What's the BP? One amp of Epi. Dump in fluids as fast as you can. Where is Foster? Get that arterial line working, something is dampening the response. Is his BP falling now?? Someone get a manual BP please." Nichols thought out loud to give the rest of the team clear, accurate orders and to let them know what he was thinking, where his thought process was headed. They responded as independent extensions of his will, moving in unison and anticipating the next step in this intense, coordinated ballet of life or death.

In a matter of seconds, the arterial blood line, a small catheter in the artery in John's wrist, was flushed and cleared. The reading was what

Nichols had feared. It was not a technical error that had made his BP tracing look weak; his heart was failing. The blood pressure was low, and the heart rate unsteady. The EKG showed the characteristic signs of a dying heart. Nichols pulled out all the stops.

"Another amp of Epi. Another amp of Bicarb. Call the cardiologist on call and the radiologist. I want to put a balloon pump in this kid. Quick. *QUICK*! *Shit!*" Nichols watched as the EKG went berserk, then became completely disorganized.

"*Stand back! Charge the defibrillator to 200 volts.* ***SHOCKING!!***" Nichols applied the electric paddles to the chest of the young man and simultaneously pressed the two red buttons, firing the device. Strahan's body jolted and his back arched instantly. The EKG continued its chaotic rhythm. Nichols waited for several seconds, then repeated the maneuver. Again no improvement. He increased the voltage and tried again.

"Another amp of bicarb. Another amp of epi. Recharge the defibrillator. How are we doing on the cardiologist and the balloon pump? Give him a minute and let's shock him again." Nichols continued the effort, but by now he knew the outcome. There was a precious window of opportunity in which to save a life. And they all knew that the window had passed.

Nichols attempted to shock the young man's heart three more times before he finally called an end to the resuscitation. The boy's skin had lost its warm color, turning a dull, mottled gray. Nichols imagined that he witnessed the precise instant that life departed the body. He gently closed the boy's eyelids over the dead eyes. He looked around, saw Foster at the side of the bed where he had been attending to the arterial line, and motioned him toward the main nurses' station to discuss the case.

"What the fuck happened with this guy? Why wasn't he intubated? Where is the plastic surgeon?" Nichols demanded. He was incensed, outraged. Minor screw-ups were commonplace in any institution, and hospitals were certainly no exception. But this seemed to be a series of major, inexcusable errors that had led inexorably to the death of a healthy young man. How could this happen? In the middle of a brand-new, clean bright hospital, in the era of technological wizardry? It had been hard enough to accept the loss of life and youth in a war far from home, but here? Now? The absurdity fell upon him like a weight.

Foster had no immediate response. He mumbled that he had been busy with an asthmatic and had tried to contact the plastic surgeon. His voice trailed off.

"Is there family here?" Nichols asked.

Foster nodded in assent.

"Get the nurses to clean up the patient and then let's go find them." Nichols looked long and hard at Foster then turned, walking toward the waiting room. He had done this so many times, but it would never be anything but painful and visceral. Life shattering news, dream shattering news, from a white-coated stranger. Rage, disbelief, fear and profound sadness all at the same instant, all with supreme intensity. The emotional blow was stronger than a physical blow, and he never knew exactly how to deliver that blow, or how the family would take it. But he was sure that his face told the tale before he ever spoke a word.

The Strahans were in the nursing supervisor's office when Nichols spoke with them. Foster didn't join them. They seemed to be expecting the news, the father slumping into a chair quickly and holding his head in his trembling hands. The mother cried quietly and then asked to see her boy. Nichols led them back to the trauma room. He explained softly what he had done to try to save their son, but he knew that they were not listening. He left soundlessly.

Mary Strahan touched her son's face, was chilled by the cool feel of his skin. Mercifully, his eyes were closed, sparing her the memory of his dull, lifeless gaze. The face that she had washed a thousand times; that she had dried the tears from in childhood, and seen the joy and love and promise as he grew toward manhood, now lay ashen and gray, lifeless. Her spirit drained from her. She held and stroked his cold hand, crying. David stood behind her and held her tenderly, his eyes closed.

Chapter 10

Tampa
One week later
May 4

Thursday was always the day that Coltrane enjoyed the most, and dreaded the most. Thursday he saw all his follow-up patients, all the trauma victims and all new patients scheduled for surgery the next week. He took stitches out, examined wounds, checked progress on post-operative patients and wrote prescriptions. He explained over and over again to patients that smoking slowed their recovery, and increased their infection rate. He replaced splints and dressings that were not supposed to be removed. He removed "special salves" that grandma had applied to cuts and lacerations to speed healing. He was amazed and frustrated at the way many of his patients totally disregarded his expert advice and instructions.

But for all the many aggravations of dealing with sick and injured people, one of the greatest joys in his life was the opportunity to lessen pain and suffering. The motor vehicle accident victim, the new patient with a skin cancer, or the woman with the recent diagnosis of breast cancer, or the victim of a serious burn; all were chances to practice his consummate skill and to comfort and assure the patient, to treat their disease and to ease their mind. This was the reward of medicine and surgery for Coltrane.

He was between patients when his nurse interrupted him with a phone call. He told her to take a message, but she responded that it was David Strahan. He picked up the extension.

"David, are you and Mary doing all right?" He hadn't seen them since the funeral a week ago. There had not been any discussion of the details of John's death.

"As well as can be expected, Bill. Thank you for the flowers, and more so for your help when John was shot. I haven't had a chance to thank you since that night. I would like to talk with you some time about why John died. I am still not sure what happened, or if I could have done anything different, or the doctors or the hospital, to save John. I need to know." Strahan paused, overwhelmed.

"You may wish to speak with an attorney about that, David."

"No, no, I am not intending to bring a lawsuit. I am on the board of directors of Citizens against Lawsuit Abuse. I just want to know what happened so I can sleep at night."

"Can you come to the office, around 5:45? I have patients all day."

"Thanks, Bill. I appreciate it."

The day went well. Patients were seen and treated. The office schedule ran smoothly, with only two or three missed appointments. Coltrane was punctual in the office, and only emergencies threw his schedule off. The staff locked up and went home at 5:30, and he retired to his private office to finish paperwork. He was there when Strahan knocked on the door. Coltrane let him in, and led him through the corridors, past the exam rooms and sparkling outpatient surgical suite.

Coltrane was proud of his private office, the inner sanctum where he could escape from the demands of private practice for a few hours. The wall behind his black leather chair prominently displayed his University of California Bachelor of Science, his enormous University of Texas Medical Degree and his Certification by the American Board of Surgery. Just to the right of these framed documents hung his Certificate of Added Qualifications in Surgery of the Hand and the membership in the American Society of Trauma Surgeons. He had always felt that all other awards and memberships were superfluous. Coltrane was formally trained as a general surgeon, but during residency had found the thrill and exhilaration of trauma surgery to be irresistible. Contrasting with the drama and intensity of trauma surgery was his passion for the intricacy and delicacy of hand surgery. He enjoyed the relative peacefulness of the long, precise surgical procedures to repair the delicate, impossibly intricate workings of the hand.

The expansive desk before him was an eighteenth century oak partners' desk made in Nottingham, England. Opposite him was an identical black leather chair, with bookcases and oriental artwork on the shelves and walls. A bronze nude female torso stood on a marble pedestal in the corner.

Strahan sat in the leather chair and leaned forward, resting his arms on the desk. He didn't speak for several moments. Coltrane asked him to slowly go over the entire night's events. As Strahan recounted the nightmare, the pain caused him to stop several times. Coltrane quietly took notes on a yellow pad. At the end, they both sat silent.

"Do the police know who shot them, or why?" Coltrane asked.

"No, but apparently it was gang-related. The boys strayed into a gang-infested neighborhood. Ballistics show that the gun was also used in another local shooting. The police want to question a known gang-member who lives on the street, but he has disappeared." Strahan answered.

"It would be impossible for me to determine if things were handled properly at this point, David. I don't know the doctors involved, or the hospitals. I couldn't give you an opinion on their reputations or skill. I guess the next step is to obtain all the medical records from Bayside immediately."

"I'm not implying that the doctors were at fault here. But I am very angry that both Bayside Hospital and my insurance carrier refused to transfer John, despite my request and your request to do so. Can they do that?" Strahan looked straight at Coltrane.

"Perhaps, but only if there's a clause in your coverage agreement that requires you to use approved facilities. In their defense, that's how they keep your premiums low. Inappropriate use of ER facilities is a tremendous waste of the healthcare dollar. Still, there is no justification for withholding adequate or appropriate care from anyone, regardless of insurance coverage."

"I'll request the records. But from what you told me that night, and what subsequently happened in Miami, I think John's case was mishandled. Had things been done differently, John might still be alive. I am sure of that. Someone has to pay." Strahan bowed his head and stared at the floor.

"You intend to file a suit?" Coltrane asked.

"I don't know. I think so. Maybe."

"David, from here onward, things will get increasingly complex. You need to find a good attorney. I think you know the lawyers in town well enough to do that. I'll probably need to discuss this with my attorney as well. If there is malpractice and you pursue litigation, you may want me to testify as an expert witness."

"Fine. I'll get the records, and keep in touch. Listen, I don't want you to think that I am just another asshole who wants to sue a doctor and capitalize on my son's death. I just don't understand why he died." Strahan shook his head, staring at his hands on the desk.

Coltrane led him back through the office and shook his hand at the door to the suite. Strahan left, and Coltrane went back to work. He reviewed the notes that he had taken with Strahan, and added notes of his recollection of the events of that night. Then he started making phone calls.

It was almost ten when he got home. Britt was pissed. She had cooked dinner, a lasagna that was not good cold. She had waited until nine, when the effects of her hunger and the two glasses of Chianti forced her to eat alone. Once again.

"I wish you could take the time to call me when you're late. I thought you would be home early. Emergency? What happened?" She didn't look up.

"Shit, honey. I'm sorry. I get so involved in what I am doing and I think I'll leave in just a minute, so I never call. I don't intend to forget." Coltrane mumbled. This was a recurring problem, and he would have to wait out her anger. The human mind is such an intricate and complex organ, he thought; why was it that he couldn't avoid continually repeating this mistake?

"I spoke with David Strahan today," He stated as he poured a glass of wine.

"Poor Mary and David. What a tragedy."

"From what I can see, the entire thing was a goatfuck from the beginning. They took him to a hospital that was not yet fully operational. Even when it does become operational, Bayside will not be the proper place to triage Level I Trauma. Then they fucked up his initial care in the ER. Then they couldn't get a plastic surgeon or a max-face guy to see him, and they refused to transfer him to JMH. They let him die in the ER of possibly preventable causes. I don't think that they did anything right all night." Coltrane paused, sipped the wine and thought about the sequence of events. He wondered for the thousandth time if he could have intervened and helped more effectively. Could he have saved the boy's life? What should he have done differently? Strahan had asked for his help in the boy's dying hours. Why hadn't he been more aggressive, demanding that he be transferred to JMH?

"You did all that you could, Bill. It was in another city, the people didn't know you, and you weren't the attending physician. Stop torturing yourself." Britt read his mind without looking up. "How is David taking it?" she asked.

"He's at the stage where he wants to address the events of John's death, and understand what happened. I asked him to get the records from Bayside, and that will take several days. I need to decide how to handle this situation; as the possible attending surgeon for John, as a family friend, as an expert witness, as an actual witness during the communications that night, or as president of the society. I'll call the FMA lawyer tomorrow to clarify my options."

"It seems like he has a case against Bayside." Britt thought out loud.

"They may have a case against the hospital, the physicians involved and the insurance company. The errors that occurred in John's care happen every day; here, everywhere. In John's case, they just all happened at the same time, to the same patient." Coltrane sat quietly next to his wife, reflecting upon the course of events that culminated in John's death.

"So sad," she said. "So very sad."

Chapter 11

May 8

Monday had never been Dr. Stephen "Steve" Hendricks' best day. He always enjoyed his weekends far more than the working week. His long standing penchant for alcohol and illicit drugs made the transition even more difficult. This Monday was like many before. He had invited a young pharmaceutical representative down from Orlando for the weekend, with promises of water-skiing and offshore fishing. But she didn't get along with his friends, or want to be around all the cocaine and pills that were everywhere all weekend long. So she took her fine young ass, untouched, back to Orlando despite the pathetic pleading of Hendricks. So he spent the rest of the weekend in the bottle, and was suffering now.

Stephen Hendricks, MD, was the first son in a large wealthy family from the Eastern seaboard. He had gone to public school, then an Ivy League college, during the drug and sexual revolution of the seventies. He had experimented with all the mind bending chemicals, LSD, mescaline, speed, mushrooms, cocaine, even heroin. But it was alcohol and cocaine that he finally settled down with, even through the brutal years of medical training. After four years at a prestigious eastern medical school and one year of family practice residency, he suffered a mental breakdown, complete with delusions and suicidal ideation. Only the intervention of an old physician family friend allowed him to finish residency, and escape southward with his problems.

Hendricks attempted to start a private practice in Atlanta, but soon found that private practice and drug abuse were incompatible. He could usually deceive his patients, but the other physicians would eventually discern his problems. His referrals dropped off, and the office overhead began to exceed his income. He was contemplating another move when he received a headhunter's letter, a recruiting solicitation for a medical director for a HMO in Florida. It was perfect. He had no requirement to disclose his prior breakdown or current drug dependence due to medical confidentiality laws, and had a chance for a new start. Within three weeks, he had closed his office, and moved to Tampa.

By now, Hendricks was in his mid-forties, and slowly coming to grips with the fact that he had let his many golden opportunities slip by. For Hendricks, the desire to avoid effort or responsibility had always superceded the desire for dignity or self-respect. The time to grasp the remaining chances for happiness seemed to be dwindling fast.

Hendricks' head was still throbbing as he entered his office, twenty minutes late. There was a lukewarm cup of coffee on his desk, beside a stack of messages. His secretary poked her head in and told him that the doctor who had called last Friday was holding on the line. Another crybaby surgeon wanting more money, no doubt. Fully three quarters of his time was spent fielding angry disputes from specialists about the low fee schedules. They would rant and rave and curse, but he knew that in the end he would prevail. They had blindly signed a contract, and had no recourse. It was all in a day's work. He sipped the tepid coffee and picked up the phone

"Dr. Hendricks, this is Dr. Coltrane. I'm a trauma surgeon on your plan. I had a patient in Miami that I wanted to transfer to another facility recently, but was unable to arrange authorization to do so. What is the policy in these situations, and how can I expedite the solution if it occurs again?" Coltrane asked calmly, using the speakerphone on his desk. He had been dictating operative reports as he waited for Hendricks' secretary to connect him. As an afterthought, he flipped a fresh cassette in and switched on the microrecorder as he began talking, recording the entire conversation.

"The policy is clearly outlined in the manual. The attending physician must contact the primary care doctor assigned to the patient and obtain authorization. Did you try to contact him?" Hendricks sighed, and massaged his pounding temples. These jerkoffs never read their manuals, or their contracts or the many letters we send them, he thought.

"What if the patient doesn't know who their primary care doctor is?"

"Then they call this office and obtain one."

"What if it is an emergency?"

"All emergency room visits MUST be cleared in advance by the primary care physician in order to be covered. You do ER work. You should know that. What do you do when you see a patient in the ER?" Hendricks asked testily.

"First of all, it is rare that I see patients in the ER except at night. And then I treat them. I assume that the ER admin staff gets all the necessary paperwork. I haven't had too many disputes, except the Avila case," Coltrane's blood pressure rose momentarily at the thought.

Coltrane remembered the aggravation of dealing with Hendricks about payment for Jesse Avila. Avila, a postal worker for twenty-five years and covered under the HMO policy that his union chose for him, had been having a couple of beers while fishing off the Tarpon Springs pier in the Gulf of Mexico. He caught a beautiful speckled trout, and while filleting it four beers later, managed to fillet his left thumb as well. He went directly to the hospital with the same name as his new HMO insurance plan. After waiting in an empty reception area for two hours, and being rudely interrogated about his drinking and lack of shoes, his wife packed him up and took him straight to the Sisters of Mercy. Coltrane had seen him there, and repaired the nerves and tendons in his thumb. Due to the contaminated nature of the wound, seawater mixed with a filthy knife and fish entrails, he had been admitted for a short course of antibiotics. The HMO insurance plan had refused to pay for any of his medical bills, stating that he had failed to notify his primary care physician when he was injured; that he had left the treating facility Against Medical Advice; and that he had been drunk at the time.

Coltrane had been outraged that the plan could be so capricious. Avila felt, correctly, that he had no obligation to pay since he had paid faithfully his insurance premiums. To further complicate matters, as a postal worker, the matter fell under federal jurisdiction. A board of inquiry would take eight months to finally resolve the issue. Over two years after the injury, Coltrane was sent a check for less than half of his fee.

"I don't remember that case. But the procedure is the same for all patients. After hours, there is a toll free number to call to help with these type of problems. Did you try to contact them?" Hendricks whined.

"Yeah, but that process takes time. It took me fifteen minutes to get through. And then the representative I spoke with didn't have the medical background to understand what I wanted or why it was important." Coltrane was up against a bureaucrat, and beginning to lose control.

"What was the patient's name, and what exactly happened?" Hendricks asked.

"John Strahan. He was shot in the face, and I wanted him transferred from Bayside to JMH in Miami…" Coltrane started.

"You weren't the primary physician in that case. I just saw something about him on my desk…Here it is. My staff has been talking with the family about his transfer. I spoke briefly with the father, I think. How did you get involved?" Hendricks interrupted.

"I was asked by his father to take on his care when he was returned to Tampa. I spoke with the physicians there at Bayside and tried to assist the family that night."

"Bayside is a fully accredited hospital, and a participating facility in our network. The hospital is brand new. Why would you want to move him?"

"Bayside is not a trauma facility and I felt that he needed to be treated at a Level I trauma center. I wanted him to go to JMH."

"That decision could only be made by the patient's primary care physician, and he could have been notified in the morning. Bayside stabilized him until that time. We will not authorize transfer of a patient because the patient doesn't like the color of the carpet in his room." Hendricks was getting tired of the debate.

"Look, Bayside is an inappropriate place to treat severe, multiple gunshot wounds. Furthermore, I doubt that many internists or family practitioners know the difference between Level I and Level II Trauma Centers. Strahan should have gone immediately to a Level I or II Center. Are any of those facilities in Miami on your plan?"

"No. The larger facilities are mostly county or state hospitals and are outside of our network."

"So HMO patients are never sent to those facilities?" Coltrane was astounded.

"Right. Listen, this is a business. We save the patient and employer considerable cost in premium expense by limiting the frivolous waste that occurs in the practice of medicine. That includes unnecessary transfers to tertiary hospitals, redundant specialist consultations and self-serving lab costs," Hendricks was getting angry. He viewed Coltrane as an arrogant, condescending surgeon with no respect for primary care physicians. Coltrane probably felt that only he was capable of caring for the Strahan boy. He continued his tirade. "I was called by the administrative center that night and I concurred with the written policy. I denied transfer on the basis that he could be treated by the enrolled facility until a HMO participating surgeon could evaluate him." Hendricks finished.

"What? Did you talk to the ER doctor?" Coltrane asked in stunned disbelief.

"No," Hendricks remembered fuzzily the events of that early morning, weeks ago. The administrative supervisor in New Jersey had called him and paged him several times, but he had been so stoned that he hadn't wanted to talk. He had finally answered and dealt with the problem in the easiest fashion. By the book, he had thought at the time.

"Unbelievable. How could you make a decision like that without even speaking with the attending physician. You had no idea what his injuries were. The only person you spoke to was the admin supervisor in New Jersey?"

"Look, I don't need to talk to anyone. The HMO policies are clearly outlined in the agreement. Maybe you should read it sometime."

"You'd better pray that the Strahans don't sue you and the HMO."

"They can't sue. It's in the terms of the contract. All enrollees agree to the rationing of health care by acceptance of the policy and premium rates. Do they think that they are going to get first class healthcare for cut-rate premiums?" Hendricks was getting uneasy about his revelation. "I have work to do. If I can be of any help, please call me in the future." With that he hung up, and instructed his secretary to take no further calls for Coltrane.

Coltrane sat in his office, still dumbstruck by Hendricks' admission. He turned off the small cassette recorder. Taking the cassette out, he broke off the tabs, making it impossible to accidentally record over the taped conversation. He couldn't believe what he had just heard.

His first call was to the Florida Medical Association. He requested to speak with Skip Watters, the FMA legal counsel, an attorney with whom he had spoken several times before. Watters was extremely knowledgeable in the complex area of medicolegal affairs, and always had answers to Coltrane's questions. Regrettably for Coltrane, the answers were rarely the ones that he wanted to hear.

"Watters here."

"Skip, this is Bill Coltrane in Tampa."

"Yes, Dr. Coltrane. How are you? Did you ever get that case with the local HMO straightened out? The problem was several different fee schedules, as I recall?"

"God, you have a good memory. No, they took the stance that I had signed a contract that did not specifically delineate the fees for all my procedures, and therefore they could pay what they liked. I just dropped them from my list of plans."

"Good riddance. We have a lot of complaints against that particular plan, but as you know, the state insurance board has a prerequisite minimum number of complaints before it investigates. And the board is staffed by insurance toadies anyway," Watters explained patiently, like a parent to a petulant child. Business is just a game, why can't doctors understand that? They always get so wrapped up, take it all so personally. Still, he had to admire Coltrane. The guy may be pissing up a rope, but he had integrity.

"Skip, I have a unique problem to discuss with you. Can we consider this privileged information?" Coltrane asked.

"Yes; part of my job is to provide legal advice to our members. Go ahead."

Coltrane gave a full accounting of the Strahan shooting and his attempts to have the boy transferred from Bayside to JMH. He related the fact that the boy eventually died in the ER, but stated that he had no knowledge of the actual medical details. He finished with a brief description of the talk with David Strahan, and the subsequent events, including the discussion with Hendricks, and the fact that he had taped it.

"Very interesting. Very interesting. Where do you stand now?" Watters asked.

"What do you mean?" Coltrane asked, uncertain of the question's purpose.

"What is your objective in becoming involved in this matter? John Strahan wasn't your patient, was he?" Watters asked incisively.

"No, he wasn't. But who else can speak for him? Only a physician would know if his treatment was or was not appropriate. As it was, his fate may have been decided by the HMO switchboard operator that night. And she may not even have a high school education. The whole system has become absurd. Physicians don't make treatment plans any more, the telephone operators do." Coltrane ranted angrily.

"I didn't realize you were a crusader, Dr. Coltrane," Watters commented dryly after Coltrane finished.

"Sorry. I recently was elected president of the Bay Area Medical Society. I get carried away."

"What about the boy's family? Does Strahan plan to litigate?" Watters continued.

"Yes, that's what the father has indicated. My feeling is that when Strahan finds out what I know, he'll file suit against the insurance company, and perhaps against the hospital and physicians as well."

"Let's assume that Strahan decides to take legal action against the parties in this case. He would probably allege malpractice, negligence and wrongful death. Do you think that he would involve you in the litigation? And if so, would you be testifying as an attending physician or as an expert witness? Actually, you could also be called as an actual participant in the events of his son's death. From a legal standpoint, this is a complex situation," Watters concluded.

"I haven't given it much thought. I've known the Strahans for seven or eight years, and have been helping as a friend. The boy's death was such a tragedy…"

"It's critical that you decide how you are going to proceed. As an attending or as an expert witness?" Watters interrupted.

"Since I never treated John, I would have to be an expert witness. I have extensive training and experience in trauma."

"Fine. And you were recently elected president of the county medical society. Good credentials for an expert witness. Now, let me tell you what I want you to do. First, do not speak any further with David Strahan other than to advise him to get an attorney ASAP. Do not, and I repeat, do not recommend a lawyer to represent him. This could taint you as an expert in the future, giving the appearance that you and the lawyer are in collusion. Make copies of the Hendricks recording and send one to me, and keep one in a safety deposit box. Then do nothing, and I stress *nothing*, until given instructions by Strahan's attorney.

"Understood. One last question. Do I have any malpractice exposure personally in this case?"

"The father asked you look into the handling of the boys' care in Miami, but you did not actually accept John or the other boys as patients. Is that correct?" Watters asked.

"Correct. I called and spoke to the surgeon and the nurse, but I don't think I accepted John as my patient," Coltrane searched his memory for his exact words.

"In that case, you have very little exposure," he stated. He paused, and continued. "An attorney who tried to involve you as a defendant would risk turning you into a hostile witness. Considering your standing in the community and the pivotal nature of your testimony, that would be a profoundly stupid tactic. I don't think that you will be sued for your part in this tragedy. I would advise you to notify your malpractice carrier, however. I will be glad to speak with you if you have any further problems. And good luck."

Coltrane thanked him and hung up. Watters had opened his eyes to the reality of the situation once again. Was he tilting at windmills? Or was this part of his responsibilities as president of the medical society? He had not seen a more flagrant abuse of trust by a health insurance company in his life. Even so, all the time and effort spent fighting this battle would not bring John back. But what he thought did not matter. The next step was in the hands of David Strahan.

Chapter 12

May 9

Medical malpractice litigation in the United States is a quagmire of claims, rebuttals and discovery, lasting years in many cases. The process is extremely stressful and emotionally draining on both the defendant and the plaintiff. Only the attorneys on both sides profit and prosper. That is the way the game is played, and that realization was being driven home to David Strahan with brutal clarity.

Strahan had spoken with a colleague who dealt solely in tax law. The tax attorney had recommended two lawyers for David, but had qualified his recommendations. He told Strahan that one of the men would be arrogant, overbearing and an insufferable prick. But he would be the most likely to succeed. He would use every dirty trick available to weaken the opposition, including investigating the witnesses' private lives, and laying bare their prior indiscretions.

Strahan had met with both lawyers and chosen the more aggressive one. The first step in litigation is the fee agreement. Most medical malpractice cases are undertaken on a contingency fee basis, the lawyer had explained. Strahan would have to pay all court expenses as they occurred, but the attorney's fee would be taken as 40% of the final settlement if the lawsuit was successful. If they failed, there would be no attorney's fees. The lawyer demanded a $10,000 deposit and told Strahan that they would meet again in one week. He requested copies of the insurance contract, the medical records and names of John's previous physicians. He explained to Strahan that depositions and discovery would take weeks, maybe months, and then they could decide if the case will go to trial.

Before they concluded the consultation, Strahan brought up the part that Coltrane had played in the events. Strahan asked how Coltrane would figure in the litigation. The attorney remarked that he could look into it.

Chapter 13

May 10

It was 10:15 AM, and Coltrane had just completed his first case of the day; the reconstruction of a wrist fracture in a twenty year old male who had been admitted that night after an automobile accident. The case had started at 7:30, and he had shared the OR with Philip Tyson, an oral surgeon. Tyson had repaired the man's jaw fracture, and wired his teeth together. They exited the OR, spoke briefly with a disinterested family, and returned to the surgeons lounge.

As the two men neared the door to the surgeons lounge, they could hear laughter and cursing echoing from within. They glanced at each other, grinned, and went inside.

Travis was holding court.

In the lounge, sprawled on one of the large couches, drinking coffee and eating a huge donut, was Randy Travis, MD. In a circle around him sat two surgeons, an anaestheologist and two male scrub techs, all laughing so hard that there were tears streaming down their cheeks. Travis was finishing a story.

"Are you off shift already?" Coltrane asked, confused. Travis was the director of the Emergency Room, and usually had the 7AM to 7PM shift. It was still morning.

"Hey, Bill. No, I had to get the fuck out of the ER before I killed someone. There is an absolute tidal wave of idiocy down there. I get in at 6AM, and the first thing that happens is this hillbilly I admitted two days ago with a Rule Out MI coded in the ICU. The nurse can't get ahold of the cardiologist, so she calls me, almost in tears. I go up there, and the guy is crashing. Hard. No blood pressure. Just a really, really faint pulse. But his EKG is fine. I grab the chart, and read it as fast as I can, check all the tests the guy has had in the past two days, look at the X-Rays, the works. I'm thinking he is going to die while I read the fucking chart. We pump his BP up a little with some meds, elevate his feet, the usual panic shit." Travis pauses, shaking his head solemnly.

"Nothing," he continues. "So I think, maybe the electronics are bad. Maybe a sensor is dead. So I grab his arm to check pulse and take a manual BP. He has an arterial line in the right wrist, so I go around the bed to the left arm. His left arm is by his side, tucked under the sheets. Odd, right? So I pull the sheet off, and yell at the nurses for not giving him a thorough exam immediately upon his coding. And guess what?" Travis starts grinning madly.

Everyone in the lounge is racking their brains to find a reason for this story.

"This guy has his index finger three knuckles up his ass. It turns out that, this morning, when he finally woke up from the week long binge he was on when he had a mysterious spell of fainting and chest pain, and found himself in the Cardiovascular ICU, the first thing that came to mind was how much his hemorrhoids were itching. So he tells the nurse about it. She pretty much ignores it, but half an hour later, she comes in and applies an inch and a half of Nitropaste to his chest, because his BP is going up. Rufus, the idiot, decides that this is his hemorrhoid medicine, since it does bear a slight resemblance to PreparationH. So he loads up this entire index finger with the Nitropaste, and liberally applies it to his asshole. *BOOM!* His BP bottoms out, and he passes out with his finger still in his ass. You can bring a horse to water, but you can't make it think."

The surgeons start laughing. The two techs look up in confusion.

"Nitropaste lowers your BP, but it is meant to be applied to the skin, and get absorbed slowly. You put it on a mucosal surface like the rectum, or mouth, it gets absorbed really, really fast. Lights out." Travis explained to the techs.

"Did he make it?" Someone asked.

"After I pulled his finger out, and cleaned his butt, yeah. That's how I started my day. Then the next patient I see is actually an entire, extended family, with no symptoms." Now Travis is becoming visibly agitated.

"No symptoms?" Tyson plays the straight man.

"Nope. Mrs. Valdez brings in her two year old boy with a cold, the nurse tells me. I go in the exam room, and there are five kids in there, sitting on the floor, playing with the otoscope, one is licking the stirrups in the gynecology exam setup. No one speaks English."

"Don't you speak Spanish yet?"

"*Mas Cerveza.* That's it. My Spanish is not good enough for medicolegal application. I don't want someone to die because I didn't get the inflection right. So I always use a translator. Anyway, I have the RN start asking about who is sick, and what the symptoms are. It turns out that Mrs. Valdez is really Miss Valdez, and none of the kids are hers, she is just babysitting for her sisters and aunt, and is not really sure which kid is sick. So since she can't leave the other four at home alone, she brought them all. And since they were all here, and it's free anyway, she decided that she would get everyone all checked out. She seems to think that we have some magical instrument or machine that looks at the kids, and diagnoses any existing health problem. I think the nurse is still down there, sorting through the kids." Travis paused, and took another deep breath.

"But wait, there's more. While I'm in with the kids from Equador, the charge nurse comes in and pulls me out to see an old guy with abdominal pain. Ever since that guy died in our ER with an abdominal aneurysm last month, everyone with abdominal pain now has an abdominal aneurysm. So I go in and start talking to him. Now, even with an intelligent, coherent male, it takes me thirty minutes to do a good belly work-up. But this guy either has Alzheimer's, or is just plain, old-fashioned stupid. I can't get an answer from him. On anything."

"'What seems to be the problem, sir?' I ask." Travis continues.

"'My stomach hurts alot,' he says."

"'What is alot?' I ask."

"'Alot,' he says."

"'Every day? Every hour? Every minute? How much is alot?' I ask."

"'I don't know. Alot.' He says."

"'Did you vomit?' I ask."

"'I had a BM,' he says."

"'Was there blood on your stools?' I ask."

"'Blood? I don't know. I don't look,' he says."

"'Did you ever vomit with the painful episodes?' I ask."

"'My doctor told me I had a fever,' he says."

"'Your doctor. Good. What is his name? Now we are getting somewhere," I say."

"'I forget. But I have my pills,' he says. He pulls out this one inch by three inch, yellowed piece of paper with his medications written on it. Only the writing is five years old and in old person writing, like he held the pencil in his mouth and wrote out the list by moving his head. And I read the list, and it reads:

> *yellow pill 1 a day*
> *green and white pill 3 a day*
> *square pill 4 a day*
> and so on."

"'What are your pills for?' I ask."

"'Christ, Doc, don't you know what the yellow pills are for? You're the damn doctor.' he says. That was it. I couldn't take it any more, I had to leave. Please don't make me go back."

"Are things really that bad, Randy? At least you don't have to take call. Or maintain an office." Coltrane was jealous.

"Seriously, Bill, the situation is getting really bad. All our experienced, bright, senior nurses are leaving. They are all burned out at the patient load, and the paperwork load. The nursing supervisor tells me that the average age of RNs is forty-two years old, and that half will be leaving the profession within eighteen months. Nursing school enrollment is way down; women have many more options open to them now. Who wants to empty bedpans all day and night?

"Plus, I'm losing docs, too. This week I lost two neurosurgeons from the call list. They can't afford the malpractice premiums for trauma anymore. I don't know how the hospital can keep the ER open. Only one in six patients has any insurance. That's even counting Medicare and Medicaid, which don't pay shit."

"Come to the society meetings, give a speech. The members need to know all this, Randy."

"I'm just going to close the ER and send all the patients to the fucking chiropractors."

Tyson and Coltrane laughed, and went to the table to pour themselves a cup of coffee. They both sat down in the little cubicles to dictate the operative reports, discuss the treatment plan for their patient, and write orders in the chart.

"I hear that you are now the illustrious president of your society, Coltrane. Why would you want to get involved in that bullshit?" Tyson got right to the point, laughing.

"It really was a spur of the moment thing, Phil. I got fed up with the pompous crap that goes on in the society and thought that we should be doing something to improve the private practice of medicine. It seems that every year the intellectual rewards as well as the financial rewards of practice diminish, and the aggravation increases. Did you hear the family out there? They didn't ask about how the surgery went, just complained that they didn't get a TV in the room. The satisfaction of caring for the ungrateful. Unbelievable…" Coltrane trailed off, tired. They had both been up since the patient arrived in the ER at 2:30 AM.

"I heard that you were involved in the lawsuit for that boy's death in Miami. Is the father suing the hospital?" Tyson asked. Bad news travels fast, even in big cities.

"How did you hear about that? I can't discuss the case because I am involved as a witness, but I can tell you that insurance companies run roughshod over patients and physicians with impunity. I told you about the different fee schedules in town, didn't I? There are five hand surgeons enrolled on the plan, and we are all paid at different rates. I'm pissed for obvious reasons. My fee schedule pays at the lowest, half of what Bookman is getting, and he never takes ER call and never even passed his boards. So I do all the shit work, all the burns and ER trauma, while he does the office surgery for the plan and gets paid twice my fees. I almost blew a blood vessel in my brain when I found that out. I called that idiot medical director and he said that it was my fault for not negotiating a good contract. How can I negotiate a contract? The HMO refuses to tell me what the fee schedule is, and it's illegal to ask another doctor what he is charging for a given procedure. I'm fucked. We're all fucked. The whole profession is fucked." Coltrane cursed.

"I have much less of those headaches, because fortunately the government and the large insurance companies have stayed out of dentistry and oral surgery so far. But I can see the writing on the wall. The HMOs are recruiting dentists now. It won't be long before we are in the same situation." Tyson reflected quietly.

"Maybe I can do something as president of the society. What we really need to do is strike, or organize a work slowdown. Every physician in Tampa should close his office for three days. Go to the beach, go hunting. Cover the hospital ERs so that there is coverage for emergencies, and shutdown the rest of the medical delivery system. Force some necessary changes in our healthcare system," Coltrane pondered the possibility. "But it would never happen."

"You're right. The idea goes against the ethics of most doctors. And it's a federal offense. Anti-trust violation. You could all go to jail." Tyson responded.

"Well, that's what they told Jimmy Hoffa, and look what he managed to accomplish." Coltrane argued.

"And look what happened to him. He's part of the New Jersey Freeway." Tyson laughed.

"Good point," Coltrane smiled and stood up. "I have two more cases to do, but thanks for the help with that kid's jaw. I'll keep you posted on my political progress." Coltrane finished the paperwork and headed back into the operating room. But the germinal thought of a labor action involving physicians stayed with him. He called his office from the phone in the OR while his next patient was being put to sleep. His office manager, Cindy Kessler answered the phone.

"Cindy, would you call the medical society and find out who is assigned to the president as an administrative assistant, and arrange for a meeting with her on Wednesday? Is Wednesday still open?" Coltrane asked.

"Yes, Wednesday is free as of now. Would you like me to block the entire day, Dr. Coltrane?"

"Yes, please. And see if you can find the phone number of that group in California that is trying to organize doctors. The article is on my desk in the recent American Medical News. Thanks, gotta get back to work," Coltrane turned around, and went to scrub. He was smiling under the surgical mask. He loved a challenge.

It was late afternoon when Coltrane made it back to his office. Cindy had found the name of the group in California, but that would have to wait. He called the medical society and asked to speak to Susan Kerr.

"Susan Kerr."

"Susan, this is Dr. Coltrane. I guess that you know that I am the new president of the society. Cindy tells me that you will be my administrative assistant."

"Yes, doctor. I have some other duties, but my primary assignment is to liaison with the society president." Susan sounded tentative.

"Good. I would like to meet with you this Wednesday at my office if that is possible. I have a great number of ideas that will require some running down. Will that work for you?" Coltrane asked.

"Certainly. What time?"

"Nine AM. I have the entire day, so we can start at my office and maybe go to the society in the afternoon." Coltrane discussed further details and then hung up, satisfied. Maybe he could get something accomplished, after all. Then he had an inspiration.

He called Hendricks, bypassing his secretary by using the private number that was listed in the HMO handbook. Hendricks answered.

"Dr. Hendricks."

"Hendricks, this is Bill Coltrane. I apologize for using your back line, but I would like to discuss something with you. I am now the president of the medical society in Tampa, and I am in the process of attempting to improve the way insurance plans and medical providers interact. Prior to your arrival in Tampa, I had some disagreements with the plan regarding the fee schedules for hand surgeons. I think that there are many injustices in the current system, and I hope to be able to make some changes, at least here in the Bay area. Would it be possible to meet with you in the next week to discuss some of the society's concerns?"

"I think that you know our position with regard to fee schedules," Hendricks tried to end the conversation.

"Yeah, I have your predecessor's comments regarding the matter on tape. But I was…"

"What? You taped him?" Hendricks interrupted shakily.

"I tape all conversations with insurance plans, both for my protection and the patient's. It comes in handy when people get forgetful and claims get lost or mislaid," Coltrane explained matter of factly.

"Did you tape our conversation about the Strahan case?" Hendricks shrilled.

"Yes."

"That's illegal," Hendricks shouted.

"No, actually in Florida it is illegal to tape other people's conversations, but anyone can tape their own conversations."

"You bastard, you didn't tell me you were recording that conversation!" Hendricks lost control. His voice cracked with emotion.

"I don't have to tell you shit! So you planned to deny your hand in this? You don't have the balls to admit to the patient's family how it really happened. Are you hoping to pin the blame on the ER doctors? Your conduct is reprehensible. I'm resigning from your HMO, effective immediately. I'll send fax confirmation and letter by mail," Coltrane hung up as Hendricks continued to curse.

He typed a short letter on his computer, then printed and faxed it to the HMO office. He was still angry when he left his office for home an hour later.

Chapter 14

May 10

After the phone call from Coltrane, Hendricks went straight to the strip club where he knocked back four bourbons in thirty minutes. The gnawing in his stomach would not go away; and the slow, artless bump and grind of the dancers could not tear his thoughts away from the sudden and disastrous turn of events. He left the bar and found his way home, continuing his drinking in his empty apartment.

Hendricks tried to understand the events of the past three weeks. The details of the evening John Strahan died were not clear to him, even now. He had called to the New Jersey administrative center after the death, hoping to get a transcript of the events, with times and details of his responses. All that he had yet received was a printout that showed that he had refused the request for transfer. In the ensuing weeks that followed John Strahan's death, he had waited every day with gutwrenching terror; waiting for the accusations to start. But nothing had happened. The family had questions, but seemed to accept that the death was unavoidable, and no lawyers had served documents to the plan. No one had called him except Coltrane, and that discussion had seemed benign enough. Until today.

His whole life was in the balance. He had failed so many times in medicine in the past. If he lost this position, he would surely never work as a physician again. With his prior private practice indiscretions and his drug problems, he would never get another state license. And if the truth about Strahan's death was revealed, he would be black-balled from any administrative position. For Hendricks, the conversation with Coltrane had been catastrophic.

He felt that his world was swirling, moving inexorably downward, faster and faster. The tension rising, the momentum gaining. He snorted a long line of cocaine, then went into his bathroom and splashed cold water on his face. He had to act, and fast. He picked up the phone, calling the only friend he had. His drug dealer.

"Carlos, this is Hendricks."

"You out of shit already, man?" Carlos was stoned.

"No, no. I need your help. Right now. Come over right now."

"I can't, man. My car is busted. I got no ride."

"I'll pick you up in ten minutes. Straighten up."

Hendricks met with Carlos Ochoa down in the alleyway behind Carlos' apartment complex. They talked in his car for an hour before a plan was chosen. It would be easy to break into Coltrane's office; there were many master keys floating around for the medical office building. Ochoa told him that he could hire a burglar to do the work, but the expense would be great. What Ochoa didn't tell Hendricks was that he regularly broke into the offices there, taking narcotics and cash from the doctors' and dentists' offices. He had inside help in two offices, making the job even easier.

"Getting in will be easy." Ochoa told Hendricks. "But how will my man know which tape is the one you want?"

"It may be labeled with my name or the name Strahan. Or the HMO's name. It will be in his desk, locked up for sure. Or in a safe. Tell him to take anything that he sees. And then take the cash and checks to make it look like a burglary. Tell him that I will give a bonus if he finds the tape. And wear gloves. I don't want him caught and led to me and you," Hendricks rambled erratically.

"He don't need you to tell him what to wear. And this will cost five thousand up front, even if he can't find the fucking tape." Ochoa was thinking that he could slip in and get the tape before the weekend. He had looked in Coltrane's office before, but there had been nothing of interest. And he would need time to get a boom box like his brother had, so he could copy the tape before he gave it to Hendricks. Whatever was on it, this asshole thought it was very valuable. "Maybe he can do it tomorrow night."

"Tonight. It has to be tonight." Hendricks pleaded.

"Not tonight. Maybe this weekend. What will a few days change? It's there or it's not. It's already three in the morning anyway. Christ, man, don't worry. And if he can't find it, he can torch the whole place. Just get my cash. I will meet you here after the job." Ochoa got out of the car and smiled as he walked back to his girlfriend's apartment. Life was good in Florida, like the beer ad went.

Chapter 15

May 10

Coltrane was looking forward to his meeting with Susan Kerr. He made early morning rounds, and returned to his office to prepare. There were many things that he found frustrating in the private practice of medicine, and he knew that some things had to be changed. Perhaps he could change them.

Remembering the article he had read about a physicians' labor action in California, he paged Cindy on the intercom to see what she had unearthed. She brought back her research. It was not good. The organization had begun with high aspirations, but the legal obstacles proved to be insurmountable. Federal and state injunctions had immediately been filed which effectively blocked any cooperative bargaining by physician groups. Coupled with widespread hesitancy by California physicians to become involved in such a radical movement, the association was broken. Not unlike early labor unions, Coltrane mused.

Susan was early. She was ushered back to Coltrane's private office by Cindy, and sat across from him at the partner's desk. She seemed unsure as to what Coltrane had planned for the society; she had seen so many grand visions come and go.

"Susan, let me give you a little background that has bearing on why we are here today. I have been elected president of the county society as the result of a short speech that expressed my profound disgust and dissatisfaction with the way that medicine is managed today. I suspect that many physicians share these feelings, but have not expressed them, save in the doctor's lounge. My election has given me a mandate to improve the delivery of healthcare in the Bay area."

Coltrane paused, noting her quiet, non-committal interest. He continued. "The critical, key element to our success is that we are relatively isolated geographically. The nearest major city with comparable medical facilities is Orlando. In addition, we have a very competent and well trained medical community, with remarkably uniform capabilities. It is my plan to organize the medical community in such a way as to bring the hospitals and major insurance providers to the table for serious negotiations, and make some necessary changes in the way that they manage healthcare in Tampa."

Susan Kerr was silent. She knew that nothing of this nature or scope had ever been discussed, even considered before. Her interaction with the local hospitals was limited to providing copies of medical diplomas and other documents for credentialing purposes. And she had no experience at all in dealing with the huge interstate insurance corporations that provided a maze of health insurance plans.

"I have never done anything like this before, Dr. Coltrane. I wouldn't know where to start." Susan responded.

"Not a problem, Susan. This is all new to me as well. We'll go nice and slow. There are federal anti-trust laws that prohibit certain actions by doctors, and any collective action will be closely scrutinized by the Department of Justice. We will need to be very careful not to go afoul of the law. But that's down the road. The first thing that I need to know is that you will be behind me in this, and that you have no reservations about my goals and direction. Furthermore, it is my promise to you that if you feel at any time that you are uncomfortable with what we are doing, that you can freely return to your present position at the society, without repercussions."

"Of course I'll do everything I can to help. I agree that changes should be made, but whether I agree or not doesn't matter. Assisting the president is my job." Susan replied.

"Excellent. Then what I want to do today is get organized and compile basic information about our membership. The members that were present and voted for me comprise maybe a third of the total membership. We will need to poll the entire society to determine what their primary concerns are, and what their suggestions for change are. I have my solutions, but I want to hear other ideas as well. I also need basic information about the capabilities of each physician's office, for example who has an adequate computer system and medical office management software, who is doing electronic submission of claims, who is enrolled on what plan,... and so on. I assume that information is available easily at the society's office?"

"It's in the membership database, Dr. Coltrane. But it'll take time to produce." Susan answered immediately.

"How many people do we have working in the office?" Coltrane asked.

"Myself, four secretaries, and the chief administrator."

"How much power do I have as president?" Coltrane wondered.

"You can do whatever you want, within reason."

"Good. I want you to select the two brightest and most motivated of the secretaries, and detail them to our project. Use them to run down the details, and research the database. Don't be afraid to delegate work. I want you doing all the in-depth research. I don't have time to spare during the day to run down answers. I'll review your findings in the evenings. Furthermore, I want you to suspend all further expenditures except essential overhead expenses. Cancel that idiotic yearly retreat we have for the society officers.

Freeze the budget. We need legal advice, and it will be costly. Nothing gets spent unless I personally approve it. Understood?"

"Yes, doctor. The chief administrator will not like it, but he has no choice." Susan smiled.

"Finally, I want to schedule a series of meetings. I want to meet individually with each of the administrators for the major hospitals, as soon as possible. Then I want to meet with the medical directors of the top five health plans in the Tampa area. Once we've had those meetings, I want to schedule a meeting of the society. Hopefully by that time we will have the results of the membership poll, and have some basic information in hand. We need to be able to present the results of our research, and formulate a plan for the future. We need strong attendance, so schedule the meeting in the evening, on a weekday, probably Tuesday or Wednesday," Coltrane finished.

"Tuesdays have the best turn-out rate," Susan replied.

"Good. Make it next Tuesday then. Can we go over to the society office now? I want to meet everyone and look at your computer database," Coltrane smiled as he stood up.

Susan finished her notes, and rose.

"They have been anticipating your visit," she said. But, she thought, they have no idea what is coming their way.

Chapter 16

May 15

Hendricks was living a nightmare. He had only two hours of fitful sleep before getting to work late, as usual. His secretary told him that the home office had called three times already, looking for him. He could sense her fear, and his stomach tightened. He felt weak, sick. He limped into his office, closed the door and was startled as the phone immediately rang. He told the secretary to take a message.

Instead, she opened his door and entered.

"The call is from national headquarters in Jersey. It's a corporate lawyer on the line. He says if I don't get you on the phone immediately, I will be fired. Answer the phone; it's line two." She scowled at him until he lifted the receiver.

"Dr. Hendricks here."

"Dr. Hendricks, this is Richard Abbott. I am the lead risk management attorney for the plan and I need to clarify some details about a case with you. I am speaking on a recorded line. Is that understood and accepted?"

"Yes," Hendricks was dazed, and too intimidated to object.

"The plan has been served papers in a lawsuit alleging that the HMO failed to provide adequate, necessary and appropriate care to patient John Strahan, resulting in his death. Are you familiar with that case?" Abbott spoke in a monotone, as if reading from a script.

"Yes," Hendricks replied weakly.

"Describe in detail your recollection of the events, please."

Hendricks was physically shaking, and had difficulty keeping his voice from breaking. He gave a very vague, and very brief account of the phone calls that night. He did not mention the later contact with Strahan, or the call from Coltrane.

"Is that the complete extent of your involvement with this case? You spoke with no other individuals in regard to this case?" Abbott paused.

Hendricks mind screamed in confusion. Did Abbott know about the call from Strahan? Did he know about the taped call from Coltrane? If he lied, was it a trap? He knew that admission of the conversation with Coltrane would mean his immediate dismissal. His only hope was to stall and hope that he could get the tape, and that this lawyer didn't know the whole story yet. Either way, he would have to move fast. The truth would not likely stay hidden long.

"That's right," Hendricks lied.

A long silence ensued.

"I want a complete, written narrative describing the entire case, signed and dated. Fax a copy to me within 24 hours. Send the hard copy to follow. Then take a two week administrative leave. Do *not* discuss this case with anyone but myself. Is that clear?" Abbott demanded.

"Yeah," Hendricks resented the man's tone. But he clung to the hope that his lie would stand, and he would be able to salvage his job and his life. He hung up, angry and bitter.

He sat at his desk for half an hour before rising. He dictated a brief letter to the attorney, vague in detail and content, but covering the key points of the telephone conversations with the insurance coordinator that evening. He omitted the fact that he had ignored the initial and final beeper pages and requests for instructions. He also omitted the discussions with David Strahan and Dr. Coltrane. He knew that by the time those conversations were revealed, it would all be over, one way or the other. He started to clean out his desk, but before he left he had one more thing to do.

He sent his secretary on a wild goose chase to allow him uninterrupted time on the main computer terminal in his office. Moving with shaking hands, he unlocked the secure terminal and input a chain of security codes. He took a stack of blank CD-Rs and began to feed them, one by one, into the Philips burner. He copied the contents of a series of files onto the blank discs, but the process was slow and cumbersome. The software application that he was forced to use was not meant for copying data, and he had to string the data to burn it onto the discs. He had filled two discs and started on the third when his secretary burst unceremoniously into the office.

She saw immediately that he was copying confidential corporate data. She openly sneered at him, turned and went to her telephone. As she dialed security, he grabbed the two completed discs and ran out of the office, down the hallway and out the back of the building. The die was cast.

Chapter 17

May 15

Hendricks spent the rest of the day in an alcohol and cocaine induced blur. He was a dissolute man, he led a dissolute life. He knew that Ochoa would try to get into Coltrane's office that night, and if he succeeded perhaps he would be able to salvage his job, and his life. If Ochoa failed to find the tape of their conversation, then he had the discs as a last resort. He wasn't even sure what he could or would do with the information on the discs. Probably the insurance company would never submit to extortion with the data. He would never be able to go back. But he could exact a costly revenge if they did fire him. Everything was happening too fast, without time for him to think, to figure out what was happening to him. Nothing to do but wait for news from Ochoa. He went home briefly to modify and encrypt the data, and saved it to his hard drive. Then he spent the rest of the night drinking, and waiting to meet with Ochoa.

Ochoa was in a foul mood when Hendricks pulled up to him in the alley, late that night. He had not found the tape, and had been forced to end his search prematurely by the security officer making his rounds. He had left behind evidence that there had been a break-in, and was worried that he might be traced to the crime. The failure to find the tape, and with it, the chance to squeeze more cash out of this gringo asshole, was burning him.

"No luck. My man didn't find nothing." Ochoa was surly.

"Fuck. Fuck. I am screwed. I lose my job unless I get that tape." Hendricks was almost crying. He opened his car door, but was too drunk to climb out of his Mercedes.

"No tape. He went through the whole fucking place. And he wants his money, now." Ochoa lied.

"Fuck him. No tape, no money." Hendricks whined.

"Listen, chief. You pay him, or he'll just kill you. He knows who you are, where you live, what you do. You'll be dead in a week if you don't give me the cash we agreed. Now." Ochoa hissed.

"Here's thirty eight hundred. You'll get the rest later." Hendricks held his head in his hands, rocking back and forth. He pointed to a pair of CD-R jewel cases in the console tray of his sedan, and looked at them through bloodshot eyes. "This is all I have. Whistleblower."

"What are you jabbering about?" Ochoa was absorbed in counting his cash.

"Never mind. I'll call you when I get the rest of the money. Give me some time." Hendricks sat in the driver's seat for a while. Then he shut the door and drove off.

Ochoa watched the car weave slowly away, thinking that it would be a miracle if he made it home without an accident. Quickly, he finished counting the cash in his hand. Then he turned and, whistling, made for his woman's apartment. Despite a very close call, not a bad night's work.

Chapter 18

May 16

It was heralded as an auspicious evening, and it had certainly started that way. The membership meeting was scheduled for seven PM that night, and Coltrane had started rounds and surgery early to have time to organize the agenda. That had all fallen apart when Cindy had paged him during his first case. She had arrived at work to find that the office had been broken into, and trashed. Equipment was strewn about, and files rifled, and Dr. Coltrane's desk broken into and searched.

Coltrane was able to return to the office during lunch, and canvassed the damage. Nothing had been stolen, but the disarray seemed to indicate that the thief had been looking for something. The police detective thought that they were looking for narcotics. Coltrane thought otherwise.

Coltrane had no time to waste today. He returned to surgery and had Cindy give an inventory of damages to the detective. The rest would have to wait until tomorrow to be sorted out. After surgery, Coltrane spent the remaining hours preparing for the meeting.

The conference rooms were full and the excitement was palpable. Attendance was higher than any meeting, except for the Christmas party. The physicians trickled in, mingled and socialized with colleagues and referral sources. These interactions were euphemistically referred to as the "food chain". All specialists, medical and surgical, from cardiologists and nephrologists to heart surgeons and orthopedic surgeons, rely on good will to bring them patient referrals. Theoretically, the family physician or general practitioner refers his patients to the specialist who is the best suited to treat that particular patient, with that particular illness, at that particular time. In actual reality, this decision is made based upon many things, and actual technical skill and ability was unfortunately only one of the considerations. Specialists were constantly cultivating and courting their referral base, and a case of fine wine at Christmas or a private fishing charter offshore went a long way in establishing a successful practice. So the social aspects of the society meetings were very important, and Coltrane allowed time for this ritual before inaugurating the session. When he rose, the physicians gradually made their way to their seats as Coltrane approached the podium.

"Ladies and gentlemen, I wish to thank you in advance for taking the time to attend this meeting. I have a great deal to report to you, so if we can all be seated, we will begin. Please hold all your questions until the end of the session, and we can have an open discussion at that time." Coltrane began.

"It has been my intention since my election to make a serious attempt to address the problems facing us as private practitioners. To that end I have sent out a questionnaire to the membership, and it was returned with many insightful ideas and comments. In addition I have met with representatives of the regional hospitals and the primary insurance plans in the Bay area. And society has retained the services of a St. Petersburg law firm that specializes in labor law, medicine and anti-trust issues. That firm will be guiding us as we negotiate and deal with the plans.

"In analyzing the response to the questionnaire, I found that the primary concern of this membership is the lack of physician input in medical decisions at the hospital and insurance plan level. This concern was expressed by eighty seven per cent of the responding physicians. The problems were the physician's inability to control the medical decision-making process of his patient's care, due to bureaucratic interference by the hospital administration or the insurance plan. This includes DRG related demands for early discharge from the hospital, refusal to cover certain medical or surgical procedures, lack of availability of certain drugs and antibiotics, and the delays imposed by red tape and the constant need for pre-authorization of treatment. The recurring, underlying theme was that critical medical decisions were being made by middle and lower level insurance personnel with absolutely no medical knowledge.

"The second most common concern was the increasing complexity of practice management. Concerns in this area ranged from the need to hire and train additional personnel just to handle the rapidly expanding volumes of spurious paperwork demanded by HMO insurance plans, to multiple claim forms for each plan, to the ludicrous demands upon ER patients and physicians to notify the family doctor prior to admission to the ER, to the actual hard costs to participate in HMO style plans such as membership fees and dues, to the myriad mazes of approved and non-approved labs, X-ray facilities and hospitals that patients are allowed to use. We all know that a great portion of our time is now spent in unnecessary and frustrating clerical work, rather that attending to our patients needs.

"The third concern relates to medical malpractice. Everyone is seeing a dramatic increase in premiums, in the face of decreasing insurance and Medicare reimbursements. We initially saw a decline in lawsuit filings and awards in the late nineties, but that trend has been reversed in the past five years. In 1994, the average award was $375,000. In 1999, it was $800,000. Now it's over a million dollars, and climbing. I can tell you that my personal malpractice premiums have gone from $40,000 to $200,000 over two years, and I have never had a suit or a loss. Miami is having trouble keeping trauma surgeons on staff at the Level I Trauma Centers. This is a horrific situation, with dire consequences for all of us, not only as physicians, but as patients as well. I'm a trauma surgeon, but even I can't operate on myself.

"The final theme that ran thorough the poll was a sense of frustration and impotence in dealings with the plans and the hospitals. The insurance industry had a banner year with phenomenal profits last year. Still, they have cut back the reimbursement schedules to hospitals and physicians dramatically. The hospital industry is doing well, as can be evidenced by the expansion and construction of new facilities across the country. But as physicians, we feel isolated and individually weak. Medicine is the most regulated of all fields by the federal government, and physicians are the most regulated in medicine. We cannot organize, we cannot negotiate or collectively bargain, and we cannot discuss fees without breaking federal law. The insurance companies send us thick, incomprehensible contracts with no fee guidelines, and we dutifully sign on faith. But I think that we are all reaching the point where we must make some changes, both for our patients and for ourselves.

"So there we have the problems, greatly simplified. The challenge facing us as a society is how best to remedy the situation. I have had meetings with the hospital administrators over the past weeks, and there is agreement on many issues between the hospitals and the medical staffs. Hospitals and physicians have traditionally worked well together. To further increase the cooperation, we will be forming committees that coordinate the various medical staff presidents with the society and with the administrators. I do not foresee any problems in that arena. The problem seems to be with the insurance plans.

"I asked for meetings with the seven largest insurance plans here in Tampa- St. Petersburg. Only two agreed to meet with me, and they sent the public relations officer rather than the medical director. The meetings were short and very non-productive. Essentially the message was that they had no intention to make any changes, and that things would in all likelihood get worse rather than better for physicians. Again the attitude was that if you don't like the plan, then leave.

"At this point, I formed a committee of physicians representing the major medical and surgical specialties. All members are volunteers, and will act as spokespersons for their respective specialties. We met and drafted a resolution that lists the major changes that we feel are critical, and you will find that list in the materials at your table. The issues are the ones discussed earlier, ranging from fixed uniform fee schedules, to listed covered procedures, to physician participation in medical decision-making policies by the plans. This list will be polished and presented to all insurance entities licensed in the three county area within one week.

"That's the good news. Now the bad news. From the poll, I was surprised to find that only sixty per cent of our membership have a Pentium 4 computer in the office, and of that number, only half can use it themselves. That has to change. We all need to enter the twenty-first century.

"Included in your materials is a list of the minimum computer equipment that all of us must have within one month. The gear must be IBM/PC compatible for ease of software applications. You must have a state of the art fax-modem to communicate with the insurance companies and more importantly, with the society. I am in the process of establishing an Internet website, and this should be operable within one month. The website will be like a news service and bulletin board, allowing all the membership to converse, leave messages and view progress as it happens. It will allow secure and instantaneous communication among all of us. The technology here is incredible. For those of us that are not computer literate, there will be clinics on topics from choosing equipment to operating the online network at the society office.

"One final word about the Internet online network. You will all be given password to enter the system, just like using a cash machine. These passwords will identify you to the system, and maintain the confidentiality of the system. The codes are not to be given to office staff, secretaries or even your wives. The system should be used only in private, and viewed with the same security as medicolegal records. Were someone to gain unauthorized access to the system, severe damage will result.

"Lastly, this effort will be expensive in both time and money. Our budget is based on the costs of the yearly directory and the Christmas party. The committee, on my recommendation, has canceled all social events in order to use these funds in a more productive manner. Even with these savings we will need a voluntary donation of one thousand dollars from each member to finance this effort."

There was an immediate low rumble of disapproval and much shifting in the seats.

"I will start by donating five thousand myself. I would remind those of you grumbling that in the last election, there were law firms in this city that donated hundreds of thousands of dollars to candidates that support their views. This should be even more important to us. This is the future of our profession."

The rumble subsided somewhat. They knew that physicians as a group were notoriously cheap when it came to political and professional donations.

"Thank you very much for your gracious patience. I now open the floor for discussion." Coltrane finished.

"Bill, we have been crying about these problems for years now. How are you going to force the plans to change with some computer game?" Dr. Fredericks challenged loudly from the rear of the room.

"Listen, the website is not a game. The Internet site is a tool; it will allow us to communicate quickly and disseminate information instantly. We have always been isolated in our individual practices, rarely sharing information or experiences effectively. With a website we can inform each other about problems with the financial aspects of our practices, our interfaces with payers, anything that impacts medicine. We have to end our isolation. We have to have a dialogue addressing the critical issues that affect our ability to deliver healthcare to our patients."

"We have a long road to travel." Coltrane continued before someone could interrupt him. "But I feel that we will succeed because we have much more power and influence than we realize. Despite the seeming erosion of the image of the physician, our patients still respect us individually. No one knows better how medicine should be practiced than doctors. The public knows that. I think that we can make some great changes; maybe not in the national picture, but surely here in the Bay area. But nothing will happen if we don't try."

"Will we be in violation of the federal anti-trust statutes by these actions?" Jack Ferrara asked calmly.

"Nothing I have proposed thus far is illegal. But the attorneys in St. Pete will be guiding all our moves, and their advice will be printed in complete form on the network. Everything will be done absolutely by the book and to the letter of the law."

There were several other comments rising from the group, but Coltrane ended the meeting with the recommendation that all further discussion be taken up with the specialty representatives. He quickly left the podium and the meeting room with Susan Kerr. She struggled to keep up with him as he made for the elevator.

"Quick exit, Dr. Coltrane. You afraid of the questions?" Susan asked with a smile once they were safely in the elevator.

Coltrane laughed. "Yeah, I actually am. But that's the way I want to run the meetings from now on. No alcohol, no open bar and hors D'oeuvres, and no thirty minutes of bullshit and discussion at the beginning and the end. There are always a few guys who love to hear the sound of their own voices. You know who I am talking about." Coltrane remembered a psychiatrist who had rambled on at a meeting non-stop for twenty minutes about nothing. Coltrane and Ferrara couldn't figure out what he had been talking about. Or why. They decided that it was his revenge for having to listen passively to people's problems all day.

"But what is this about an Internet service? I don't know anything about that." Susan had been surprised at that announcement.

"That idea just came to me as I was speaking. You would think that if ten year olds can organize international bulletin boards to play Final Fantasy, we should be able to set up a local system. That we'll have to check out tomorrow."

"Hope you're right. Nice speech though." Susan commented.

"I don't like public speaking, and that address was a big step for me. Especially the request for money. They will be cursing me for a year. Hopefully we will get some donations from the group. Thank you very much for your help. See you tomorrow at the society office. We have a great deal to do to keep this effort moving." Coltrane saw her to her car and left for home.

Coltrane slept poorly that night, unable to rest as problems and possible solutions continually crept into his consciousness. He made rounds early, and was in the society office at seven AM. Susan arrived at eight, and they started soon after. Coltrane reviewed the capabilities of the society's outdated computers with Susan, and they decided to purchase a new Intel based computer with a state of the art communications interface for the sole purpose of running the Internet service. The old computers could be used for all the routine database applications. Coltrane had recently equipped his own office with a new computer system, and was familiar with the currently available technology.

"We'll need a high speed Pentium based computer to act as the brain of our website, one with a huge hard drive, maybe dual hard drives, and 512 megabytes of memory. And to communicate with the computers in the offices of the members, we need high speed, continuous Internet connection. Probably a cable or satellite modem. I think that the rest of the interface is done at a remote location, maybe a huge mainframe computer or a server somewhere. We can have IBM or Gateway or Dell provide the actual website hosting. I really don't know all the details on how to set up a website. You'll have to make some calls and find a consultant to help us with that."

"No problem," Susan replied, making a note in her daily planner.

"Actually, I think that Dell can set the entire thing up for us. But make some calls and get several bids. We will need to establish a very secure website, with limited access by the public. The public access section will have society members' information, such as medical school, Board Certification, office phone numbers, and insurance plan affiliation. Nothing too complex. Maybe some general health tips, useful information about clinics and blood drives and so on. I want ninety-five percent of the website to be restricted to physician access only. The website should allow physicians to get current medical research, Medline articles, and current drug and prescription information. I want to provide a substantial continuing medical education component. In addition to that database, I want the website to allow secure communications between the society and the members, and among the members themselves. And I want to gather information about the membership and about the insurance plans."

"What kind of information?" Susan raised her eyebrows in interest.

"Health plan policies. Covered procedures. Fee schedules. Complaints. Disciplinary actions. Anything and everything that pertains to the way that insurance plans and HMOs do business." Coltrane turned and looked intently at Susan to gauge if she comprehended the intent of the website.

"I see," she answered quietly.

"Excellent. Our priorities must be the cash donations first, then the computer service, then the in-depth discussions with the attorneys, then the listing and presentation of our demands to the insurance plans." Coltrane paused, thinking.

"Demands?" Susan was taken aback by the term.

"Yes. We have to look at this as a labor versus management dispute, even though it may not be technically classified as such. I want to stress that I will not do anything that is illegal; however this is a gray area in the law. If you have any legal or ethical concerns, you may step down and I will find someone to replace you. You will of course remain at your prior duties at the society." Coltrane allowed her to consider the possibilities. He wanted her to understand fully the ramifications of the course that they were planning.

"As I said before, this is my job. If anything changes, I'll tell you." Susan was enjoying the challenge.

"Excellent. I am going to go to St. Pete this week to meet with the lawyers. What we should do in the next week is pressure the membership for the dues, and obtain as much information about the Internet service as possible. I will leave that up to you. Pick up the checks personally from the doctor's offices if you have to. I am going to spec out and order the office computer tonight, and also two Pentium V notebook computers with cellular fax-modems so that you and I can communicate easily. Let's get them set up and functioning as quickly as possible." Coltrane was happy with the immediate plan.

"Great. I'll see you when you get back." Susan took her notes, and started to get up.

"One more thing. See if you can arrange a meeting with Dr. Hendricks for next week. He may be our weak link, a good place to start negotiations." Coltrane was hoping that Hendricks' compromised position might be the chink in the armor that he needed.

"Sure. Oh, by the way, do you have a name for our website?"

"*Caduceus*."

The ancient Greek symbol for the art and science of medicine.

Chapter 19

May 18

Coltrane had been busy for a solid week with a backload of surgery resulting from his taking time away from the practice for society duties. He had two wrist reconstructions and a severely burned patient that took all his time for that week, and little was done on society business. Finally, late in the afternoon, he got out from under the workload and was free to contact Susan.

"Susan, this is Coltrane. How are things coming along? I have been very busy lately and delinquent in the society duties. Fill me in." Coltrane apologized.

"Everything is going very well. We received the computers; thank you very much. The Pentium main station is running well, and its sole function will be the input of data for the Internet service. We have put in a dedicated cable modem line for that computer only, and I am trying to learn how to use my notebook computer as well. I got multiple bids from Internet consultants, and went with the Dell proposal. I have been meeting with them all week, and things are moving very rapidly. *Caduceus* is one week from being operational and online, and seems to be very simple to use. I want to show you how they organized the home page and the site map, but I feel that you will like the design. The membership should adjust to it well."

"Very nice job, Susan. How are the donations coming in?" Coltrane asked.

"Pretty well. We have a total of five hundred seventy-three members, and we have received twenty percent of the members' dues. Still, that amounts to over one hundred thousand dollars, and that should keep us running for the next several months. I have an idea how to speed up the cash flow, but you may not like it." Susan hesitated.

"Go ahead."

"When we go online, the introduction graphic can be anything we want. I thought for the first few months, we could show who has and who hasn't made their contribution. That may embarrass the holdouts."

"Outstanding, Susan. You really have a flair for this." Coltrane laughed. That tactic would be very effective, but most certainly piss off the recalcitrant physicians. Good, he thought. He didn't want anyone riding on his coat-tails.

"Thank you. I have another idea. I've spoken with the major distributor of computers here in town, and they will give the society a significant discount if we buy fifty or more units. I told him that we have over two hundred doctors who need office computers. That's the figure that we derived from our poll last month. He will set up and program the computers in the doctors' offices, instruct the staff how to use the computers and install all software that we select. The electronic claims submission software is available through Medicare at no charge, and some of the insurance plans also offer free software for that purpose. Those services alone are worth the dues, and if you include the computer savings, it is a very sweet deal for the members," Susan finished.

"Great. Do it. I have a medical office management software system that I will see if we can get as well, and you should send out a letter immediately about your idea. This will accelerate our communication network. Soon we will be like the Hydra." Coltrane rambled, out loud.

"Hydra?" Susan was confused.

"The Hydra was a mythological beast, with many heads, and one body. Sorry. The point is that if we can be connected instantly, we can let each other know what is happening to our profession much more effectively than ever before. We will know when drugs are removed from the pharmacies, when patients are being dumped from hospitals, when individual doctors are concerned about medical matters. Up to now, we have all been living in our own cocoons, and find out about these disasters only too late. The possibilities are endless."

"What did the lawyers say down in St. Pete? I got their bill before you got back to town." Susan brewed.

"I think it was a very worthwhile meeting. I want to discuss the details with you because we need to insert some language in the welcoming page on the Internet service. We will make a simple warning that every member will have to see before going online, to remind them what is legal and what is not. But basically the attorneys said that so far we are in the clear. We will have to be very careful when we get to the phase where we negotiate with the third party payers. Speaking of the insurance companies, have you made contact with Hendricks yet?"

"Very strange with him. His secretary first told me he was at a meeting, then two days later she started saying he was sick. Now it appears that he is on leave, or has been fired. All the medical matters have been referred to the main office in New Jersey." Susan had been unable to arrange a meeting with Hendricks, or anyone else from that carrier.

"He is in trouble about the Strahan case, if I am correct." Coltrane reflected on that tragedy. He hadn't heard anything from Strahan or his attorney since the last meeting in his office. Coltrane wished that he could contact them and see what was happening. He finished his discussion with Susan and started going through the piles of messages and mail on his desk.

He found no messages from Strahan, and several from an attorney that he did not know. Then he found the letter he was looking for. It was a certified letter, on heavy linen paper, with the telltale letterhead of twenty or thirty names indicative of a large, powerful law firm. The first three partners were long dead. He began to read it, and saw that Strahan was listed as the plaintiff, and that there was a very long list of defendants: Bayside community Hospital, some New Jersey hospital corporation, the HMO insurance company, Dr. Hendricks, Dr. Foster, Dr. Meyer, Dr. Nichols and,... the name jumped off the page at him...*Dr. William Coltrane.*

Coltrane was stunned. He was being listed and sued in the case? Why? Attached to the legal document was a letter informing Dr. Coltrane that he was being named in a malpractice action involving the wrongful death of John Strahan. The attorney was demanding copies of the records.

Coltrane felt a knot in his stomach that was physically painful. He tore the papers in half and cursed, then threw them on the floor. He sat in his chair, and hoped that this was a mistake on the lawyer's part, and that Strahan would correct him. He got up, found the letter and taped it back together. He dialed the number on the letterhead.

"Perth, Lawton and Perth." a young woman's voice answered sweetly.

"John Alistair, please."

"Who shall I say in calling?"

"Dr. William Coltrane."

After a short pause, Alistair came on the phone. "Dr. Coltrane, it is not usual that I discuss cases with the defendants except in the courtroom. What can I do for you?"

"I was never involved in this case, how can you list me as a plaintiff? Does Strahan know he is suing me?" Coltrane was angry, and spoke quickly.

"Of course he knows. He initially didn't want to proceed against you, but he now realizes that you were at fault along with the doctors in Miami. I will not discuss this with you any further. Send me your records as soon as possible." Alistair demanded curtly and hung up the phone.

Coltrane could barely control his rage and frustration. He slammed down the phone and cursed bitterly. He had done everything he could have done, and more. He would have done more if he had known more about John's medical condition. But he had been told nothing until the boy died. What reasonable person would blame him for the death? He felt sure that he would be vindicated in the end, but one could never tell. And he would surely suffer during the trial. The media would name all the defendants, and that would taint his name irreparably. The trial and the depositions and preparations would take weeks out of his schedule; and the cost to defend the case would be staggering. Not to mention the physical and emotional stress and damage that a jury trial would engender. He had seen friends' spirits broken by long, arduous and petty lawsuits. He sank lower into his chair, and felt the strength fade from his body.

He thought about the medical records request. He had no records, nor had he made any notes about the discussion with Strahan or the hospital that evening. He had seen no need to do so. Now he realized that he would need an attorney. He knew that he would have to discuss the matter with his medical malpractice insurance company, something he had not yet done. He looked up the number in his electronic organizer, and called. He was directed to the Risk Management Department, and spoke to a case worker. She told him that an attorney would call him within the hour.

Coltrane sat back, and tried to make some sense out of the situation. He asked Cindy to hold all calls other than the lawyer's. He tried to understand why Strahan would want to sue him, if not for the money involved. Certainly Alistair would have done his best to enflame Strahan. The more plaintiffs, the more money. But he could have been a friendly witness for Strahan. Why throw away a friendly witness to the events? And what should he do with the tape? He had not had a chance to tell David about the discussion with Hendricks, and now the circumstances were drastically different.

Cindy buzzed him to let him know that the lawyer was on the line.

"Dr. Coltrane here."

"Dr. Coltrane, this is Mark Roland, with Florida Southern Malpractice Company. I understand that you received an Article 533 letter today?" Roland sounded calm. Roland referred to Article 533, recently enacted by the Florida Legislature, requiring that all physicians named in any suit be notified immediately upon filing of the action.

"I got a letter from an attorney requesting records on a patient who died in Miami several weeks ago." Coltrane went into the details with Roland, sparing nothing, and discussed the problem with Hendricks and the conversation that they had. He mentioned that the content of the discussion was damaging to the HMO, and that he had taped the conversation.

Roland listened quietly, taking notes, and occasionally interrupting to clarify one detail or another.

"What do you think?" Coltrane asked, completing his story.

"First, John Strahan was never a patient of yours before the shooting? Correct?"

"Correct," Coltrane answered.

"And you never sent a bill or charged for your assistance the night of the shooting?"

"Correct."

"Well, first of all, this is clearly covered by your malpractice insurance even though the child was not truly a patient of yours, and you never treated him. Therefore, the company will provide legal defense for this claim under your existing policy. I do not think that it will be difficult to prove that, under Florida law, you did not fulfill the legal requirements of a treating physician. I think that we will very quickly get you dropped from this suit. Secondly, I think that under the new statutes that the Republicans have enacted in the State legislature you may have a strong potential for a countersuit. That, of course, would be up to you, and you would have to assume all legal fees yourself." Roland was confident and unperturbed.

"Then why would that idiot name me in the suit?" Coltrane was angry.

"Probably he is hoping that we will settle, rather than fight it in court. Your legal fees in a case like this usually run about seventy-five to eighty thousand dollars, and most companies will settle out of court to minimize costs. But, as you know, we are a doctor owned entity, and we have always maintained an aggressive policy in this regard. We will not negotiate or settle unless you specifically request us to do so. When the attorney discovers that you are insured with us, he will probably drop you from the defendant list."

"This is absurd." Coltrane was becoming even more outraged as he learned how the game was played.

"Listen. Off the record, there is an option that you may want to consider. The taped conversation that you have is valuable to the case, and Strahan's lawyer would be a fool not to use it. But you have no reason to give it to him, and he does not even know that it exists. Am I correct?" Roland moved slowly with this line of thought.

"That's correct." Coltrane followed along.

"You may be able to finesse a significant expert witness fee from Strahan's attorney by holding your testimony over his head. It amounts to legal blackmail, but it is done every day. You will bargain with him, using the testimony that you described to me as your trump card. But I must warn you, don't try to do this by yourself. You'll need to retain another attorney to help you with this action. And I suggest an attorney who does not routinely involve himself with litigation. Whoever represents you will not engender any love in the trial lawyers' society in the Bay area."

"But once he knows that I spoke with Hendricks, can't he just force me to testify to that effect?" Coltrane liked the concept, but did not understand how to pull it off.

"Let your lawyer work that out. It is all in the use of attorney client privilege. Sleight of hand. It may work, and if it does, you will probably be able to split the contingency fee, maybe get ten per cent of the total award. Lawyers are always doing this kind of deal. In fact, there are lawyers who specialize in finding and farming out cases to other attorneys. They never try a case themselves, but get a hefty percentage of any settlement."

"Amazing." Coltrane liked the idea of stealing from Alistair. He was silent.

"This whole thing is a sad story. I have a teenage daughter, and I empathize with Strahan. But you did everything that you could, didn't you? Keep in touch with me about the case. And since we will maintain that you at no time accepted John Strahan as a patient, do not send any records or material to his attorney. Send me all correspondence from them and do not discuss this with anyone, except your private lawyer. Best of luck, Dr. Coltrane." Roland left his fax number, and hung up.

Coltrane sat in his office for an hour and thought about the recent turn of events. His staff had gone home long ago. Only the arrival of the night janitor roused him, and finally he headed for home.

The house was empty when he arrived, so he ate some cold leftovers, and turned on CNN. The world is still as fucked up as it was yesterday, he thought. By the time Britt returned from her workout at the gym, he had finished two drinks and was getting philosophical.

Coltrane followed his young wife into the master bath, and watched her slip out of her running bra and spandex shorts. He set down his glass of wine, and ran an appreciative hand along a smooth thigh, admired her taut belly. Her skin was hot, flushed from hours of exercise, her muscles full and hard. He pulled her close, held her hard against him and kissed her lightly on the mouth, tasting her full, wet lips, feeling the heat of her body. She pushed him away, annoyed by the attention while she was still sweaty from the workout. Coltrane laughed as he took off his scrubs and followed her into the shower. She feigned coyness as he bathed her, caressing her breasts and nipples through the slippery lather, running his hands over her coltish legs, cupping her buttocks in his palm.

Their bodies clean and still wet, they went from the bath to lay on the bed, and made love. Wordlessly, with the intensity and passion that comes only from years of tenderness, they pleased each other.

Spent, Coltrane collapsed back and luxuriated in the sensations coursing through his frame. Britt showered again, and he joined her. Afterwards, as they lay in bed, he told her about the tactic that Roland had proposed. He was unsure if it could succeed.

"The only attorneys that I know personally are unlikely to help. They are all relatively high profile in litigation and personal injury and will be vulnerable to retaliation from Alistair sooner or later." Coltrane explained.

"What about the lawyers in the group against lawsuit abuse? Aren't there several attorneys involved in that coalition?" Britt asked. She had been to some of the organization's meetings, and remembered those present.

"Most of them are politicians, judges and public officials. They probably do not practice this type of law, and may not be willing to go against David Strahan because of his involvement with the coalition."

"Can you think of anyone who just doesn't like this guy? What's his name?"

"Alistair."

"Maybe some lawyer who has been beaten by him in the past?"

"Shit, they don't take lawsuits personally. I see them in the club all the time, drinking and bullshitting about the day's proceeding. Winner and loser, laughing over drinks. It is just a game to them. The only one who loses is the client. The attorney always gets paid." Coltrane sneered.

"Someone must have suffered a loss somewhere along the road. This is a small town. People remember." Britt paused, and then sat up. She looked at her husband and smiled. "What about one of the hospital attorneys? Aren't they always opposed to the trial attorneys?"

"You're a genius. Maybe our kids will have a chance after all."

"If you ever decide you have time for children." Britt responded softly.

"All in good time, my love. Soon. Maybe if I can get a partner in the practice."

"I know, sweetheart. When we are both ready. What about Davis Clark?"

Coltrane considered her suggestion. There were three major hospitals in town, and he knew one of the hospital lawyers personally. Davis Clark was a wily attorney, and a friend. Coltrane had repaired a chin laceration on his youngest son years ago. Tomorrow he would give him a call. Satisfied, he went to sleep beside his wife.

Chapter 20

May 19

It took five phone calls and three hours before Coltrane contacted Davis Clark, the St. Mary's Hospital attorney. Clark, as always, was cordial. He saw the daily workings of the hospital and its physicians and nurses, and was frequently asked to defend them in court. Over ninety percent of the time, he won.

"How are you doing, Bill?" Clark asked sincerely.

"Not so well, Davis. I have a problem that I want to discuss with you. You heard about the Strahan boy, didn't you?"

"Yeah, that is very sad. He and my boy were in school together. He was often at the house, nice kid." Clark was silent.

"Really? Your boy is a teenager already?" Coltrane was surprised how fast time had passed. "How does his chin look?"

"Great. Whenever you ask about his chin, I know you want me to apply pressure to someone, Bill. You got a lot of mileage from that one inch cut, Doc." Clark laughed.

"Yeah. Did I ever charge you for that, by the way?" Coltrane knew he hadn't.

"What can I do for you?" Clark laughed.

"I have been named in David Strahan's suit against the HMO and the hospital…" Coltrane started.

"As a defendant? I didn't know anyone here was involved. How did you get named?" Clark interrupted.

"David Strahan called me the night of the shooting, asking for help. I did what I could from here. I don't know why they named me. I thought Strahan was a friend. But the reason that I called is that I have damning evidence against the HMO, and I need legal advice on how to use it. Britt thought of you. Can you come to my office? It should be discussed in private." Coltrane finished.

"No problem. How about five o'clock?"

"Good."

Coltrane saw patients until four o'clock, then closed the office early and sent the staff home. They enjoyed the time off, and he had time to organize his thoughts and notes. Clark arrived late, but in good spirits. They retired to Coltrane's private office, and sat opposite each other across the desk, upon which rested all the legal documents that Alistair had sent Coltrane.

"I see that one of my colleagues has been hard at work." Clark smiled ruefully.

"John Alistair."

"The prick. I had to settle a bullshit case with him last year. Obstetrical disaster related to a drug abusing mother. He wanted to pin it on the hospital anesthesiologist. Despite the fact that the mother was so high when she delivered that she didn't need anesthesia. We had to put her in detox for a week before she could go home. But they demanded a jury trial, and the administration guys didn't want the negative publicity. So we settled." Clark's face was contorted with distaste as he recalled the incident.

"He's suing me for the Strahan death." Coltrane went straight to the point. He laid out the history of the boy's death, and his involvement. He related the opinion of his malpractice attorney, and then paused. "I really don't think that I am at great risk regarding malpractice in this case, but…"

"I agree. You didn't formally accept Strahan as your patient." Clark interrupted.

"Right. But there is a different reason that I asked to speak with you. Before I received the letter naming me as a defendant in this suit, I had assumed that I would be a friendly witness for Strahan. And I spoke to the HMO that Strahan was enrolled with at the time of John's death. There was some question about whether or not to transfer the boy that night."

Coltrane went into detail about the attempted transfer, and then about the discussion with the HMO physician, Hendricks. He explained that he had taped the discussion, and then played a copy of the tape for Clark. Clark sat quietly, but was obviously stunned.

Coltrane paused, allowing all the elements of the situation to sink in. Then he recounted the strategy that Mark Roland had suggested. He gave Clark time to contemplate the tactic.

"Roland has a copy of the tape?" Clark questioned.

"No, this is the only copy. He knows about the conversation, but didn't want the tape. I want to keep it as a last resort tactic."

"The tactic is borderline, but legal. You are under no legal obligation to volunteer that tape, as this is a civil proceeding, not a criminal one. I could approach Alistair and demand to be made a part of the legal team, with a fee based on a percentage of the award. I would have to convince him that your evidence is so damning that it would significantly increase his chance of winning, or increase the amount of the award. The problem is that I would have to do that without revealing your name. Once he knows that you are the source, he can simply interrogate you on the stand. And that would cost him nothing." Clark sat back and thought for several minutes.

"Well, first of all, would you be willing to try this?" Coltrane asked.

"Hell yes. The beauty of this is that Alistair will get screwed, but the award to Strahan will not be reduced. Your money would come straight from Alistair's fees. I'm assuming that the case was taken on a contingency arrangement. I'm sure that it was. I suppose I could do my part for a straight hourly fee. But a stiff hourly fee, Doc." Clark smiled.

"Fine. I can always stop if the cost gets prohibitive, right?"

"Sure. You should know that this is a long shot. But there will be very little time involved here. We will try to get papers filed, a lien on the award, as soon as possible." Clark stopped, seeing the puzzled look on Coltrane's face.

"A lien is filed with the presiding judge who is handling this case. It will be signed by myself and Alistair, and it guarantees that we will be paid first from the settlement award. There are usually many liens on cases like this, for attorneys, medical bills, court reporters and the like. The money that is left will be divided by Alistair and Strahan. You can pay me from that settlement. Fair enough?" Clark seemed delighted at the idea.

"Very fair." Coltrane reached across the desk and the two men shook hands.

"The next thing I will do is meet with Alistair and present the proposal. I will create the impression that the witness is an internal HMO source, someone who came to me asking advice on how to proceed with insider knowledge. Maybe Hendricks' secretary? I will not mention the existence of the tape. It may or may not be admissible, but certainly with Hendricks and the HMO aware of its existence, your position will be greatly strengthened. You had better give me the tape for safekeeping in the hospital vault. I'll ask for sixteen percent of the award. That'll be one third of his fee. Not bad, you think?" Clark grinned an evil grin.

"I don't know..." Coltrane's voice trailed off.

"What?" Clark queried.

"That seems inappropriate somehow."

"Listen. If you didn't have this tape, you would be looking at seventy-five, maybe a hundred thousand dollars to defend this suit. That prick knows that you were not guilty of malpractice, or even misconduct. Your conduct doesn't come even close to fulfilling the legal requirements for medical malpractice. In fact, because you didn't charge for your help, you may even be covered by the State of Florida under the Good Samaritan Statutes." Clark was vehement. "I would ask for twenty percent, if I were in your place."

"You're right. You handle the negotiations. I have never been very good at that."

Coltrane and Clark talked for several minutes further, and then concluded. Coltrane gave the cassette to Clark, who carefully slipped it into a manila folder, and placed it in his briefcase.

Life is so complex, Coltrane thought as Clark left the office. He felt guilty at the thought of profiting from this tragedy. And it seems that they could profit handsomely indeed. But at least his motives had been good from the start. He wondered how some lawyers could sleep at night. He turned off the lights, and headed for home, weary.

Five blocks away, Clark pulled into a convenience store and pumped seven quarters into the payphone on the wall. His conversation was animated. Twenty minutes later, he hung up. He was smiling.

Chapter 21

May 22
4:33PM

Davis Clark called Coltrane late in the afternoon three days later. He had spoken in detail with Alistair, and described the content and the critical value of his client's testimony. Alistair had been very interested, especially as the insurance plan had the deepest pockets of all the defendants. But unfortunately, Clark said, he laughed outright when the fee split was introduced. He countered with an offer of five percent. Clark had refused. He suggested to Coltrane that they sit on the offer for a week and then meet and discuss the possibilities. Coltrane agreed.

Chapter 22

May 30

Things were moving rapidly at the medical society office. Susan Kerr had completed the initial software installation for the Internet service, and a trial run was planned for later that afternoon. The computer system had been set-up via downloading the required data in minutes. Somewhere in the United States, a huge powerful mainframe computer would handle all the incoming data from the individual physician, and process it back to them at the speed of light. All that remained was for Coltrane to upload the final components of the website from CD-Rs he had painstakingly created, and brought today in his briefcase.

Caduceus was organized into two primary sections, one for the general public, and one for the physician membership. The general public had access to updated health information, hyperlinks to appropriate and credible health information sources, and basic information about the medical community. Doctors' office hours, addresses and training or specific areas of expertise were listed to help the patient choose a physician. Health fairs, and other public services of the society and state and local health agencies were listed.

But the critical content of *Caduceus* was for physicians only. This area was secure, and comprised of three primary sections; medical education, society positions, and political actions. It opened with a strong and clear warning relating to the confidentiality of all communications on the service, and admonitions not to allow non-members access to the material in any form. From the medical education menu that followed, the physicians could select from a library of current medical periodicals, short texts on late pharmaceutical developments, and even access MEDLINE, a vast compilation of medical knowledge spanning decades in thirty languages. On the society position menu, Coltrane listed in short form the position that the society took on the major matters that were discussed in the recent meeting. There was a synopsis of what the membership felt was wrong with medicine as it was currently practiced, and how to best remedy the situation. The wording was very carefully chosen.

But it was the political action section that was the keystone of the system. The other two areas were just window dressing to Coltrane. All that information was available elsewhere. He wanted to organize and motivate and strengthen the medical community with political action. When the society had elected him president, he had thought that seeking significant change would be a futile effort. But he had felt that he should make that effort. Now, as the system materialized before his eyes, he realized its full potential. He knew that if he could successfully harness the tremendous power of the physician community, he could enforce their demands upon the insurance plans.

He sorrowfully reflected on the decline of medicine in his professional lifetime. He had entered medical school in the seventies, with a great intellectual hunger and a strong urge to understand medicine and excel in it. He, like all the other students in the entering class, had absolutely no knowledge of the realities of medicine, of dealing with the sick, the infirm, the dying. They, like all that preceded them, were attracted by the challenges: physical, spiritual and intellectual. They were proud of the intense and arduous training that they endured and overcame. They were the pinnacle of the educational process, enduring the most lengthy training sequence, and the most demanding. Competition simply to enter American medical schools had been brutal. Four years of college with majors in the sciences, chemistry, physics and mathematics. All the time, aware that among his classmates, only one in two hundred would get a place in medical school.

Then four years of medical school, and the gradual immersion into the clinical sciences. Anatomy, microbiology, pharmacology, biochemistry. Working on the hospital wards, drawing blood, taking stool samples, doing scut work for the nurses, the senior medical students, the interns and the residents. Slave labor. He had deeply resented that aspect of his training, and in retrospect, he still wondered what the medical school administration hoped to prove by the ritual. Finally, graduation and the pride of his parents and family. Embarking on a great journey, an opportunity to wield his newfound skill and talent.

Seven years of residency awaited him after medical school. Few laymen realize that in modern American medicine, a medical degree is only the beginning of the training. He used to think that the purpose of medical school was to weed out the weak, the vain, the dreamers and the posers. He and his surgeon friends would joke that they never used anything that they learned in medical school, anyway. But post-graduate training was another matter. He spent five years in general surgery residency, learning the skills and diagnostic wisdom to earn the right to violate the sanctity of another human body with a knife. He had extensive exposure to general surgery, cardiothoracic surgery, orthopedic surgery, pediatric surgery, urological surgery, trauma surgery, hand surgery, head and neck surgery, vascular surgery and plastic surgery. It had been trauma surgery that had thrilled and amazed him. It was a period of spectacular advances in surgery, and trauma surgery in particular. New techniques of burn reconstruction, synthetic skin substitutes, advances in the treatment of multiple trauma and pharmacological techniques for pulmonary and vascular support of the critically injured patient and a technological renaissance in plastic surgery. Coltrane had loved being a part of it. Despite an almost irresistible urge to start practice, Coltrane took an additional two years in fellowships in Trauma Surgery and Hand Surgery. Then, after over a decade of medical training, he established his private practice.

For almost two decades, Coltrane had a rewarding and distinguished career. He had the respect of his patients, and his referring physicians. He practiced honest and ethical medicine, avoided excessive treatment and perfected his art. He prided himself on the rarity of his surgical complications, in a specialty where complications were routine. His professional and personal life was beyond reproach.

Then the rot had set in. Tremendous amounts of time were spent justifying surgical procedures to insurance companies. The arrival of HMOs and managed care further oppressed medicine. The government programs were thoughtfully designed by accountants and bureaucrats to minimize the funds expended on health care. As all this was happening, the public was demanding that healthcare be considered a fundamental right. Coltrane had lived through it all, and hoped every year that it would get better, that people would realize that health care is not a commodity, but a service. That healthcare does not respond to an economic model that some Washington political appointee tries to place it into. Volume discounts do not work in medicine. There are only twenty four hours in a day. Any family practitioner will tell you that. But just when he thought it could not get any worse, it would.

Physicians had clearly lost their self-determination and power. While the public always saw them as the most expensive part of healthcare, in fact physicians' fees were less than seventeen per cent of the total costs. The waste and the excessive profit taking was by the middlemen, the parasites of the system. The fraud in healthcare revolted Coltrane. He felt that physicians, and only physicians, had the knowledge and experience to govern the system. That was the goal that drove him.

And *Caduceus* and the political action segment was the weapon that would make collective bargaining a reality. Coltrane was one of the few physicians that fully realized the enormous power that they held. He often contemplated the effect of a mass labor action by doctors. The result would be paralyzing. Almost incomprehensible.

It further amazed him that physicians themselves never considered this as an option. Many felt that any such action would violate the Hippocratic oath. Maybe they were right. But as medicine became corrupted by outside influences to an intolerable level, perhaps it was the only way to address the situation. Drastic situations require drastic measures, he thought.

Coltrane had spent weeks organizing and collecting the database for *Caduceus*. Now, he took a stack of CD-Rs from his leather briefcase, and carefully stacked them on the table next to the computer tower. In the exact, specified sequence, he uploaded the data from the CD-Rs into *Caduceus*. In the political action subsection of *Caduceus*, Coltrane input a massive compilation of information. He entered the five primary insurance HMO plans, and the basic forms of their administrative structure. This explained the protocols that every participating doctor must adhere to in the process of treating patients. It covered the procedures mandated to order tests, request a second opinion or consultation, to admit patients, and to transfer or discharge patients. Then he input the lists of all the participating doctors on each plan. He added the fee schedules for each plan, and how the fees related to the Medicare fee schedules. Lastly, he described in concise but brutally clear terms the financial and legal risks that all participating physicians would incur if they strayed from the HMO's rules.

Coltrane knew that none of the physicians in private practice ever read the fifty page contracts that they got from HMOs. He knew that they signed if their colleagues were on a plan, or if one of their referral sources was a provider. Many times they signed because they were afraid that if they didn't sign, they would lose their patient base. Further he knew that they never read, or could hope to have the time or legal vocabulary to understand, the three hundred page bylaws of the plans. And if they were on several plans, and most of his friends were on ten or twenty HMO group plans, they were lucky to even have space to store all the paperwork and notebooks of directives.

Lastly, he loaded a separate document that listed the concerns and demands of the society pertaining to improving the efficiency, standards and quality of healthcare in their community. He left the changes that each doctor and medical office must be willing to make as the final segment. As he input the information, he reviewed it thoroughly. Satisfied, he saved it to the *Caduceus* memory, and ran tests on the service with the staff and Susan Kerr. They connected the dedicated line, and inaugurated the system with an interaction through Susan's notebook PC. Everything worked beautifully. Now it was up to the society. Coltrane thanked the staff, and asked Susan to arrange for meetings with the insurance executives in the next several days. Then he left to finish his hospital rounds.

It was nine-thirty before he got home. Britt had eaten, so he grabbed a plate of cold chicken and sat down in front of the television. A teaser for the ten o'clock news caught his attention. A local physician had died in a boating accident. Details to follow. He shouted to Britt in the bedroom if she knew who the victim was, but she hadn't heard. She came out, a look of worry on her face.

The pretty female anchor came on, and ineptly related the story. The body of Dr. Stephen Hendricks was found in the channel between the Bay and the Gulf of Mexico late this afternoon, after being in the water for several days. His boat was missing from his condo dock. Apparently his death was the result of a boating accident. She immediately went on to a story about the need for a traffic light at a downtown intersection.

"How very sad. You said he was an unhappy man. Do you think he killed himself?" Britt looked at her husband.

"Very likely. Susan said that she couldn't contact him, and he was on leave or possibly had been fired. At any rate, when the tape that I made gets revealed, he certainly would have lost his job. Poor guy, he had problems." Coltrane leaned back and closed his eyes. The realization that his actions may have resulted in Hendricks' suicide tormented him.

"It is not your fault, Bill. You didn't do anything to him. You just exposed what he had done to himself. And to John Strahan."

"Both deaths were unnecessary." Coltrane shook his head slowly.

They watched the rest of the news in silence.

Chapter 23

June 2
2:07AM

Coltrane was awakened from a sound sleep by his cellphone's soft tone. The number on the display was unfamiliar. He got out of bed quietly to allow Britt to get back to sleep, and called from the kitchen.

"Dr. Coltrane here."

"Dr. Coltrane, sorry to bother you. I lied to the answering service or they wouldn't call you. I need to talk to you about Hendricks."

"In the middle of the night? Who are you?" Coltrane was still sleepy, but the mention of Hendricks instantly revived him

"Juan Resendez." Ochoa lied easily.

"What about Hendricks?" Coltrane asked.

"He's dead."

"Yes, I know that. A boating accident."

"It was no accident. He had to be murdered."

"What?"

"Hendricks didn't know shit about that boat. There was no way in hell he would take it out, not at night. He had that boat just to get pussy; he couldn't find his way out to the channel without help. I always drove the boat anyway." Ochoa was rambling, obviously stoned.

"How do you know this? How do you know Hendricks?"

"Hendricks and I partied together a lot. We were friends." Ochoa lied again.

"Why tell me? This is something the police need to know. Where are you?"

"I ain't talking to no police. They be more interested in me than Hendricks."

"But why call me? You can call the anonymous tip line. Maybe get a reward."

"Them stupid cops won't find nothing. These guys were pros. I know." Ochoa was talking faster now, becoming excited. "I went to the condo Friday, after Hendricks disappeared. Someone searched it good. It was different, things in the wrong places, and torn up. They were looking for something."

An electric shock jolted through Coltrane. His office had been rifled as well, for the same reason? What could they have been looking for? But this didn't fit together quite right, he thought. Something was wrong, but he couldn't pinpoint it.

"Juan, wait a second. I have to change phones, my wife is trying to sleep." Coltrane placed the kitchen phone down, and ran upstairs to his library. There he noted the name and phone number on his caller ID unit, and wrote them down. He quickly set up a tape recorder, and continued the discussion through the speakerphone.

"All right. What do you think that they were looking for?" Coltrane knew that the man knew more than he was offering.

"Hey, your voice sounds like you are in a tunnel." Ochoa was suspicious.

"I'm on a portable phone. Talk to me. What were they looking for?" Coltrane pressed him.

"I got what they wanted. It is a disc, some kind of computer thing."

"A CD?" Coltrane was relieved immediately. If all this was true, at least no one would be after the tape of him and Hendricks. But then who had ransacked his office?

"Yeah, a CD. Like with music on it."

"A compact disc. What's on it?" Coltrane was increasingly interested.

"Fuck, I don't know. It don't play no music in my boombox, and I don't have a fucking computer." Ochoa was getting angry about the questions. The bargaining was not going as he had planned.

"Then how do you know that it is what the killers were after?"

"Because Hendricks showed it to me that night...the night I saw him last. He said that it was all he had left. It was his "horn blower" he said. And I figure that it is worth something to someone, for sure. So I went back to the condo and found it in his car, in the CD rack." Ochoa paused for effect.

"You need to give that to the police. That is evidence, in a murder case." Coltrane was still missing something in the chain of events, but he didn't know what.

"I ain't giving this to anyone. I will sell it to you, ten thousand dollars. Cash. I think this disc is very bad news for you." Ochoa bluffed, praying for luck. The loss of his main client would have serious effects on his life style.

"Why do you think that? And why did you call me? You never answered that."

"I called you because Hendricks was always talking about you, like you had something on him. I figure that this disc is his revenge, something on you." Ochoa was getting flustered. He was stoned, and tired, and this doctor was much more trouble than he had anticipated. Only greed kept him on the phone.

"Listen, Juan. I don't know what is on that disc, maybe some computer game or Hendricks' financial records. But it is useless to me. No one has anything "on" me. I am clean as snow, amigo. And what they were looking for is not a computer disc. They want a tape of a conversation that Hendricks and I had about three weeks ago. They broke into my office and searched for it. Maybe they thought Hendricks had a copy." Coltrane was now very concerned for his wife's safety, if someone was willing to murder for possession of that tape.

"It ain't the tape, Doc. I was the one who broke into your office. And I didn't find no tape. Hendricks told me to look for the tape. It's not the tape. It's this disc. If you don't want it, I'll sell it to someone else." Ochoa still hoped he could cash in on the disc.

"You're the guy who trashed my office?" Coltrane thundered in disbelief.

"Yeah."

"I don't believe it."

"You got a picture on your desk, you and a girl on the beach with some boat in the background. And you got two of them Chinese balls in your top desk drawer. Right?" Ochoa was back on track, his hopes up.

"Shit." Coltrane felt a chill run down his spine. "You have big balls calling me and admitting that, then trying to shake me down for ten grand with a disc you haven't read." Coltrane was beginning to realize that he was dealing with a stupid thug. But if he was the thief, then the story about the disc may be true. Certainly this guy didn't seem clever enough to fabricate the entire sequence of events.

"Well, you don't know nothing about me."

"Wrong. I know that you are calling from the phone of Guadalupe Herrera, and I have a tape recording of your voice, and this conversation. I am sure that will be enough to find you. But you had better consider that if the guys that killed Hendricks think that you have the disc, then they will kill you as well. Whoever those guys are, if they exist." Coltrane was thinking that he would like to see the disc anyway.

"I'll take my chances." Ochoa concluded the conversation.

"Juan, you give me the disc now, and I will see if there is anything on it. If it turns out to be worth anything, I will give you twenty percent. Otherwise, I call the police as soon as you hang up, and either they get you or the killers do. Your choice." Coltrane was thinking of where to make the exchange.

Ochoa cursed slowly. The disc was worth nothing to him, and maybe this doctor could make something out of it. What else could he do now, anyway?

"Fifty percent." Ochoa was pissed.

"I'll give you thirty percent. You're lucky to get anything, you broke into my fucking office, for Christ's sake. Now decide. Now or never."

"Fine. But you better never cheat me. I can find you." Ochoa growled.

"Thirty percent of any profit from the disc. Meet me at the south ER entrance of Doctor's Hospital. It is well lit, with security guards. Come alone, and no bullshit. I will be in the doctors' parking lot, in a white Expedition."

"Give me twenty minutes." Ochoa grumbled.

"Fine. I'll give you twenty minutes, then I call the police." Coltrane hung up.

Coltrane threw on a pair of surgical scrubs and told Britt that he had to go to the hospital. He left a brief note explaining the meeting in the event that he didn't return. Then he opened his safe, and pulled out a stainless steel Walther PPK/S. The small, heavy gun felt reassuring in his palm. He checked the clip, and chambered a round. He slipped it into a black ballistic nylon holster, and left the house.

Judging from the address of Guadalupe Herrera in the phone book, Coltrane knew that he would get to Doctor's long before Juan. He hoped that this extra time would give him a chance to prepare. He sped along, taking the short cuts that he often took to the ER. He arrived and parked the Expedition near the front of the lot, in the shadow by the brightly lit ER doors. Then he got out, and moved quickly to the back of the lot, where the concrete walls ended in a blind alley. From that position, no one could get around behind him. This is the best I can do, he thought. He released the safety on the Walther, and felt in the darkness for the protruding metal pin on the top of the weapon, assuring him that a round was chambered. Then he settled into the shadows in the corner, and waited.

Ochoa was late, but not by much. He came from the visitors' parking lot, stumbling on a curb as he entered the doctors' lot. Coltrane could see that his hands were empty, but he wore a baggy jacket that covered to the knees. He went straight to the white Expedition, and knocked on the tinted glass. He squinted, and put his face and palm up to the glass to see in. When he saw that the car was empty, he searched the lot in confusion.

Coltrane called to him softly. Ochoa cautiously made his way toward the end of the lot, looking to the right and left as he walked. When he was within three paces of Coltrane, he halted.

Coltrane's heart was racing. As he stared into Ochoa's bloodshot, mindless eyes, he wondered what the fuck he was doing, playing this deadly game. Still, he had come this far…

"Could anyone be following you?" Coltrane asked.

"If they thought I had this, they would have grabbed me days ago." Ochoa stated, grimly.

"Is that the only copy?" Coltrane asked about the slim CD case Ochoa produced cautiously.

"This is the disc Hendricks had. I be surprised they didn't torture it out of him first. Maybe he was tougher than I thought." Ochoa coldly reflected. He handed the jewel case to Coltrane.

"Here's two hundred bucks. You would be wise to get out of town for a while. If there is something on this disc, things will get very hot, very fast. I'll remember our deal. Goodbye." Coltrane backed up, and moving around a parked car, headed into the hospital. Before Ochoa could act, he was gone. Ochoa shrugged, turned and shuffled off towards his distant car.

On the opposite side of the visitor's parking lot, a tall man sat in the driver's seat of a rented sedan. He watched through a set of fourth generation night vision goggles as the two men separated, and the man in green scrubs entered the hospital. Then he watched Ochoa walk back to his car, get in and drive away. He sat for a moment, then followed Ochoa as he left the hospital complex.

Chapter 24

June 2
4:45AM

Coltrane went into the hospital, straight to the nearest stairwell and climbed as fast as he could to the fifth floor. He exited onto a medical patient wing, and walked to the far stairwell. He then went down three floors, and ducked into the operating room. He turned down a corridor, opening a security door after punching in the passcode. He slumped on the sofa in the surgeon's lounge and sighed, long and low.

During the drive to the meeting, several disquieting thoughts had occurred to him. Since there was evidence that Hendricks' place had been searched, it was possible that Hendricks had died before giving up the disc. If that were true, then the killers may still be searching. And Resendez may have been seen coming and going from the condo. They may be watching him, following him now. Coltrane had cursed himself for not thinking of that. He should have had Juan drop the disc in the mail. But it was too late to change the meeting by the time Coltrane realized the danger. So he had attempted to make the meeting seem to be a drug sale, between Juan and a hospital employee, a lab technician or any of many specialists at the hospital that wears scrubs regularly. Hopefully anyone observing the garage meeting would reach that conclusion.

Coltrane waited for forty minutes in the lounge, reading the recent journals laying around. Then he changed from his green scrubs to a pair of the hospital blues, and went downstairs to the medical records section. He went to a cubicle and switched on the computer there. He pulled the CD from the Mariachi music jewel case that Juan had put it in, slipped it into the CD-ROM drive, and opened the file. It was an unlocked file, and opened easily. Inside was an endless stream of numbers, like a book, reading from left to right, no punctuation, no identification, just number after number after number. He scrolled down and down and down. Nothing but numbers. Finally, he skipped to the final page of the file. There the numbers ended. No explanation.

Coltrane pulled the disc out of the CD-ROM drive, pocketed it and headed out the ER door. It had been two hours since the meeting, and he felt safe enough to leave. He climbed into the Expedition, and drove out. He took the long farm road route, and doubled back twice to check for a tail. When he was sure that he was not followed, he headed home. I have been watching too much television, he thought to himself as he drove into the garage. Once up in the study, he carefully took the CD-R out of its jewel case, and slipped it into the D drive of his desktop computer. He booted up his Philips CD burner, and made a duplicate copy of the disc. Then, handling the original by the edges, he replaced it in the Mariachi jewel case, and put it in his fireproof safe. Tomorrow he would move it to the safety deposit box at his bank. Then he tore up the explanatory note on his desk, and turned on the security alarm. As a second thought, he put the PPK/S on the nightstand before he got into bed. Britt didn't awaken.

Chapter 25

June 2

Morning rounds were never ending. He visited all his hospital inpatients, traveling a circuit of all three main hospitals, finishing with the County Hospital. It seemed to Coltrane that each of his patients had developed a dozen new symptoms the preceding night, but he carefully evaluated each problem, and documented them in the charts. He changed dressings, ordered some tests and asked his favorite nurses to check on the patients' progress for him. As he left the hospital for his office, he thanked the Lord for the nurses. They truly were angels, and devoted to a difficult and often thankless job.

Halfway to his car, Coltrane thought about what the caller had said last night. Ochoa was sure that Hendricks had been murdered. If that was the case, it would have to be investigated. That meant an autopsy. He turned around, and headed back into County Hospital.

The Pathology Department and County Morgue were located together in the hospital basement, partly because of the cooler subterranean temperatures and absence of direct sunlight, but also to avoid interaction with mainstream hospital employees, visitors, patients and family. It was not a cheerful place. The gray concrete floors, pervasive smell of formaldehyde and chemical reagents, and the heavy presence of death weighed heavily on anyone who ventured into the realm of the death and disease that existed below the main hospital floors.

Coltrane had moonlighted in pathology labs during his medical training, and was knowledgeable in the art of tissue fixation, H&E staining, and microscopic examination of tissues. Often, in his practice, he would have a patient with a suspicious lesion that required excisional biopsy. He would take the patient to the operating room, surgically remove the tumor, and then hand carry it down to the pathologist. He could then review the tissue sections immediately with the pathologist, and get far better information about the size, depth and extension of the tumor than if he waited for a report to be written and mailed a week later. It took a little extra time, but in the long run was worth the delay. And it generated him friends in the path department.

When Coltrane walked through the heavy stainless steel doors into the pathology section, the technician was confused.

"Are we looking at a biopsy for you, Dr. Coltrane? I haven't gotten it from surgery." The tech sat behind a microscope, preparing and examining a series of breast biopsy frozen sections.

"No, Steve, I am just here to see Ken. Is he around?"

"Yep. In his office."

"Thanks." Coltrane nodded and headed for Jasper's small corner office. The door was open, and he found Dr. Kenneth Jasper hunched over his microscope, totally engrossed in the examination of a tissue slide. Coltrane gently closed the door, and the sound of metal on metal got his attention.

"Hey Bill, what's up? Do I need to pull some slides?" Jasper assumed that Coltrane was there to review a patient case.

"Nope. Got a question for you, though. Are you still assistant coroner?" Coltrane asked quietly.

"Yeah. That honor goes with being the Chairman of the Pathology Department at County. The County Coroner is a politically appointed position. He's not a physician. Why?"

"You remember Steve Hendricks? Died in a boating accident. Did you do an autopsy on him?"

"No. Not yet. As you may know, state law requires an autopsy in any cases of suspicious death, or death of unknown etiology. He was just a drowning, wasn't he? I don't know anything about it, and I haven't heard from his family about disposition of the body. He's still in the morgue, as far as I know. Why do you ask?" Jasper was now very interested, leaning back in his gray metal swivel chair, looking directly at Coltrane.

"Can you do me a favor? Can you take a look at him? Just see if there is anything unusual?" Coltrane avoided answering Jasper's question.

"You suspect something." Jasper said.

"Nothing specific. Just a bad feeling about it." Coltrane lied.

"Well, it is not unusual for a guy to kill someone, and dump the body in the Bay. Every criminal genius in Tampa thinks that the gulf water will cleanse all the evidence from the corpse." Jasper laughed. "No problem. I will make a cursory exam of the body this afternoon, and if anything sends up a red flag, I'll call you. But I gotta take care of the living first. Breast biopsies. You understand."

Coltrane nodded, stood and shook Jasper's hand, and left the office. He didn't know what the exam might turn up, and hadn't thought about the ramifications of his involvement if Hendricks had indeed been murdered. How could he explain his miraculous insight into a murder without becoming involved in a very serious way? In any case, it was too late to worry about that now, he thought as he climbed the stairs to the hospital main floor.

He made it to his office with an hour to spare before his first appointment. He called Susan Kerr.

"Susan, what have you been able to line up with the insurance plans."

"Dr. Coltrane, they refuse to meet with you personally or on the phone. The response I was given is that the contracts are binding, and will not be renegotiated."

Coltrane was silent for a moment.

"Those arrogant bastards. They are not even interested in hearing what our concerns are?"

"No."

"Susan, send out a letter today to all our members requesting an emergency meeting next week. Make it a mandatory meeting. State that our request for a dialogue with the insurance companies has been rejected, and we need to take further steps. And make it a full day retreat. I want the best resort conference facility in town. Try the Excelsior Saint Petersburg, that's where the Florida Medical Association always holds their meetings. We can do it next Friday, and make it a long weekend. Tell them to close their offices...no, no, no... just tell them to plan to be at this meeting all day."

"I can put that on *Caduceus* as well." Susan offered.

"Good, but not everyone is online yet. Then contact the chairman of each specialty group and have him arrange for citywide hospital coverage by his specialty. I don't want someone to die of a heart attack because all the cardiologists are at this meeting. Any questions?" Coltrane was agitated.

"No. I assume that this has priority over all else."

"Correct. I will be in the office if Cindy or I can help. Call me if there are any problems or questions. Oh,... and Susan... Put in the letter that roll will be taken at the meeting, and all those who do not attend will be listed prominently on *Caduceus*."

Susan understood and Coltrane could tell from the tone of her voice that she grasped the significance of what was evolving. Hopefully the membership will be as astute, Coltrane thought. He set down the phone, put on his starched white coat, and strode out to the exam rooms to examine the first patient of the day.

Coltrane was adjusting a splint when Cindy interrupted him with a call from Davis Clark. He finished the splint, admonished the young man not to use it to strike his little brother again, and went to his office to answer. Clark was clearly excited.

"Coltrane, did you know that Hendricks died in a boating accident a couple of days ago?" Clark asked quickly.

"Yeah, I saw that on the news."

"You realize how that affects your testimony, don't you?"

"No, I hadn't thought about it. I suppose it makes it worthless."

"*Worthless*? No, it makes it *priceless*! Hendricks cannot repudiate it, and now we have a legitimate reason to request to enter it into evidence." Clark patiently explained.

"That doesn't do much good if Alistair is not interested."

"Ahh, Dr. Coltrane. You seem to be in such a sour mood this fine day. Let me cheer you up. Hendricks' death puts us in a far better position to negotiate with Alistair. From my initial discussions with him, I am confident that I can get us a percentage of the award. And that's not all. I told him that a condition of the deal is that no action be brought against my client in this matter. I led him to believe that my client is an insurance company employee who is partly responsible for the errors that resulted in Strahan's death. He didn't think twice. So at the worst, you're out of the lawsuit. And at best, you will get a nice settlement from Alistair's fee." Clark laughed outloud. He was very proud of the way that he had finessed Alistair.

"You're a genius. Just getting me off that suit is a godsend. My sincere thanks, Davis." Coltrane felt the relief wash over him.

"You'll get my bill, amigo. Oh, by the way. You can't tell anyone, *not a single soul*, about our arrangement. It is *absolutely* critical. If Alistair knows that you are my "client", the deal is off, and you are back on the defendant list. Understand?"

"Sure."

"And another thing. Are there any other copies of the tape? Other than the one you gave me?"

"Nope."

"Okay, I will dupe it, and keep them both in the hospital vault.

"Thanks."

"Listen, this process with Alistair will take some time. The lawsuit is in discovery, and it will be at least a year before it goes to trial. Maybe longer. So don't worry if you don't hear from me or Alistair for a while. Just stop worrying about the case. Everything will be fine."

"I really appreciate this, buddy," Coltrane thanked him again.

"No problem. Talk to you later." Clark hung up.

Chapter 26

June 5

The two men sat at the small hotel room table, and looked out at the bay. The hotel was one of the finest in town, and suited their needs well. There were multiple floors, multiple exits and several parking garages. Their comings and goings would be very difficult to observe and trace.

The tall man was an Anglo, wiry and weather-beaten from years in the Florida sun and wind. Across the table sat a short, squat Cuban. The Cuban was angry. The tall man, known only as Johnny, had just told him that he had lost the tail on Ochoa, that Ochoa had disappeared.

"How did you lose that stupid fuck?" he cursed.

"Sorry, man. He must have slipped out the back and down the alley while I was out the front. He took his girlfriend's car. He must be gone twenty, thirty hours by now." The tall man cursed his luck.

"His girlfriend is still here?" the Cuban asked.

"Yeah, I saw her an hour ago."

"He must be the one then. Hendricks' girlfriend is still here, nothing odd about her behavior the last week. Hendricks' secretary is not doing anything unusual either. But why wait until now to split? He must have met with someone. He must have sold the disc or hidden it somewhere. Fuck."

The Cuban sat quietly and reviewed the events of the last few weeks. He was a professional, once a senior captain in Castro's intelligence network. Events of a personal nature had forced him to leave Cuba on a small fishing boat several years ago. He quickly found that his talents were needed and very well compensated for in the murky Florida underworld of drugs, guns and money. He had been contracted via phone to rush to Tampa and retrieve computer discs stolen by a company doctor. His only mistake was to hire this idiot gringo to back him up. His usual associate was face down in a shallow grave in the Everglades, having paid the price for failing the Cuban one time too many.

The job had been bungled from the beginning. They had found the doctor easy enough. He was sitting in his condo, drunk and stoned when they politely knocked on the door, dressed in overalls and carrying toolboxes. Hendricks had let them in when they told him that the condo below had water coming from the ceiling.

When they were inside, they shocked Hendricks with a small, hand held stun gun. He went down hard on the floor, twitching uncontrollably.

Johnny had cuffed him and taped his mouth, hands and feet quickly with duct tape. Then they looked very carefully and thoroughly throughout the entire condo for the discs. They searched for what they had been ordered to find, two CDs with data relating to insurance plans on them. They found Hendricks' computer, and all the discs that were on the table with the computer and the printer. But they found only one unlabeled CD. The Cuban had put it into the D drive of Hendricks computer, and opened it. He found nothing but numbers, page after page of numbers. He knew that this was what he was looking for. But he needed the second disc.

After half an hour, Hendricks had begun to regain consciousness. His eyes filled with wild terror as they hogtied him and moved him into the sunken whirlpool tub in his master bath.

"Don't want to bloody up your nice clean rug, eh, Doc?" Johnny had drawled.

They used a favorite technique of the Mexican police to extract the location of the discs from Hendricks. The beauty of the technique was that, if the victim survived, there would be no incriminating signs or marks. They repeatedly submerged Hendricks head, drowning and reviving their victim until he had defecated and urinated and defecated again. But he was so drugged and coked up and tortured that he probably never understood what they wanted from him. He just kept nodding when they asked him where the other disc was. No answers, just moronic nodding. Finally Johnny kept him under too long and he vomited into his taped mouth. By the time they realized what was going on, he had choked on his vomit and strangled to death.

They cleaned up the condo, removed the hard drive and all the loose CDs from Hendricks' computer and dragged the body down to his boat. The Cuban easily motored out past the channel where they cleaned, stripped and dumped the body. The Cuban personally melted and dumped the disc into the gulf, along with the hard drive and all the CDs. Then they sank the boat and dinghyed in, with the Cuban cursing Johnny all the while in Spanish. He made Johnny carry the deflated dinghy back the three miles to their car while he slept on the beach. They had barely finished by daylight.

Now, the Cuban sat and reflected upon whether he should kill this inept gringo now, or after the job. They had not needed to kill the doctor, but that they had was of no consequence. What was of great consequence was that he had died before surrendering the second disc. Now he had to backtrack and find where and with whom Ochoa had made contact.

"Order something up to eat. This will take some time. We have to go over every move Ochoa made in the last week. Your memory better be good, Johnny."

"Yeah, sure. I want some beers too, I am dry from sitting in that car all day."

"No beers, you fucking idiot. I need all of your limited concentration to try to find where Ochoa passed off that disc. He would not just leave town like that. He met with someone, or called someone before he left. He is a punk drug dealer, he is too greedy and stupid to play it smart. Start with the last day that you saw him."

Johnny sullenly ordered room service, then sat down and wrote notes, day by day, on the activities of Ochoa. The Cuban glared at him from the desk as he did the same for the two women that he had tailed. Hendricks' secretary had been mentioned by the man on the phone, as well as an occasional tittie dancer and barmaid that Hendricks dated when he had cash. Fortunately for the Cuban, the secretary worked in the daylight, while the dancer moved at night. He had watched both and neither showed any promise, and stuck to very predictable patterns and habits all week. Still, he didn't want to miss a connection.

Johnny finished a day's journal, and handed it to the Cuban. The Cuban read the notes, and questioned Johnny about details. This went on, day by day as they traced Ochoa's deals back through the week. Then the Cuban sat upright in his chair.

"What is this? He made a deal at a hospital?"

"Yeah, he sold some dope to a guy in a parking lot." Johnny nodded, sleepily.

"That was the guy. That was no dope deal, that was the disc. A hospital, man. Did you forget that doctors are around hospitals?" The Cuban was livid.

"No, man. It was just some hospital employee, in the middle of the night. He was working in the hospital, in a hospital uniform."

"Maybe. But we still have to track him down. Tell me exactly what you saw." The Cuban started to gently interrogate Johnny, knowing that he was too obtuse to recognize critical information.

"Ochoa drove to the hospital from his girlfriend's…"

"Was he excited or moving faster or slower than he usually did?"

"Faster, I think."

"Did he stop anywhere after leaving the apartment?"

"He went to his brother's house."

"Inside the house? For how long?"

"No. He just went into the garage. I think that he keeps his dope in the garage."

"Why? Why do you say that?" The Cuban knew now that Ochoa had had the disc.

"He went in the garage several times, but usually after he talks to his brother. This time he went straight to the garage."

"Then what?"

"Then he looks around, as usual. But he can't see me, I'm a block and a half away, with the night scope. Then he takes off for the hospital."

"You followed him into the hospital parking lot?"

"No. He turned into the main entrance, which was too good lit up. So I went to the next lot and watched from there."

"Tell me exactly what you saw." The Cuban was gently coaxing Johnny.

"He went into a parking garage that was real well lit, but I couldn't see him good, because he was facing away. The other guy was with his back to the wall and in a dark corner. I couldn't see him good, neither."

"Then what happened."

"Ochoa talked fast, and speedy like. He gave him a packet of dope, and the guy gave him some cash."

"Are you sure it was dope? Could it have been the disc?"

"It looked like a plastic baggie of some shit."

"And you saw the cash?"

"Yeah, and I saw Ochoa count it after the guy left."

"*After he left*, not *before* he passed him the dope?"

"Yeah."

"When he usually made deals, did he count the cash before or after he gave the junkie the dope. Think hard. This is important." The Cuban was excited.

"Always he counted the cash, then reached in his pants for the dope."

"So this deal was different, *si?*"

"Yeah."

"Then what?"

"Then Ochoa walked to his…"

"Slow or fast. Did he walk slow or fast?"

"Slow."

"Where did he go?"

"Back to the girlfriend's apartment."

"He stayed there all night?"

"I don't know, I watched til sunup, then came here for a rest."

"What about the guy? What happened to him?"

"I just saw him go into the hospital after Ochoa gave him the packet. I wasn't paying him no attention."

"Describe him."

"He was about six foot, medium build, short hair. That was all I could see."

"White, black, hispanic? Could you tell?"

"White. Or hispanic, maybe."

"What was he wearing? What kind of uniform?"

"Those green pajama things."

"Scrubs?"

"Yeah. Scrubs."

"How about his walk? Did he walk fast or slow?"

"Fast."

"So he was young, or old? Did he walk like an old man or a young man?"

"Young, I guess. He could move pretty quick. I just figured he didn't want to get caught off the job."

"Maybe you're right. Maybe he works at the hospital. But I'm sure that he's our boy. Ochoa must have given him the disc. What did Ochoa do after that drop?"

"He went to just one place, then home."

"Let me guess. At his brother's?"

"Yeah. He stopped at his brother's garage. How'd you know?"

"Cause I use my fucking brain, that's how. And he left town the next day?"

"Yep," Johnny answered sullenly.

"Didn't say bye to his brother?"

"Nope."

The Cuban had it now. Ochoa sold the disc to the man at that hospital parking lot, picked up his stash and headed out of town. His brother probably knew nothing. He would never catch up with Ochoa. But the other man was a different matter.

"Get ready. Get the Starlight scope. We are going to go to that hospital."

"Right now?"

"*Right fucking now.*"

The Cuban was quiet on the drive over. He was blind with rage at Johnny for missing all the signs that a fool should have seen. The urgency of this contract, and the unanticipated loss of his hand trained associate, had forced Johnny into his employ. In Cuba, he had shot men for less, much less. Wars are won, lives are lost by small, sometimes insignificant things. This was the wisdom of the warrior general, Sun Tsu, as translated in "The Art of War". The ancient text was believed to have been written in 500 BC, and has survived thousands of years, remaining the definitive treatise on the waging of total war. Sun Tzu had said that the use of spies is perhaps the greatest tool of a warrior general. The Cuban had read the Art of War many times, demanding that his subordinates memorize it in its entirety. There were few doctrines that he had not personally employed during his bloody career, and he revered most the section on defeating the enemy without fighting. For that was the section dealing with the use of spies.

They found the hospital, and parked in the exact spot that Johnny had been in that night. They looked at the area through the scope, and found the parking lot where the deal went down. The Cuban got out of the car and strolled over to the area, passing through the ER waiting room as if he was with a patient. He casually walked to the spot where the transaction occurred, then walked toward the ER doors. Then he returned slowly to the car.

"Do you know why that lot is so well lit?" He asked Johnny.

"No."

"That's the doctors' parking lot. That guy was a doctor, I am sure of it now."

"Wait a second! Wait. Ochoa walked up to a car before he met with the guy. Right on the end there. He looked into the car, then saw the guy." Johnny was excited, knowing that he may be able to redeem himself for his fuckup. He had to remember the car.

"Is the car there now?" The Cuban felt the thrill of the chase, the kill.

"I don't think so…it was a Suburban or a Expedition, maybe a Yukon. Full size."

"What color?"

"Light color. Tan, light blue, white maybe."

"Solid, or two tone?"

"Solid, and it had to be a Expedition or a Suburban. Big, four doors." Johnny was beaming.

"You sure?" The Cuban didn't know one American car from another.

"Yeah."

"Alright. Tomorrow, you go back to watching Ochoa's girlfriend. He may come back. I'll get some phone tapping gear flown up from Miami, and tap his girlfriend's line by tomorrow. I want you listening to that line twenty four hours a day. If Ochoa shows, shock him fast and take him out of town in his car, then call me. Don't think twice. And if you accidentally kill him, I'll kill you. It will be easier to find that guy from Ochoa than hunt him down. I'll watch this parking lot. He'll have to come here sooner or later. Now take me back to the hotel. I need some sleep."

Chapter 27

June 8

The Cuban sat low in the sedan, watching the doctors' parking lot. He was uncomfortable, his ass hurt from sitting for hours. He had a headache and he was hungry. On a long term surveillance with primitive techniques, he had to remain very inconspicuous. The hospital security people would eventually start to notice him.

These fucking doctors get up too early and work too late, he thought. He found that the day and night long procession through the lot began at 5:30 AM and lasted well past 9 PM. And he found that there were many sport utility vehicles: Yukons, Expeditions, Excursions, Landcruisers, Land Rovers, Suburbans, Pathfinders. So far he had found seventeen trucks that fit the description. Out of the seventeen, there were five men who could match the physical description. He got their license plate numbers. He could get them run in Miami later.

The first physician he had found that matched Johnny's description was a well dressed man in his fifties, slightly balding, but with plenty of hair left. He went into the hospital and emerged fifteen minutes later. He had walked quickly, with a powerful stride. The Cuban thought he might be the one. He had followed the doctor to several hospitals, all over town, each time stopping for periods of time ranging from fifteen minutes to an hour. Then the doctor went into a hospital, and didn't come out. The Cuban had followed his trail into the hospital, but found nothing. He had wasted an entire day. Frustrated and angry with himself, he returned to the pattern of simply watching the lot, and taking license plate numbers. He prayed that Ochoa would get stupid and return to Tampa, and daydreamed about finally killing Johnny.

Only one good thing had come out of the day. All the hospital employees wore blue scrubs. The ER docs, ER nurses, even the orderlies. They all wore blue scrubs. Johnny had been sure that the man in the parking garage had worn green scrubs. At least that fucking idiot wasn't colorblind, the Cuban thought.

But now he was absolutely positive that the man they sought was a physician. And a surgeon.

Chapter 28

June 9

The meeting didn't go as planned. But that was no surprise for Coltrane. All he wanted was a good turnout of the membership. He guessed that maybe sixty percent of the active membership attended the session.

They chose the Excelsior Saint Petersburg for the venue, both for the large conference facilities and the security. Coltrane was concerned about media interference and the confidentiality of the proceedings. Susan arranged for the third floor of the premier hotel on the bayfront for the conference, and had hired extra security as an added precaution. No one was allowed onto the third floor who was not an active medical society member.

The meeting began tumultuously, with angry complaints about the disruption of members' practice routine. Coltrane had stayed out of sight until the furor died out, then made his way to the dais. He took the podium and remained quiet as the questions began again. When everyone had calmed down, he opened the meeting.

"Ladies and gentlemen, I thank you for taking the time to attend today. I asked for this meeting because our attempts to reach an agreement with the insurance companies have failed. Not a single plan has offered to speak with us, not even on the phone. Their attitude is that we are locked into our contracts, and that if we are dissatisfied, then they will find other physicians." Coltrane spoke quickly and forcefully.

"As physicians, we have a fiduciary responsibility for our patients' healthcare interests. We, alone, are responsible for safeguarding their care. We have to place their interests above the interests of the HMOs."

"Our first duty has always been to our patients. There is only one thing I remember from the version of the Hippocratic Oath that I took upon graduation. That is the admonition:

Primum non nocere.

Above all else, do no harm.

"In Hippocrates' time the true nature of disease was not understood, and physicians were not always successful in treatment. Sometimes the treatment was more dangerous than the disease. Our predecessors thought that disease was caused by an imbalance between the four bodily humors, so they would drain the patient of his toxic blood. Ancient surgical bloodletting was not quite as precise as it is now. In fact, we surgeons were not even considered physicians. Those are days you swamis probably long for, as near as I can tell." There was mixed laughter from the internists in the assembly. "But I digress."

"The chances of an ill outcome in today's medicine is very slight. Less than one percent. We are not failing our patients in our practices. We are failing them by allowing outside entities to come between us. By allowing third parties to intervene in the relationship between doctor and patient. Third parties originated simply as insurance entities. Now the "third" party has become the dominant party. Making decisions for the doctor and the patient, instead of simply disbursing funds from a common premium fund. Why do we allow insurance entities to determine the course and specifics of our medical treatment plans? Does a car insurance company tell you what kind of car to buy? Where to gas up? What kind of tires to buy?"

"What has happened to the profession of medicine has been so slow, so insidious, so gradual that we haven't noticed the decay. Just fifty years ago, medicine was like any other profession. You complete your training, and open your practice. You provide care to your patients, and they repay you. Not always in full, but as best as they can. The profession was honorable, and respected, and we all contributed to the community. Then Medicare came along, and for the first time in history, a government regulated fees charged by individuals for their services. But the idea was noble, providing care for the elderly and disabled, so we gladly accepted the arrangement. Then came Medicaid, with fees much lower than even Medicare. But this program was for the poor, so again we accepted the fractional payments. I never made the obvious conclusion that these programs were simply transferring the expense of medical care directly to us, the physicians. All these years, we physicians have been personally paying the costs of healthcare for the indigent, uninsured and elderly. By providing free or heavily discounted services to this huge population. I didn't realize that hospitals and medical supply houses and pharmaceutical manufacturers were still getting good reimbursement. Then came HMOs, PPOs, and other managed care entities, all decreasing the reimbursement even lower than Medicare, and adding red tape and restricting care as well."

"We, as physicians, need to regain control of our profession. We will take control from the insurance companies. From the federal, state, and local governments. From the trial lawyers and the haphazard justice of our antiquated legal system. From the misguided talking heads of the news media. From politicians seeking to cull favor with political action groups of all kinds."

"That is what this conference is about. The practice of medicine is the pinnacle of education and training. Everyone in this room has endured decades of sacrifice and schooling to be here today. The absurdity of having to request permission from a telephone attendant to admit a patient to the hospital *has* to end. *NOW*. It is because of our complacency that we have arrived at this crossroads. It is time to act. On behalf of our patients. On behalf of our profession."

"As you know from reading my reports on *Caduceus*, we are very limited in the collective bargaining that we can legally attempt. I feel very strongly, however, that we do not have to continue in a relationship with inflexible, financially motivated bureaucracies that care nothing for the welfare of their clients, whom are our patients. I feel that if an insurance plan is providing sub-standard or inferior healthcare, then we have an ethical and moral duty to withdraw from involvement with such an entity. Physicians, and only physicians, can determine the standards of medical practice." Coltrane was very precise in his choice of words. The group became silent as they followed his implication.

"The purpose of this conference is to divide our active members into groups based on specialty, and discuss thoroughly the problems that they have encountered with the five main plans. Based on today's discussions, we will formulate a recommendation for the society as to whether to continue participation in these plans."

The society's members were stunned by the implications of the president's statement. As they went over his words in their heads, they realized that nothing had been said directly about any boycott, or collective action, or strike. But they also realized that if enough physicians dropped off a plan, or stopped taking new patients enrolled in that plan, or simply shifted appointment schedules against that plan, soon the plan would suffer. The patients would be inconvenienced somewhat because they would have to find a new doctor, or go outside the list of approved doctors. They would pay an extra fifteen dollars per visit. But the cost to the plan would be astronomical. They would be obligated to pay full normal fees to the new treating physician and hospital, and also incur the wrath of the patient who would also have slightly increased costs. Coltrane knew that only financial considerations would bring the plans to the table. They had shown time and time again that quality healthcare was not their prime consideration.

There were several physicians who left the meeting at once. Coltrane knew that some of them were in conflict with the ethical issues, some with the legal exposure, and a few hoped to profit by the possible opportunities.

Scabs. The rest hesitated, and began to discuss the situation among themselves. Susan quickly took the microphone and organized the members into groups based on specialty. Internal medicine, surgery, pediatrics, obstetrics and gynecology, family and general practice, and the subspecialties were all organized into committees. Among their peers, the doctors found support and empathy. Soon they began to list and describe the incidents that they had previously decried only to their wives or husbands or office managers. They found that there was a strong common thread of duplicitous practice and sub-standard medicine being promulgated by two of the plans, far more so than the other three. This was the case in all specialty groups, and by an overwhelming margin.

Coltrane went from group to group, watching the proceedings and assuring the members that they were within the bounds of the letter of the law. The previously appointed chairmen of the specialty committees were present during the session, and kept a record of the findings. Coltrane didn't interfere or comment on the discussions of each group as he moved around the ballroom. Twice his beeper went off, and he saw the number of the pathology department on the display. That would have to wait. Everything went smoothly until midafternoon.

Coltrane was interrupted during a conversation by loud angry voices from the corridor. He saw Susan moving to the door, and motioned for the security personnel to join them. The scene in the corridor was tense. Wilson Andrews was a high profile local television reporter, known for aggressive journalistic techniques. He stood at the top of the escalator platform with his video cameraman and sound man, trying to enter the conference area. A stout female security officer stood in his way, and refused him entry. He was loudly protesting that the freedom of the press was being violated, and that the hotel would regret assaulting him. The security officer was intimidated and giving ground. He was pressing home his advantage.

Coltrane had anticipated this confrontation, and planned for it carefully. The private security people were chosen for physical presence and height, and one of the officers moved ahead of Coltrane toward the group at the escalator platform. Coltrane let the officer crowd close to the reporter, and had him shield Coltrane from the camera's lens as Coltrane spoke in a low voice to the reporter.

"Mr. Andrews, I see you are on top of things as usual. I'm Dr. William Coltrane, the medical society president." Coltrane soothed him.

"What is going on here, Dr. Coltrane? All of the doctors' offices are closed today. I have the right to interview your members." Andrews demanded.

"This is the private conference of a society limited to members of the medical profession. I doubt that you would find anything going on here interesting. Furthermore, this is the hotel conference floor, and you and your cameras have no more right here than you would have in the hotel room of any of the guests here." Coltrane stopped and smiled. The huge security guard towered over the reporter and continued to obscure the cameraman's view.

"You can not stay here, nor will I allow you to disrupt this meeting. Security is entirely within their rights to escort you physically from this building if you do not leave immediately. I will give your station a personal interview within forty-eight hours, however, if you like. If that is acceptable, you can arrange it with Susan Kerr." Coltrane smiled, stepped back as the security officer stepped forward into the face of Andrews, who sullenly withdrew, bumping into his soundman.

Coltrane and Kerr walked back down the corridor, listening to the voices of the television crew fade away.

"Damn, that was sweet. Planning pays off again. I knew that little weasel would show up sooner or later. Let him spend the rest of the day looking for a car accident to tape." Coltrane was satisfied by the handling of the reporters. The security people had been briefed on the appropriate defense against this intrusion, and how important it would be to avoid bright lights and cameras on the doctors as they left the meeting. And he didn't want anyone trying to be the spokesperson for the group without knowing what to say and how to say it. That was his job, and hopefully he would do it well, he thought. But now he would have to win Andrews back to his side, if possible. One thing at a time.

The rest of the day's meeting was anti-climactic. The findings were supported by other incoming physicians, and a consensus was reached to censure the two plans. Coltrane closed the conference with a warning not to discuss any of the proceedings with anyone, and not to reveal any of the findings, especially to the media. With that, the assembly dispersed, and Coltrane was relieved to head home. As soon as he was in the car, he took his cellphone out of his pocket, and dialed Jasper's extension.

"Doctor Jasper." The pathologist answered on the second ring.

"Ken, this is Bill Coltrane. You paged me?"

"Yeah. Jesus, have I got news for you. Sorry it took me so long, I have been busy as hell. Your hunch was dead on. Pardon the pun. I found enough evidence to call this a murder, no question." Jasper was clearly excited.

"What did you find?" Coltrane felt a chill go up his spine, the tiny hairs electrified on the back of his neck.

"Anyone who has ever seen *Quincy, MD* knows to check the water in a drowned man's lungs. Of course we analyzed that first. Turns out to be freshwater."

"Then he didn't drown in the Bay." Coltrane interrupted.

"He didn't drown in the Bay or anywhere else. The preliminary findings are that the cause of death was asphyxiation, secondary to aspiration. Vomitus."

"Drunks are always aspirating and dying on their own vomit. Maybe he was a heavy drinker. That's not murder, is it?"

"Maybe not. But the presence of freshwater in his lungs is clear evidence of foul play."

"Maybe he died at an inopportune place or time. Say a married woman's house. And she dumped the body in the Bay."

"Maybe, but not likely. I found something else." Jasper paused. He considered the wisdom of releasing further information to Coltrane. How had Coltrane had such insight into what was, on the surface, simply a boating mishap? He shook off the ill ease, and continued. "Hendricks had multiple hemorrhagic petechiae on his peri-oral area, ankles and wrists. As well as gray adhesive, probably from duct tape. This means that he was bound and gagged, prior and during death.

"Christ."

"Someone tried to remove the adhesive, probably with rubbing alcohol, and there is evidence of that attempt as well. But duct tape adhesive is like radioactive uranium, it stays around forever. I have a piece on my garage door that has been there for three years, I just can't get it off."

"Damn." Coltrane exhaled slowly.

"Bill, listen to what I am going to tell you now." Jasper lowered his voice, and his tone became serious and concerned. "I assume that our discussion last week was based purely on your intuition, not on any actual involvement in this tragedy. I have known you since you started practice here, ten years ago."

"Fifteen, actually." Coltrane said, quietly.

"Fifteen, then. I cannot imagine you murdering anyone, and if you had, you certainly would not want the coroner investigating the circumstances of what was initially presumed to be an accident. But I have questions about how you obtained your information, and if the police question me *specifically*, I have to be honest. And forthcoming. As much as I would like to, I can't conceal our conversation. Do you understand?"

"Yes. Don't hide anything. Just be entirely truthful. I can explain the circumstances to the police if I have to. And I appreciate you sharing your findings with me. I won't call you about it again. Thanks." Coltrane sensed the hesitancy as he hung up the cellphone. He would have to repair his reputation at a time in the future.

Chapter 29

June 12

The work didn't end when the meeting adjourned. Susan called Coltrane's office the following Monday to tell him that Andrews had phoned three times to arrange a meeting with him. Coltrane asked her to call back, and talk to the reporting staff. He instructed her to talk with the reporters on staff, and find one who she thought would be sympathetic and knowledgeable. Preferably a woman, because she would be more likely to have had problems with the healthcare system's obstetrical bureaucracy. Women usually selected and paid for their family's health insurance anyway, he explained. Coltrane wanted above all else, a reporter who was knowledgeable in the field. And under no circumstances, did he want to talk to Andrews. He also asked Susan to find a newspaper reporter. She knew instantly who she wanted for that role. He stressed that the media exposure that they received would be critical in achieving the society's goals.

"I'll arrange for the interview at your office tomorrow at three o'clock, if that's acceptable." Susan went over some details, then hung up.

Coltrane sat down at his desk and looked at his office schedule. He would be seeing patients until six tonight, and had surgery in the morning. That meant that he would have to work all night to get a position paper ready for the interview tomorrow. He called Britt and told her not to make dinner for him. He would be home late tonight.

His office was a wonderful place to work late at night. The staff was gone, the exam rooms dark and quiet and the entire building silent. Coltrane sat at his computer and composed a simple and clean position paper for the press meeting the next day. He wanted to express the feelings of the medical community in a positive way, without accusing the insurance plans or the hospitals. He didn't want to slander or accuse. He only wanted to start some form of discussion and start the process of reforming what he felt was a grossly corrupt and inefficient system. Coltrane knew that the media could be a powerful ally in the reform, or a destructive enemy.

Chapter 30

June 13

The meeting came sooner than Coltrane would have liked. He barely finished with his two morning cases by lunch, and had his position papers ready by the time that the media circus began to arrive.

To represent the newspaper, Susan had invited a neophyte reporter, recently assigned to the medical bureau. Elizabeth Volk graduated from the University of Florida just two years earlier, and had moved to Tampa because of the city's great newspaper heritage. With a major in political science and a brilliant academic record, she had anticipated a posting to the paper's active political bureau. That was not to be. She soon realized that to earn a byline meant years of toiling in obscurity and paying her dues, far from the spotlight. After a six month tour reporting on the city's social scene, she was moved to the health and medical bureau. She had run into Susan Kerr at a local health fair, and the two had hit it off immediately. She came to rely on Susan as a dependable source of factual information on the many health topics that she covered in the paper.

After several calls to the television station, Susan selected a seasoned reporter who had just had her second child, and was still angry about the early post-partum discharge that the HMO plan had mandated for her. It would be better to have the media sympathetic, Susan thought as she hung up the phone.

Coltrane had given Susan instructions on how to manage the interview. Only the reporters would be allowed into his private office for the actual meeting. The sound and light people, and the cameramen would have to wait in the reception area. They could take cosmetic shots later. Coltrane had learned the hard way that he didn't need cameras and lights and surprises. He also knew that most people lose fifty IQ points when they are on camera. While he was now somewhat accustomed to television cameras, they still unnerved him. And he was well aware of news producers' penchant for editing and portraying comments out of context. If there was any manipulating to be done, Coltrane was going to be the one doing it. The technicians complained, but Susan handled them well and ushered the reporters into Coltrane's private office.

"Ms. Elizabeth Volk, Ms. Barbara Farrell, this is Dr. William Coltrane." Susan made the introductions, and quietly left the office, leaving the door half-open.

Coltrane sat down behind his massive desk, and waited as the reporters got settled. His suntanned face stood out against the starched, bright white doctor's coat and green scrubs. Behind him, the wall was covered with awards, certificates and his enormous University of Texas diploma. He smiled confidently at them, leaned forward, and rested his arms on the desk.

"Ladies, I want to thank you very much for taking the time to meet with me, and hope that I can answer all your questions. But first, let me give you some background as to why I asked you here. I think that you would agree that our healthcare system can benefit from change. As president of the medical society, I have the responsibility of presenting the proposals of the medical community to the public and other healthcare entities, such as insurance plans and our hospitals. In order to be successful in that role, I am seeking the aid of the media. I believe very strongly that we must educate and inform the public of the condition of their healthcare, the importance of which cannot be underestimated for it impacts their very life. Together we can do great things, effect great changes.

"My purpose in selecting you is simple. I offer your paper, and your station", Coltrane nodded to each respective reporter in turn as he spoke, "exclusive access to our position papers and press releases. All I want in return is an honest and thoughtful analysis of the issues, and accurate journalism. I do have one rule. I have been misquoted and quoted out of context more times than I care to recall. If that happens, I will never deal with you again. And I will tape all our interviews, just for the record." Coltrane smiled sweetly as he placed his microcassette recorder on the desktop, and switched it on. He leaned back in the leather chair, and waited for the questions to begin.

"Dr. Coltrane, what was the aim of your citywide slowdown of medical services and the closed door conference?" The television reporter got right to the offensive.

"First of all, there was no slowdown of medical services. All medical specialties are providing full coverage, and all emergency rooms were advised in advance of the conference. Patient care was not compromised in any way. Secondly, conferences like this occur daily, all over the country. Continuing medical education is mandated by Florida law, and physicians and dentists have meetings going on all year long. And by the way, they are always closed to the public and the media."

"What did you have to hide at last week's meeting?" she persisted.

"Nothing at all. You must understand that in medical meetings, patient cases are often discussed, and patient confidentiality would be violated by opening these proceedings to the press." Coltrane continued, "The purpose of our meeting was to evaluate the patient care protocols of the five major health insurance plans in Tampa-St. Pete. We are trying to make a significant change in the way that physicians and insurance entities interface here."

"What do you see as the problems?" Elizabeth Volk asked.

"There are many problems in the healthcare industry today. Our immediate goal is to address the inability of the attending physician to implement his or her treatment plan for the patient. The insurance industry policies are obstructive and dangerous. The HMO, PPO, and other similarly styled plans are by far the worst in this area, but our hope is to evolve guidelines that can be enforced statewide."

"What policies do you feel are obstructive and harmful, Dr. Coltrane?" the television reporter asked.

"The list is very long and oppressive. The most controversial policies you have no doubt read about. These would include mandatory discharge of mothers from the hospital on the second day after childbirth, discharge of patients from the hospital when their stay exceeds the national average for their particular disease symptom, the deletion or substitution of certain pharmaceuticals on the basis of cost, refusal to pay for certain lab tests, and the refusal to cover certain surgical procedures. These are only a few of the countless, absurd examples of bureaucratic interference in the practice of medicine by the insurance industry."

"These obstructions are only the most glaring," Coltrane continued. "In addition to the obvious meddling, there are volumes of absurd protocols and procedures that the physicians must follow in order to treat the patient, and have that patient's treatment covered under their policy." Coltrane paused.

"So you are concerned about your fees, Dr. Coltrane?" again the television reporter went on the offensive.

"Fair and uniform reimbursement is one of many issues, yes. But when I speak about non-coverage of treatment, you realize that the patient then becomes solely responsible for the entire bill. If the HMO deems that their protocol was not followed, the costs will fall upon the patient. Hospital bills, ambulance, lab, all the bills." Coltrane paused again. He knew that very few policyholders ever read anything but the monthly premium invoices. He let the thought sink in. "Are you aware that if you are on many HMO plans, before you go to the emergency room you must contact your family doctor? The plans want you to call some telephone exchange at three in the morning while your husband is having a heart attack, and ask to speak to your family doctor to get permission to go to the ER. It's outrageous."

"If you don't like the policies of the HMO, then don't participate. Why are doctors always whining about HMOs when all they have to do is quit?" Farrell charged.

"Well, it's not that simple. Even if you are not a participating provider, invariably you will have HMO patients in your practice. And the way that..."

"Sure it's simple. Just refer the patient to a participating physician. How hard is that?" Farrell interrupted.

"Let me finish. You don't understand the way referral patterns work. If I see a patient that has severe lung disease, I will refer them to one of three pulmonary specialists for evaluation. I know each doctor well, I have worked with them for years. I know what their areas of expertise are, and what they do best. Now, if that patient with the severe lung disease was your father, would you want me to choose his physician based on who I feel is the best suited to treat him, or on who is on some HMO panel? I select the physician whom I feel is the best qualified. I don't have the time nor the inclination to carry around a manual from every HMO in Florida listing who is and who isn't on each plan. Furthermore, doctors jump on and off those plans monthly. I can't keep track of who is participating. And when I am on call, covering the ER or emergencies, should I refuse to see anyone who is not on my participating health plans?"

"It gets very complex." Coltrane paused.

"I agree. I had to change my obstetrician three times during my pregnancy due to insurance plan changes. And supposedly, I have the best of the four plans the station offers." Farrell fumed.

"But there is more to it than just that. As the referring physician, I am morally and even legally responsible for the actions of my consultant. The patient trusts me to provide him with quality care, not only by my own hand, but also by the hand of any consultant that I bring into his care. A perfect example of this tenet is the selection of an anesthesiologist for surgery. In twenty years of surgical practice, not one of my patients has ever met with their anesthesiologist prior to the day of surgery. Few of them even remember the doctor's name or face the day after surgery. I choose the doctor, and I do it very carefully. There are only a few people I use, and they are the *only* people I use. I know who the best is, but there is no way the patient could ever know that. Now I guarantee you that it is better for the patient to have me making those decisions than to have the HMO selecting the referrals."

"Are you inferring that your elite circle of colleagues are the only competent doctors in Tampa?" Farrell asked, her voice dripping with sarcasm.

"Of course not. But I do know far more about the capabilities of the local physicians than any outsider could. I see their patients in consult; I watch them treat in ICUs and in ORs; I sit on several hospital committees that review quality of care. I have intimate knowledge of the workings of the medical community of the Bay area. There are brilliant physicians, many good ones, and some inadequate ones. Just as in any human endeavor."

"I still don't understand why you are so opposed to HMOs. The only constant thread that I hear from you is that your reimbursement is too low. But you can't deny that HMOs have had a powerful effect on the rising cost of medical care in this country, and been instrumental in keeping health insurance affordable for American families. Do you really believe that the greed of surgical specialists should have precedence over the basic healthcare needs of working families, the working poor?" Ms. Farrell accused.

"Of course not. Now, let me ask you a question. Do you do your own research?" Coltrane asked quietly.

"What do you mean?" Farrell fired back.

"Where did you find that HMOs have kept costs down? Where did you get that data?" Coltrane queried.

"It is published information. We get it from our research department," she answered, hesitantly.

"If you think about it, you will realize that it is an absurd statement. To prove that assertion, you would need two identical populations of patients, exact same age distribution, same disease incidence, and a static medical delivery system over a period of years. The cost of medical care, in the real world, goes up every day as new treatments evolve, new drugs are synthesized, CAT and MRI scans are readily available, and so on. What HMOs do is keep *premiums* down. That's all they do, and to do that they just limit availability of care, and minimize payments to providers. Insurance companies are having banner years, making billions. Patients aren't saving money. They are simply getting less medical care for a smaller premium. But of course, patients don't see it that way. They expect world class healthcare for their half price premium. Everybody is unhappy but the insurance company."

"Do you want to abolish HMOs in Florida?" Volk asked.

"No, not at all. I think that there is room for the HMO model of healthcare delivery, but I feel that *all* medical decisions must be made solely by physicians. The fundamental and tragic flaw of the HMO system is that far too many of these decisions are made by people ignorant of the issues involved."

"Look, I don't claim to be an expert on everything," Coltrane continued. "I don't understand why we send billions to Japan in currency loans when they haven't paid us for the Gulf War yet. I don't understand why taxpayers give billions to support tobacco and sugar commodity prices, or why we subsidize those moronic "Got Milk?" ads. I don't understand how the military can pay three billion dollars for a bomber but couldn't put a few tanks on the ground in Somalia. I don't know why a television producer of those insipid sit-coms makes one hundred thousand dollars a week, or why a policeman who risks his life every day makes twenty-six thousand dollars a year. There may be facts that I am unaware of that explain these things. I don't know. But I know medicine like the back of my hand. I know why things work, and why they don't work. I have been doing this for twenty years, every day, fifteen, sixteen hours a day."

"It is an easy matter to criticize the free market system. What's your solution to the problems you raised?" Farrell picked up her note pad to copy his response.

"First of all, the American healthcare system is not even *remotely* close to a free market, laissez-faire economy. It is the most regulated industry in the world, by bureaucrats from the federal to the state and local levels. Not to mention the omnipresent, constant, insidious regulation by the insurance industry. That aside, I think you would be surprised to hear my personal opinion is that we need a single payer, government run healthcare system." Coltrane answered.

"Like Canada? Canada has a model system, with free care for all Canadians," Volk agreed.

"No, not like Canada or Sweden or England. Canada's system is a disaster in many ways, and the waiting list for surgery is months long. And it's not free. Canadian taxes are very high, over fifty percent at relatively low income levels compared to American marginal rates. I prefer a Medicare style system, funded by federal tax revenue and perhaps administered by private insurance entities. It could easily be done, and universal care provided to all Americans, but there would have to be some changes."

"Underlying all the problems that I have named is a much more serious situation in American medicine. The practice of medicine has always been rigorous and stressful, demanding much from its practitioners. But the onerous federal and state and insurance interference coupled with medical malpractice and increasing workloads and decreasing reimbursement is leading to an exodus of the most experienced and successful physicians. Doctors in their fifties are retiring, going into less stressful and demanding professions. Or cutting their stress by working two or three days a week.

These are physicians at the peak of their experience, wisdom and productivity. And the new crop of young physicians are more interested in nine to five positions than in private practice. The cumulative effects of these trends will negatively impact the quality of healthcare for years to come."

"But are your tactics justified? By closing doctors' offices for your meeting, the ERs all over town were flooded. Patients suffered." The television reporter continued.

"As I said before, medical services were provided without any interruption. ERs are always flooded. The emergency department is the most abused sector of medicine. People use the ER for colds, for headaches, for symptoms that have persisted for weeks. They use the ER after hours so they don't have to pay for an office visit to their family doctor. Only *ten percent* of ER visits are actual emergencies." Coltrane began to get irritated by the reporter's insistence. The microcassette clicked, signifying the end of the tape. He picked it up, flipped the tape, and set it on record again.

"Are you aware that PatientsChoice has filed a charge against you for a COBRA violation as a result of your slowdown?" the reporter spat.

"What?" Coltrane was jolted. A COBRA violation was a very serious charge. He had heard nothing of this before.

"The HMO alleges that you dumped a burn patient inappropriately on the day of the meeting. You refused to admit a burn victim from a chemical plant, is that right?"

"No." Coltrane thought back quickly.

"Are you Chief of Surgery at County?" she quickly followed.

"Yes."

"The plant physician called County and requested that the patient be transported to your burn unit. Apparently the plastic surgeon on call could not be located. Who was that?" The reporter smelled blood.

"I do not know. I wasn't on call that day. Nor was I contacted." Coltrane wondered if she was fabricating the entire story.

"The patient was then flown to Orlando to some hospital there, against the family's wishes. They and the insurance plan are planning to file federal charges against you and the hospital immediately," she finished, and smiled smugly across the desk at Coltrane.

"Patients are often transferred to other hospitals for many reasons. I do not know the details in this case, but I will find out. But I can assure you, on the record, that it had absolutely nothing to do with our meeting." Coltrane was emphatic.

"Let's hope so. For your sake…"

"I will have an answer for you tomorrow. Thank you both very much for your time." Coltrane was visibly concerned. The reporters finished their notes, and left the office. The television journalist smiled as she left. She had done her homework for this meeting, calling the hospitals and insurance plans about Coltrane and his reputation. She only regretted not having the camera on his face when she sprung that COBRA violation at him.

Coltrane waited until the reporters and media people had left the office, then asked Cindy to close the office. It was past five anyway. He sat at the desk and looked up who was on call the day of the meeting. It had been Bookman. He called the office number and was switched to the answering service. He asked for Dr. Bookman to be paged. It was twenty minutes before Bookman called back.

"Dr. Bookman."

"Ralph, this is Bill Coltrane. Do you know anything about a burn case two days ago? A severe chemical burn?"

"Yeah, I was in the OR at the time, just starting a long case. I referred it to you."

"Why did you refer it to me? You knew I was at that meeting all day. Why not one of the six other guys?" Coltrane was pissed.

"I'm sorry, *your highness*. I momentarily forgot that you are our president. I was going to be tied up for hours with a breast reconstruction, and there was no way that a seventy-five percent burn could wait. Why didn't you see him?" Bookman shot back. He and Coltrane had never gotten along.

"No one called me about him. Apparently he went to Orlando."

"Probably the ER doctor's decision. I am sure he went to the Burn Unit. They'll take good care of him."

"I am told that a COBRA violation has been filed against the hospital and myself, and you too, I am sure."

"By who?" Now Coltrane had Bookman's attention.

"The HMO and the family."

"Fuck that. The Orlando burn unit is an appropriate transfer for any burn, much less a seventy-five percent total body surface burn. The HMO is just pissed because it will cost them more. And since when do we let family members decide where to treat third degree burns? Fuck that."

"I hope that you're right. Who called you, do you remember?"

"No." Bookman had nothing more to say.

"If you hear anything, call me."

"Right." Bookman hung up.

Coltrane got his briefcase, locked up and left his office to finish evening rounds and go home. One more thing to worry about. He needed a vacation. Britt had planned one soon, he remembered. It couldn't be too soon.

Chapter 31

June 14

Coltrane called the Federal District Office in Miami. He knew that there were only two investigators on the COBRA staff, and if a complaint had been filed they would know of it. Neither man was in the office, but he left his name, number and his message on the voice mail. Then he went back to seeing patients. It was three hours before the call was returned.

"Dr. Coltrane, this is Rueben Perez at the Miami COBRA office. I got your message to call. How may I help you?" the voice dryly asked.

"Mr. Perez, I understand that I have been charged with a COBRA violation. Could you give me the details?" Coltrane was fishing.

"Certainly, Doctor. I'm investigating that particular case, and I have not called you because you have been completely cleared by our investigation."

Coltrane sighed audibly on the line. While he knew that he had done nothing wrong, the allegation had hung on him like a cloud.

Perez continued. "The complaint was brought by an insurance company and the family of a burn patient, and pertained to inappropriate transfer of the patient to another facility. I spoke to the hospital, and that decision was made by the ER physician based on sound medical criteria. You were not involved in any way. I am unsure why the charge was even brought. But you don't need to worry about it at all." Perez paused.

"I have never heard of an insurance company filing a COBRA charge. Usually the patients are uninsured, aren't they?" Coltrane knew that the COBRA legislation levied stiff penalties on hospitals accused of transferring or dumping uninsured patients to other medical facilities.

"Yes. But if one of a HMO's patients is transferred from a participating hospital to a non-participating hospital, the HMO must pay the full fee for that patient's care. At the participating hospital, the HMO would pay nothing, the costs are already covered. So they lose quite a bit of money. In this case, the burn patient may be in the burn unit for weeks, maybe months. They want to keep their enrollees in their hospitals." Perez had already processed five such complaints by insurance plans that morning. He was frustrated by the extra workload, and began to tell Coltrane more than he should have. "I think that the HMOs are using the COBRA charges as a means to bring their participating hospitals and doctors in line. I get frantic calls like yours constantly now."

Coltrane thanked him for the information and hung up. He went back to seeing his office patients, profoundly relieved to know that he was not involved in a COBRA charge. It would not be until hours later that night before the significance of the conversation became clear.

It came to him as he sat in front of the television that evening, mindlessly channelsurfing. Clearly the HMO kept a very close track of their expenses on a patient-by-patient basis. And it had been hurt by the transfer of just one patient to an outside facility. Coltrane realized that he had been trying to reason with the plans using medical logic, which they didn't comprehend or value. But he knew that they would understand dramatically increased expenses. Financial logic was something they could understand.

Coltrane called out to Britt, who was sitting in the adjoining living room reading.

"Britt, listen to this and tell me what you think. None of the plans are responding at all to our requests for reform. If we can't reason with them, then maybe we can make it too costly for them to continue the present system. My guess is that by disrupting the normal tedious maze of referrals and paperwork they have arranged, we can hurt them financially."

"You mean stop seeing HMO patients? You can't do that without breaking your contract. Or arranging some kind of physician strike." Britt was wary of any radical approaches.

"Not a strike. Not even a slowdown. All that we have to do is hold another conference, maybe two or three days, maybe a week. During the conference, everybody continues to see patients, but we arrange a crossover of HMO coverage." Coltrane was getting excited. The plan was brilliant, he thought. There had to be a flaw somewhere.

"What do you mean, crossover?"

"Okay, let's say there are three neurologists in town, one on HMO A, one on HMO B, and one on HMO C. Ordinarily, all HMO A patients go to Doctor A, and so on. Well, during our conference, the call rotation will be every third day for each doctor. Therefore, every day, two HMOs are going to be hit with high bills as their patients go to a non-HMO doctor. And patient care will not be compromised at all. There are details to be worked out, like call schedules so that the town is well covered and the doctors don't get exhausted. But computers can do that easily." Coltrane sat back, his mind flying, trying to find an Achilles heel to the plan.

"Can you single out the worst HMO offenders?" Britt asked.

"Brilliant. The membership database in the society computer can sift through the plan enrollment, and tell me who is on each plan in town. We then pick the two worst HMO offenders and make sure that none of their providers are on the call list for two or three days. We will make them active participants in the seminar. Nice touch."

"Make damn sure the lawyers have cleared this before you do it. You don't want to be breaking federal law."

Coltrane went to his computer, and went to his online *Caduceus*. He went straight to the introduction page. He entered his password, and began to compose the bulletin that all members would soon be reading. The text was short and very clear. It declared that the initial conference had delineated two HMO plans as being egregious, and that attempts to redress the problems have been met with failure. Therefore, a second, longer conference is planned for the immediate future.

Details to follow.

Chapter 32

June 15

The next morning, Coltrane was on the phone first thing with Susan Kerr. He outlined the idea to her, and asked her to do a quick check into the feasibility of running a computer analysis of the physician membership, by HMO contracts.

"We have that data from our questionnaire, you know. It asked everyone to list the HMO and insurance plans that they had contracted with." Susan replied.

"Good. What you need to do is break that list down by specialty and by HMO. What were the two worst offenders again?"

"AthenaHMO and PatientsChoice Florida, by a wide margin," Susan replied without hesitation.

"Good. Then what we need is a list of all the doctors, by specialty, and by HMO participation. I will need that list today, so I can make a new call schedule. I am going to have to personally call each doctor for their permission."

"I can have that list in thirty minutes." Susan answered.

"Then the next thing will be to set up a time to have a third conference. Schedule it for one full week. Same hotel, and even tighter security arrangements. And send a nice letter to all the HMO medical directors, informing them of the dates and inviting them to attend." Coltrane was on a roll.

"Wait. Wait. A week long conference? And invite the insurance trolls? I am totally lost." Susan hadn't had time to digest the essentials of the strategy.

"Get us the list and then come on over to the office. I'll lay it out for you." Coltrane hung up, then wondered to himself how much she should know. Maybe he should keep her in the dark. The less she knew, the better for her sake, he concluded. And maybe his.

Their meeting was short.

Chapter 33

June 16

Ochoa had been gone from Tampa for two weeks. It was all he could take. He had run out of dope by the fifth day, and living on the floor of his cousin's trailer wore thin fast. He had called his girlfriend several times, but she was never home, even late. He wanted to know where the fuck she was. At two in the fucking morning.

Chapter 34

June 18

Coltrane was working late, alone at the office when the back line rang.

He immediately recognized anxiety in Susan Kerr's voice. "Dr. Coltrane, you need to meet with the media representatives again, and soon. Somehow, news of the weeklong conference has leaked to the press, and I'm being deluged with media requests for the details. The television coverage has been very negative, and it is causing panic in the community. And Wilson Andrews is going after the society with a vengeance. We need to respond."

"Alright, call Elizabeth Volk and arrange an interview. I can meet her at my office anytime tomorrow."

"What about Barbara Farrell?" Susan asked.

"To hell with her and television news. She just wastes my time. I spend three hours talking to her, and she's just looking for a sound byte and a meaningless ten second piece to get ratings. Look how she ambushed me with that COBRA allegation. She wanted to ask me that question on camera to see how I'd react. Our local news isn't journalism, it's a form of entertainment. Car crashes, violent crimes, sordid details of the lives of our public figures. I want to present the community with an in-depth explanation of our positions. Only the newspaper can do that. See if Volk can meet me tomorrow."

"Fine. She has been calling me daily with questions. I'm sure she will interview you. I'll call you with the time."

"Any response from the HMO plans?" Coltrane asked hopefully.

"Nothing. It is virtually impossible to get answers from those people. I can't even find out who is in charge of physician relations at the plans. No one ever calls me back, and they all defer to the corporate offices when I ask about policy matters. I'm getting nowhere."

Coltrane set the receiver down, and questioned whether he should subject her to the travail that was sure to come as the conference progressed. Unsettled, he closed his briefcase, shut off the lights, and left his office for home.

Chapter 35

June 19
10:00AM

Coltrane drove the short route to his medical office building, and was relieved to see that the parking lot and lobby atrium was relatively empty. When the conference was announced by the news media, scores of anxious patients had flocked to their doctors' offices to be seen. When many realized that treatment was going to be available, and that their out-of-pocket costs would remain the same, the hysteria had evaporated. He took the elevator to his level, and entered the office suite by the private door.

Today was a day normally scheduled for surgery, so the waiting room was empty. The office was quiet, with the girls doing paperwork, and submitting electronic claims. Coltrane walked past the admitting desk and greeted the receptionist. As he turned down the hallway to his private office, Cindy followed him with an armful of charts.

"Good morning, Dr. Coltrane," Cindy smiled. "Elizabeth Volk will be here at one o'clock. I ordered up lunch for you, your usual. I need to review some charts and CPT codes, and discuss what you want to do with the surgery schedule for the next few weeks."

"How are our patients taking this?" Coltrane looked up from his desk as Cindy sat down across from him.

"Very well, actually. The vast majority of our patients are loyal, and have great respect for you. I truly believe that they would continue coming here even if it meant a slightly higher out-of-pocket cost. You'll be happy to know that our accounts receivable has dropped dramatically since the conference. Everyone's sending in their overdue balances. Even the deadbeats are sending in their money, some even coming to the office to pay. I guess they think that you won't see them unless they pay. What a novel idea." Cindy smiled sarcastically. It had always amazed her the way people had the gall to expect treatment without payment, even their deductible. You don't go to the grocery store and walk out with food without paying, or to a restaurant and walk out without paying the bill. Only in medical offices, some patients were indignant about paying their bills. It continually astonished her.

"You know how I feel about billing, Cindy. Please be careful not to create the impression that we will not see anyone based on their ability to pay. That's a violation of state and federal law."

"I know, Dr. Coltrane. But I can't stand to see any more of these women on Medicaid digging in their beautiful Dooney & Bourke purses pretending they left their checkbook in the car. And last week..."

"I don't want to know. Tell me about the surgery schedule." Coltrane interrupted her, holding his palm up to stop the tirade he knew was coming. Cindy was the office administrator, and took her job seriously. She also took personally the many patient attempts to avoid, delay and otherwise refuse to pay for services rendered. Coltrane appreciated her dedication, but he couldn't listen to the details. He had learned long ago that there were aspects of private practice he didn't want to handle. Financial reimbursement was one of those things. He found that when he was aware of an absurdly low reimbursement, or non-payment of a patient's bill, he came to resent the patient and the time he spent with them in follow-up. Usually it wasn't the patient's fault, usually it was the HMO's fault. But, human nature being what it is, it colored Coltrane's interaction with the patient. So he had decided that Cindy would handle all financial matters, and keep him isolated from those issues. She maintained a database on the reimbursement of each of the plans that Coltrane participated with, and advised him as to whether the practice should continue on the plan. It was a compromise and a loss of control of the practice, but he trusted her completely, and the solution had been a good one for years.

"Okay, you have twelve patients scheduled for the week of the conference. I can postpone eight, they are purely elective procedures; scar releases, removal of lipoma, and three delayed tendon reconstructions. But the remaining four I need your approval to reschedule. Schuller and Jackson are tendon repairs," Cindy paused for a response.

"Move them up immediately. I've only got a two week window in which to repair those tendons."

"What about Mitchell and De La Garza?"

"Reschedule them. I've been after Mitchell for a year to have that biopsy. He can wait a week. Anything else?"

"Nope. All is well in the front office, and we are enjoying the little break. Volk will be here in a while. You want your lunch back here?"

"Yes, please." Coltrane thanked her and began to work on his comments to the newspaper reporter. This interview had to go well. An in-depth article in the major daily paper for the Tampa-St. Pete area would make or break their effort. He reviewed the recent articles Volk had written, and the editorial comments in the paper. The letters to the editor section was devoted entirely to the society conference, and the majority of the sentiment was anti-physician. It would not be easy.

Coltrane's intercom rang to tell him that the reporter was here. Cindy brought the young woman back, and seated her across from Coltrane. Elizabeth Volk was in her mid-twenties, attractive and athletic. Her conservative skirt and blouse could not conceal her lithe body and long legs. After asking if she would like coffee or a cold drink, Cindy left, leaving the door open behind her.

"Good afternoon, Ms. Volk," Coltrane greeted her as she opened a leather portfolio and extracted a yellow pad with her questions neatly arranged in sequence. She leaned back in the black leather armchair, and surveyed the office, and Coltrane's diplomas and certificates. As she crossed her legs, Coltrane heard the gentle rub of her nylons.

"Thanks for seeing me again, Dr. Coltrane," she started. "I've been given twelve column inches on the front page for this article, if the editor approves." She smiled at the thought. "I appreciate the exclusive you are giving me."

"You should thank Cindy for that. But this is a two-way street. I am dealing with you and your paper because I strongly feel that a newspaper can give far more comprehensive and in-depth coverage of an issue than a fifteen second videobyte on the TV news. All we want is a fair and accurate story."

"That's my goal. I have no prejudices in regards to this dispute." She paused, and looked at her legal pad. "If you don't mind, I have a series of questions that I would like to ask."

"Go ahead." Coltrane reached over to the microcassette recorder on his desk, and clicked it on. The tiny machine whirred softly.

"The primary concern of our readership is that your proposed 'conference' is a thinly disguised labor action, the goal of which is to extort higher physicians' fees from the HMOs. Some people feel that all the gains that HMOs have made over the years will be lost if you are allowed to succeed. How would you respond to that statement?"

"First of all, I must make it clear that our conference is not a physicians' strike or a labor action. Any such action would be a violation of the Sherman Act, and punishable by civil or criminal penalties. Are you familiar with the Sherman Antitrust Act?"

"I remember it was used against AT&T when Ma Bell was broken up into the Baby Bells. And didn't the attorney general use it against Microsoft?"

"Right. The Act was passed in the 1890's, after the industrialization of the US. Huge companies like Standard Oil, DuPont, US Steel and American Tobacco were formed by mergers, and held strangleholds on commerce. There emerged "captains of industry" who presided over empires that dominated the entire spectrum of production. These huge monopolies ruthlessly destroyed smaller businesses, and eliminated competition. In response, the Federal government passed a series of laws that established the Federal Trade Commission as the watchdog agency to protect the American consumer and small businessman from unfair trade practices of large, monopolistic corporate entities. Somehow, somewhere along the way, someone decided that these laws apply to healthcare providers, despite the fact that there are hundreds of thousands of us, each in our own little office, each with our own little practice. It's absurd."

"How does the law affect physicians?" Volk asked, writing as she spoke.

"It effectively blocks any attempt by physicians to organize. The risk of antitrust litigation is so great, and the legal costs so high, that physicians have been barred from organizing PSO networks to compete with the HMOs. The net effect of the laws, or perhaps I should say, the net effect of blind enforcement of the Act, is that competition is actually stifled. The insurance entities, both the traditional forms and the HMOs, are delighted to have the FTC do their litigation for them."

"I never hear about any of this in the media, nor have I found reference in my research. Are these theoretical concerns, or has the government ever taken action against physicians?"

"The government is taking a very active stance in the prosecution of these cases. Three Arizona dentists were indicted on *criminal* charges for allegedly trying to increase their patients' co-payments. Criminal charges carry a three year jail time, and $50,000 fine. The charges were eventually dropped or reduced, but these guys' practices were ruined. Eighty Salt Lake City pediatricians were taken to a grand jury for possible price-fixing in their IPA. The government has gone after OB-GYNs in Georgia, and a group of Boston allergists as well. Can you imagine the effects of a five year federal lawsuit? If you get hit with a federal lawsuit, you have to pay all the court costs yourself. Malpractice insurance won't cover a penny. The legal fees alone would bankrupt you. And add that to the lost work time, and the down time for your practice. It is a virtual death sentence for your practice. And your life. That threat alone has kept many physicians from attempting to form any managed care entity."

"Price-fixing should be illegal."

"Absolutely. I agree. But how do you define price-fixing? Medicare has a standard fee schedule that is implemented nationwide. If you ask for that fee schedule, is that price-fixing? If there were only two physicians in town and they both agreed to charge five hundred dollars for an office visit, that's price-fixing. But there are over a thousand physicians, just in the immediate Bay area. How am I going to get all of them involved in a price-fixing scheme? Impossible."

"Are you campaigning for changes in the antitrust laws or freedom to organize a physician owned managed care organization?"

"I honestly don't know where this process is headed or where it will end. My goal is to streamline the healthcare delivery system, here in Pinellas and Hillsborough Counties. I have no ambitions beyond that. Physicians have tried this type of organization in Texas, New Jersey, Pennsylvania, Washington and Louisiana, with mixed results. There are regional differences in law and competition. All I know is Tampa, and we will see what happens here."

"Enumerate for me your three main goals." Elizabeth Volk placed her pad on her lap, and waited for Coltrane's answers.

"Three goals? We have more than just three goals. But our highest priority is physician control of *ALL* medical decisions. By that I mean choice of treatment, duration of hospitalization, type of medication and therapy, and so on. I spend far too much time and energy on the phone requesting pre-authorization for a procedure from someone who doesn't have the slightest idea what I am talking about. We are demanding an end to drive-by mastectomies, drive-through deliveries, and all the cost-cutting and cost-shifting tactics that negatively impact patient care. I will argue that physicians are the only authorities who should be charged with these decisions."

"Secondly, we want significant and dramatic changes in the field of medical malpractice. Again, this is an area that is so complex that it should be reviewed by *experts*. Physicians do make errors, as do all human beings. The current system is more like a lottery than a system of justice or regulation. If your claim is minor, that is, if you survived without some horrible or sensational deformity, then no one is interested in your case."

"What do you mean by that?" Elizabeth looked up from her notes.

"Let me give you a personal example. My younger brother had gallstones, and had vague pains in his stomach for weeks. His symptoms were atypical, so I never got a good handle on what was going on and since he lives in Seattle, I didn't get a chance to examine him. He went to a family practitioner who examined him several times, and eventually took an ultrasound of his abdomen. He mis-interpreted the ultrasound, partly because he had an untrained office girl operating the machine, and partly because he has absolutely no training in reading sonograms. He had recently bought the machine to boost his practice revenues. Unfortunately, what happens when you don't pay a doctor fairly, sometimes he may try to increase his compensation some other way. This bozo decided to play radiologist on my brother, and nearly killed him. Any moron can see a damn gallstone with ultrasound, they're the size of marbles, for God's sake. I tried to get his license, but the state won't act against him. He was within his rights to practice medicine. And no attorney will touch it because there is no death or brain-dead baby to enrage a jury and elicit a huge award. So this clown goes on, taking ultrasounds of anyone walking through the door."

"Report him to the Board of Medical Examiners. Can't they discipline him somehow?"

"It's a little known fact that a medical license entitles the physician to practice any medical specialty the he or she pleases. With or without any residency training or board certification. I could legally practice neurosurgery, or cardiothoracic surgery. Whatever I want. Legally. The medical board was unable to act against him. I think that our tort system is inadequate for overseeing medical practice. I think a system like the worker's compensation board review panel would be more effective and more equitable. When Texas mandated that all workmen's compensation claims go to a workmen's comp panel and took the process out of the courts, the claims dropped dramatically. We need something like that for medicine."

"You'll get plenty of argument from the trial lawyers about that proposal."

"There's no question about that. The lawyers in this town contribute millions of dollars to the political campaigns of their candidates, many of whom are lawyers to start with. It will be difficult to change the system, simply because the system is run by lawyers, and benefits their interests. But something has to be done to reform our legal system. Hold on, let me pull this E-mail up. I got it from one of our society members this morning." Coltrane turned to the flat panel monitor on his desk, and signed on to AOL.

He started reading from the forwarded E-mail:

Forwarded Message:
Subj: Make a buck
From: AllytmpaMD5
To: WmColtraneMD

The Stella Award

In 1994, a New Mexico jury awarded Stella Liebeck $2.86 million for the injuries she suffered after spilling coffee on her lap while trying to open the cup in an automobile. The Annual Stella Award is given to the most absurd and frivolous lawsuit filed in United States Courts, and the following are the final candidates. Only time and space limitations prevent us from listing the thousands of other meritorious candidates:

1. Man attempts to rob home, and in the process is trapped in the garage due to malfunctioning electric garage door opener. Subsists on homeowner's dry dog food and warm Pepsi until discovered 8 days later. Sues for undue mental anguish, and is awarded $500,000.

2. Woman has fight with boyfriend while out for dinner, throws soft drink at him, then slips on the drink and busts her ass. She sues the restaurant, and is awarded $113,000.

3. Woman breaks her front teeth in a fall while trying to sneak into a nightclub through the ladies' room window. She didn't want to pay the cover charge. She sues the owner of the club, and wins $12,000 plus medical costs.

4. Woman breaks her ankle by tripping over toddler running in a furniture store in Austin, Texas. Jury awards her $780,000, in spite of the fact that the misbehaving toddler is her own child.

5. Man buys a brand new Winnebago motor home, and on the maiden voyage, gets up to 70 mph and sets the cruise control. He then calmly gets out of the driver's seat, and goes back to the kitchenette to make something to drink. The 32-foot motorhome glides off the freeway, rolls over and crashes. He survived, and sued Winnebago for not clearly explaining that he could not leave the driver's seat in that manner. He is awarded $1,750,000 and a new Winnebago. Hopefully without cruise control.

6. Gardener finishes mowing his client's grass, and starts to trim the bushes. Since he had been out all night in a topless establishment, he had failed to return to his shop and pick up the necessary tool, an electric hedge trimmer. Improvising, he turned on the gas lawnmower, picked it up by the wheels, and tried to trim the bushes with the mower's blades. He lost three fingers in the process. He sues the homeowner and the manufacturer for negligence, and was awarded $890,000 plus medical expenses.

AND THE WINNER IS:

A Phoenix clairvoyant who claimed that her abilities to forecast the future was lost during a MRI scan during the workup of her brain tumor. She was awarded $3.2M and all her medical expenses. Despite the defense attorney's argument that if she truly could predict the future, she should have seen this coming.

"Unbelievable!" She wondered if the reports were really factual.

"I don't know how accurate this E-mail is, but I doubt anyone will argue the legal system needs to be changed. People need to realize that they are paying for these awards. Corporations have to increase the prices they charge for goods and services, governments have to charge higher taxes, and insurance entities pass on all their costs to the consumer. Homeowner lawsuits related to mold have driven Allstate and State Farm out of California. The lawyers figured out that it is impossible to prove that the plaintiff actually does not have an allergic response to mold. And that raises homeowner's insurance rates there dramatically. It's not a crusade, or David versus Goliath, like the trial lawyers like to paint it. It's just a never-ending spiral of greed and opportunism."

"It is easy to give this to my research department, and I can verify if any or all of it is true."

"Please do." Coltrane printed the E-mail and passed it to her.

"What is your final goal?"

"Thirdly, we have a far more achievable objective. In the past decade, the business side of private practice has become onerous. I have personally had to add two full-time employees just to handle the paperwork and red tape associated with being a participating HMO provider. And the vast majority of the work is unnecessary. We want mandatory implementation of the system developed by Medicare for electronic submission of claims, and electronic payment. This will eliminate thousands of hours of redundant paperwork and handling a different claim form for each insurance plan. All providers should be verified by their bank accounts, and all payments must go directly to the provider. That alone will make health insurance fraud much more difficult. Lastly, we want a uniform fee schedule or a relative value system so that we can evaluate the fees paid by HMOs more accurately."

"Ahhhh, finally we get to the matter of fees, Doctor." Elizabeth smiled cynically.

"Why is it that everyone gets a tight ass when it comes to paying doctors? Sorry. Very sensitive issue with us." Coltrane apologized for his crude comment.

"No problem. I have three brothers. I will not quote you." She laughed.

"Look, let me be the devil's advocate. When other professions get highly paid, the public approves. Everyone wants a free market economy, where one's goods and services are valued on their merit. And cash is how merit is determined. Alex Rodriguez just got a $252 million contract with the Texas Rangers. Mike Hampton got $121 million. Ken Griffey Jr. got $116.5 million. No one begrudges them their contracts. They get what the buyer, in this case, the owners, think they are worth. Shaquille O'Neal makes almost $30 million a year. Michael Jordan made over that in his best year. Michael Buffer, the 'Let's Get Ready to Rumble' guy, his empire made close to $250 million merchandising that unique phrase. I have no problem with any of that. We all love our athletes and entertainers, and admire their abilities and skills. Why shouldn't they get paid what they are worth?"

"But are they really worth that?"

"They are worth that to whoever is paying them that salary. No one has a gun to the owners' heads, forcing them to pay those incredible salaries. They pay because if they don't, another team will. Supply and demand. Pure and simple."

"But that is the entertainment industry. It's different."

"That's exactly my point. Sports, movies, television, music, theater, all these industries are essentially luxuries. Yet it seems more important to compensate them well than to compensate healthcare providers. On top of that, did you know that entertainers have a lower marginal federal income tax rate than the rest of us? I think it is 22 percent, max. Seem bizarre to you?"

"Why? I don't believe it." Elizabeth was incredulous. "Another job for the research department."

"Some things about our society and the values we place on goods and services shock me. Do you know what a 'champagne girl' is?" Coltrane asked.

"Not exactly. Sounds like sex is involved."

"They're girls that sell glasses of watered champagne to patrons of strip clubs. The champagne is cheap, and the prices very high. They aren't even dancers, just wear little outfits and high heels. The point is that they make $1500 to $2000 a night in big city men's clubs. And the dancers usually make more. There are escort services that have girls who make $4000 to $5000 a night, doing similar things. Tax-free."

"Sex sells. That's not news." Elizabeth looked mildly disgusted.

"Fine. My point is that the same guy who will pay $50 for a two minute lap dance will get angry if he has to pay $20 for an office visit. Do you realize that Americans spend $4.3 billion in herbal supplements a year? Do you realize that the cosmetics and beauty industry, and by that I mean lipsticks, makeup and hairspray, is one of the top five segments of our economy, netting billions yearly? Do you know that the US government spent $1 billion on anti-drug ads that actually may have increased teenage drug use? And since they are not sure, the taxpayer will get to fund further research into the efficiency of the ad campaign. And Americans spend $600 *billion* gambling yearly. And Medicare paid over $20 billion in incorrect or fraudulent payments last year? Do you know that a visit to a physical therapist costs $80, and a visit to the ER, with physician time, nursing time, labs, fluids, and so on, is only worth a flat fee of $95 to my HMO? I know a pair of nurses that opened a home health care company and made $600,000 each last year. All on Medicaid and Medicare patients. You probably would be surprised to know that the federal government will pay a LPN to go to your house and change your bandages twice a day. My point is this: There is enough money, public and private, to fund an efficient healthcare system for all Americans. We, as a society, simply have chosen to avoid taking responsibility for our own healthcare. Do you know that 85% of uninsured American families are *employed?* These families have the money, they simply chose to spend it elsewhere. Why pay for insurance when you can just walk into any hospital, anywhere in the country, and get care for free? Try that in Mexico. Try that in France. Doesn't work. Just here. Our system is great for most people as it stands. It puts all the burden on the physicians, the hospitals, and employers. So who cares?"

"You want to be better paid. Is that a fair representation of your position?"

"Yes. I don't think that physicians, as a group, can be accused of being greedy or avaricious. There are just too many other ways to make more money, much more easily, than medicine. Given the intelligence and discipline that it takes to survive medical school and residency, I think that is an accurate statement. You should spend a day with me, and see what private practice involves. You would be enlightened, I think."

"Do you want to implement free market economics in medicine?" Elizabeth assumed that was the logical approach.

"No, that would be a disaster. Years ago, the Shah of Iran came to the United States for treatment before he died. Should his physician have charged him more than other patients, simply because he could have afforded to pay billions to stay alive? Plastic surgeons charge whatever they want for facelifts. And a facelift in Miami or Beverly Hills is much more expensive than a facelift in Tulsa or Boise. But it is really the same procedure. I don't think individual physicians should be allowed to set fees arbitrarily; it could lead to bitterness and charges of extortion. Besides, there is already an established uniform fee schedule."

"You mentioned some relative value determination earlier. What does that mean?" Elizabeth looked up.

"There are several systems published. McGraw-Hill has the most comprehensive one. Basically, it is a huge index of procedures, each described and then given a relative weighting." Coltrane spun his chair around, and reached into the credenza and pulled out a thick, bound notebook. He turned back to Elizabeth. "Pick a procedure, any procedure," he asked with a showman's grin.

"Hysterectomy."

"Hysterectomy. Under Genito-Urinary, female. Let's see ... here we go. Bilateral vaginal hysterectomy...Code 58262 at 13.99 Units. Every procedure and billable event is listed and given a unit value in this book. Office visits, hospital visits, emergency room visits, ICU visits, surgical procedures, injections, even legal testimony and medical reports. Everything gets a unit value."

"I don't understand the purpose of the units."

"Its a brilliant system. It allows the system to be flexible, and adapt to inflation or deflation with time. To convert units into dollars, the billing physician fixes his conversion unit value at some given amount. Usually, all the physicians in a given area at a given time use a similar conversion rate. For instance, when I started practice in the early eighties, my unit value was one hundred twenty dollars. So, if I were a gynecologist, I would have charged 13.99 Units multiplied by one hundred twenty dollars, for a fee of..." Coltrane punched his calculator and said, "sixteen hundred seventy-nine dollars. And as time passes, and inflation increases costs, the conversion factor can be adjusted upward. I use a factor of one hundred eighty dollars now. Very simple."

"You want all the HMOs to use that system for reimbursement? That seems simple enough. Why don't they do that?" Elizabeth put down her pad, and seemed genuinely surprised.

"They refuse to tell the participating physicians what the fee schedule is. They claim that it is proprietary information, and they won't release it. The only time you find out what they will pay is when you get the check. And to keep things interesting, they pay good fees for some procedures, and ridiculously low fees for other procedures to keep their costs low. In effect, they cut their costs and increase their profits on the backs of the providers. We, as physicians, have been fools for years by allowing them to do this. What kind of an idiot would take a job without knowing what the salary is? We do that every time we join a HMO."

"Have you presented your demands to the insurance industry? How did you go about doing that?"

"During our last conference, we discussed and prepared position papers on all the issues I just mentioned. We have asked for meetings with representatives from the major hospitals in the Bay area, and with the insurance entities in the Bay area. All the hospitals sent delegates for ongoing meetings with our coordinating committee, and we have some innovative ideas coming out of those meetings. Despite repeated invitations, none of the insurance plans has responded. They continually refuse to engage in any dialogue. Please make sure your readers are made aware of that."

"And if the HMOs refuse to comply with your demands, what then? Are you going to stop seeing HMO patients entirely?" Elizabeth was showing that she had teeth.

"Of course not. We have retained legal counsel to advise the membership on the intricacies of terminating our associations with the area HMOs. Furthermore, we are considering organizing the society into a non-profit501(c) (3) company to provide an all-inclusive, seamless medical delivery system for Pinellas County. But how this ends remains to be seen." Coltrane sat back, turned off the microrecorder and placed his hands on the leather desk blotter before him.

"Thanks for the interview, Dr. Coltrane. I suspect that you chose me as your media liaison because of my inexperience. Even a novice can see that there is more to what you are doing than you admit. But I can see your viewpoint. I must tell you, however, that I will meet with the hospital spokeswoman this afternoon, and later with the spokesman from Athena Healthcare. I will report on all these interviews in tomorrow's edition. I hope you still will talk to me after the story." Elizabeth Volk stood and smiling sincerely, offered her hand.

"I hope so as well." Coltrane shook her hand, impressed by her forthright manner and candor.

After she left, Coltrane sank into his soft leather chair, and spun toward the windows lining his office walls. In the distance, the Gulf of Mexico sparkled in the afternoon sun. His tired mind drifted, vaguely aware of the momentous events hurtling toward him.

Chapter 36

June 20

Coltrane was very satisfied at the progress they had made. In the space of several days, Susan had organized the third meeting and he had arranged a call schedule. The announcement of the meeting's date and agenda was posted on *Caduceus* and registration was proceeding smoothly. Coltrane hoped that the membership would be able to read between the lines, and deduce the strategy.

Coltrane was examining post-op patients when Cindy interrupted him. He went back to his office with her, as she explained that the caller was from the FBI. Ordinarily, she didn't take him from patient exams, but this sounded important. Coltrane agreed.

"Dr. Coltrane," he picked up the line after Cindy left and closed the office door.

"Dr. Coltrane, this is Special Agent Scott Lynwood with the Federal Bureau of Investigation. I am conducting a preliminary investigation into allegations presented to the Bureau involving the Bay Area Medical Society. You are the current president, is that correct?" Lynwood was serious, but cordial.

"Yes, I am. What is this regarding?" Coltrane asked, his stomach sinking.

"Would it be possible to meet with you today? I have some questions to ask you, and this should not be done over the phone."

"I have patients all day, but I could meet you in my office at four thirty."

"Thank you. I'll be there."

Coltrane went back to his patients, but the conversation and the prospect of interrogation by the FBI put him on edge. His tolerance was much less than usual, and it showed. His last patient of the day was an unemployed student. The man had cut his foot by kicking in a plate glass pharmacy window during a robbery months ago. His wounds had healed long ago, but he was visiting the office to obtain a narcotic prescription and a certification of disability. Coltrane patiently explained that he could not prescribe any more painkillers and then inquired as to the nature of his disability.

"I can't work anymore, and the Social Security office needs a disabled form filled out."

"What was your job before the accident?" Coltrane asked.

"I didn't have no job."

"How do you know you are disabled if you have never had a job?" Coltrane quietly demanded.

"My foot hurts all the time, and it don't work right."

Coltrane bent down, and removed the man's plastic shoe. His foot was filthy, the sole black and the nails long and broken. He performed a thorough exam and noted in the medical record that all sensory, motor and vascular functions were perfectly normal. His resentment built as he documented accurately the physical findings. He recalled the night that the dirtball had come into the ER, drunk and refusing to cooperate with the nurses. The arresting officer wanted to take him to the county lock-up, but the suspect, who had been caught in the pharmacy red-handed and bloody-footed, knew how to play the game. He had feigned complete paralysis and thereby insured his admittance to the hospital. It had taken Coltrane and two consultants four days to evaluate all his phony symptoms before they could punt him to jail.

"I don't find anything seriously wrong with your foot, Mr. Jensen. I will, however, refer you for a disability evaluation if you like."

"I need this form signed by you for disability, man. You know my case. I got no money for rent, and payments." He stood up menacingly, and pushed the grimy crumpled form toward Coltrane.

"I can't sign that, I would be falsifying records and lose my license," Coltrane reasoned with the man, and opened the door to guide him out of the office. "Cindy will give you the name of the disability examiner. He can help you better."

"I am telling you that my foot don't work, man. You calling me a liar? Fuck you," Jensen shoved past Coltrane, screaming in his face. He charged out the door, brushing by a tall man in a dark suit who entered the waiting room as he stormed out.

Coltrane went to the staff bathroom, and washed the spittle from his face. The man's foul stench, and beer breath clung in his nostrils. He had come perilously close to reacting to his abuser. He fantasized in slow motion of forearm slamming the scumbag into the metal door frame as he passed by, cursing. He washed his face, breathed deeply and returned to his private office.

He sat and gazed out the window at the tranquil blue waters of the Gulf of Mexico. Sunlight danced on the waves, sending brilliant sparkles of white light off the surface. In the distance, a white sloop sailed smoothly away on a beam reach. He daydreamed about his upcoming trip to the islands with Britt. It couldn't be too soon. The intercom jolted him back to his reality.

"Dr. Coltrane, Mr. Lynwood is here to see you." Cindy announced.

"Send him back, please." Coltrane rose.

The man entered Coltrane's private office as if he owned it. He wore a tailored dark gray suit, and carried a well used briefcase. He introduced himself and sat down opposite Coltrane. In contrast to his stylish suit, he wore short blue socks and scuffed wingtip oxfords.

"Dr. Coltrane, as you know, the FBI is the domestic criminal investigative arm of the federal government. Along with many other duties, we handle enforcement of anti-trust legislation. I have been asked by the Miami office to personally look into this case because I am an attorney with anti-trust expertise. This is only a preliminary interview, but you should know that anything we discuss now will be considered as evidence, and can be used in court against you. Is that clear?"

"Very. What is this all about?" Coltrane asked tentatively.

"Formal complaints have been filed with the Federal District Attorney alleging anti-trust violations on the part of the Bay Area Medical Society." Lynwood paused to gauge Coltrane's reaction. When Coltrane sat impassively, he continued. "The attorneys for three separate insurance plans have all filed actions, stating that the medical society plans to stage a week long strike in an effort to renegotiate existing physician contracts with the plans. Is there any truth to this?"

"No," Coltrane was stunned. The idea for the conference was just five days old, and the letters to the HMO plans could only have gone out two days ago. They had reacted with lightning speed. How could they have gotten a guy up from Miami so fast, he thought. Coltrane realized that he had a whirlwind by the tail.

"Why would the insurance plans think this?"

"I have no idea. The accusation is ridiculous."

"Tell me about the conference," Lynwood pursued.

"We are having a strategic planning conference next week. Nothing unusual. Continuing medical education."

"The HMO plans claim that the entire physician population will be at this conference, and it is tantamount to a city-wide strike by the doctors. They claim that this action will severely affect healthcare in the Bay area and that the tactic is being used illegally to bring them to the bargaining table. How do you respond?"

"First and foremost, patient care will not be compromised in the least. Call coverage by specialty has been personally arranged by myself, and discussed with all the area ER facilities. Secondly, physician conferences and continuing medical education is routine, commonplace. In fact, it is mandated by Florida law to maintain licensure. The AMA holds meetings every year that are attended by thousands, maybe tens of thousands of doctors. Do you investigate those meetings?"

"Hey, doctor, don't take your anger out on me. I saw your last patient, he almost knocked me down too. I am just trying to get to the heart of this matter," Lynwood held his hands up in mock surrender. In doing so, his coat opened, revealing his holstered Sig-Sauer 9mm.

"Sorry. It was a long day." The sight of the gun sobered Coltrane, and brought back the gravity of the situation.

"They claim that you have presented them with a list of demands. They refused to follow your recommendations, and therefore you called this special session," Lynwood again paused.

"An aspect of the society's function is to interface on behalf of the physicians and their patients with other healthcare entities. We are very concerned with the trends in modern medicine, and this meeting will address these problems. But I fail to see how any medical meeting can be described as a strike."

"This is a very gray area in federal law, and the law is constantly evolving with time. There is no precedent to this case, and I will go on the assumption that federal law is not being violated as of now. The FBI will continue to monitor the situation, however. I would advise you, however, to seek legal counsel in regards to this matter. The costs of a federal lawsuit are crippling, and even if you win, you may regret it." Lynwood rose, shook hands with Coltrane and left the office suite.

Coltrane let the office staff go home, and locked up the doors. He sat in his private office, and stared out at the Gulf, as the sun descended into the blue waters. He felt as if he were on a thundering train, accelerating downward, downward. Hellbound. Everything was happening so fast, he thought. The insurance plans obviously had tremendous and far reaching power. Perhaps he had bit off more than he could chew. Don Quixote jousting with windmills, he visualized himself. He decided then to minimize his personal exposure. He gathered his briefcase and computer, and turned out the lights and headed for home.

Entering the underground parking lot, Coltrane looked right and left cautiously. The lot was nearly empty, and quiet. The combination of increasing rates of urban violence and too much television had made him very watchful of his surroundings. His senses were sharpened by years of bow-hunting, quietly stalking deer and wild hogs in the brush of Florida and Texas. He wondered if the FBI would place him under surveillance. He wondered if the men after Hendricks' disc were still in the city, or if they ever existed at all.

Coltrane drove home, pondering the situation in which he found himself entangled. He had to assume that the FBI would tap his home, office and car phones. Perhaps even bug his home and office as well. Up to this point, he had only discussed the truth of the strategy with Britt, and she could not be forced to testify against her husband. Their discussion had occurred before the complaint to the FBI, so there was no chance that any electronic eavesdropping could have occurred. Therefore, he reasoned, he was safe up to this moment in time. No conspiracy or intent to violate anti-trust laws could be proven. He had to keep very clean from here on.

Britt was at home when he arrived, and surprised at her husband's early arrival.

She was further surprised when he motioned her to be silent, placing his index finger over his lips. He continued making small talk about his day, and led her into the library.

There he pulled out a sheet of paper, and wrote her a message:

> THE HOUSE AND PHONES MAY BE
> BUGGED- FBI DO NOT TALK ABOUT THE
> SOCIETY CONFERENCE!!!

She read the notes and nodded, her eyes wide.

"It has been a long day, let's go out for dinner." Coltrane took the note and fed it into the diamond shredder by his desk.

"Wonderful. I'll get my purse, and we are on the way." Britt grabbed her bag and they went out to the driveway, and jumped into the Expedition.

They spoke very little on the way to the restaurant. Coltrane chose one of their favorite places, a small northern Italian trattoria that had intimate, candlelit booths. Coltrane guided his wife to a booth in the corner, facing the front doors. Anyone following them, or attempting to eavesdrop on their conversation would have great difficulty. Coltrane contemplated his options and the consequences of each different path. He concluded that the foundation had been laid for a successful conference, and that his physical presence at the conference was not absolutely essential. Susan Kerr could continue pressuring the membership to maximize attendance, and he could appoint his vice-president to run the actual proceedings. All the better, because the vice-president was completely innocent of any anti-trust conspiracy. Coltrane and Britt could take the sailing trip to the islands that they had planned for next month a little early. He desperately needed to get away.

The waiter introduced himself, produced a menu for them and a winelist for Dr. Coltrane. He left. Coltrane got up, and moved over to his wife's side of the booth, slipping in next to her and putting his arm around her shoulders. He nuzzled her and pretended to be whispering intimate suggestions while she smiled amorously. He told her the story of the day's meeting with Lynwood, and his conclusion that he was safe up to this moment in time. He also told her that they should expect that they might be placed under surveillance. He asked if she had discussed their conversation with anyone, her sister, her mother, anyone. She hadn't. He leaned back against the upholstered booth and exhaled, temporarily relieved.

The waiter came and Coltrane ordered a bottle of Chianti Classico, and they made their dinner selections. The wine came, and Coltrane filled their glasses. They touched glasses and sipped the Chianti slowly, each deep in thought. Then Coltrane bent over and whispered in her ear for a long while as she nodded slowly in assent. They finished their wine, and enjoyed a long, sumptuous meal.

Chapter 37

June 21

Coltrane was at his office at 5:15 AM, early even for him. He completed all the paperwork on his desk, and when Cindy arrived at 7:30, told her that he had been asked to deliver a scientific paper at an upcoming medical meeting. He would be in New York for a week or two. Coltrane regretted having to lie to his close and valued assistant, but it was best not to involve her. She was to tell anyone who inquired that he was attending an out of town surgical meeting. Then he asked her to shuffle his schedule, and to call all the hospitals and have his unfinished medical records pulled for his completion.

Coltrane went back to his office, and turned on his notebook computer, connecting the computer's input jack to his phone line. He reached into his briefcase and found the AOL computer disc. AOL was an Internet access service and vast computer information source that provided online resources such as sports information, news, financial reports and stock market prices. It also allowed computer users to communicate in real time from anywhere in the world. A free starter disc was provided with every new computer sold. Coltrane inserted his disc, and with the help of the simple onscreen instructions, installed the communications program and input his personal E-mail address. The entire process took less than five minutes.

Coltrane then called Susan, and arranged to meet her at the society office in two hours. He asked her to subscribe to the same online network, AOL. Finally, he called his favorite marine outfitter. He needed information about the latest marine communications equipment.

Coltrane drove down towards the marina, again feeling the allure of the sparkling blue water of the Gulf. He was a relative newcomer to boating, having been raised in the landlocked Midwest. He had always been intimidated by the mysteries of the oceans, and the blue-blood aura of sailing. A friend during his residency had introduced him to sailing on a small sloop in San Diego Bay, and he had been exhilarated by the experience. The wind, the sun, the water and the sensual feeling of speed and power as the sleek craft had slipped silently, rhythmically through the waves had intoxicated him. Over the years, he gradually had increased the range of his experience and ability to sail and navigate. He loved the annual bareboat charter that he and Britt planned to the Caribbean, in search of the perfect, desolate white sand beach.

He turned into the marina, with its sparkling water and lines of white hulled boats at rest in the slips. The marina store was on the main dock, stocked to the ceiling with gleaming brass and stainless steel fixtures. Coltrane felt like a kid in a candy store there, and rarely left empty-handed. Today he had a specific device in mind. He went straight to the back of the store to talk to the manager, Red Houghton. Red had spent twenty-five years in the US Navy prior to retiring to Tampa, and Coltrane figured he knew more about seamanship than anyone in the Yacht Club. He found Houghton at his desk, shuffling through piles of invoices.

"Cap'n Red, how are you, got a second?" Coltrane asked, sitting down in an empty chair in the cramped, smoky office.

"Sure, Doc. What can I do for you?"

"I am going sailing, bareboat in the Caribbean, and need a means of communicating with the States. Last trip in the Virgin Islands, I ran into a couple who had a PC in their boat, and they were downloading stock market quotes and managing their portfolio from the deck of their boat. How were they doing that, that far offshore?"

"They were getting realtime stock market quotes on their PC? Was it through a news service or CNN?"

"No, it was realtime, interactive. He would request a price for, say, Intel, and in a split-second it would flash on the screen.

"Then he was linked to a broker or a brokerage service via a phone or data link." Houghton answered immediately.

"By radiophone?" Coltrane asked, knowing the answer.

"No, radiophones will not transmit data, just voice transmissions. He had to be using a cellular phone. Or a satellite phone. Where were you?"

"Virgin Gorda."

"Could be a cellular phone, it depends on the power of the particular phone, the distance to the nearest cell tower and the location where it is being used. Here in Tampa, you can use a cell phone in the Gulf, for about five miles offshore, ten miles max. But even that will vary with weather and atmospheric conditions. Where will you be using the phone?"

"Bahamas."

"Where in the Bahamas? It's a big place."

"Nassau, all over."

"Do you want this link to be functional throughout your entire cruise?"

"Absolutely."

"No cellular phone will have the power to transmit that far, that consistently. You will need a satellite phone. I can show you the Motorola Iridium unit we have here."

Coltrane followed him out onto the floor of the store, past the aisles of multi-colored rope, lines and hawsers, past the fishing tackle and marine fittings and charts and books. They ended at the glass display case showcasing the pride of the shop, the state of the art electronic and optical gear that could mean the difference between life and death to a sailor in treacherous seas. Coltrane gazed lovingly at the night vision binoculars, GPS units and radar and marine communications equipment in the glass display cases.

Houghton reached up on the shelves and pulled down a compact Halliburton aluminum case. He opened the case, and spun it around on the glass to show Coltrane. The case was compartmentalized and foam padded. There was a silver gray Iridium handset, virtually indistinguishable from Coltrane's digital cellphone. Connected to the handset by a cord was a gray transceiver about half the size of a phone book, and a smaller antennae unit. The transceiver had input jacks that would receive the cable from his notebook computer and the phonejack input from his fax-modem. As he looked at it, he realized that the entire unit was only slightly larger than his carphone.

"This will work ten miles offshore?" Coltrane asked in disbelief.

"This will work anywhere on the globe. If you want a 100% reliable communications system for voice, fax and low speed data, I would recommend the KVH unit. That's what all the big yachts, freighters and tankers, commercial oceangoing vessels use. But that's a permanent, hardwired system. Not portable. You want something you can take on and off a charter boat, not a permanent installation, right?"

"Right. We charter once, twice a year, and want something we can use on the boat, then take home with us. Will this work anywhere in the world?"

"Everywhere, including the oceans and both polar regions. This is all military technology, recently released for worldwide consumer use. It is very similar to the GPS technology. By the way, how did that GPS unit work for you?"

"Beautifully, thanks. It is very accurate, maybe pinpoint. We were never more than two or three meters off course."

"The Department of Defense has GPS units accurate to within inches, but that technology is unavailable to consumers. The satphone technology is, however. You'll love it, Doc."

"I can take it anywhere I want, and it will work?" Coltrane was incredulous.

"Yeah, but it's not that simple. Satphones use a constellation of sixty-six Low Earth Orbiting Satellites, set in place by Iridium years ago. The company didn't do well, and I am not sure who is running it now. But Boeing operates the satellites, and Motorola makes the phones. A satellite phone works by uplinking to a geostationary satellite. Then the message is passed on to other satellites, and then down to the ground. Your phone has to be programmed for the area that it is intended to be used, so it will hit that overhead satellite. You couldn't then take the phone to Europe, and have it still work. It has to be programmed for the satellite that is orbiting directly overhead. But they work great, and you can send fax and data transmissions just by plugging into the port in the transceiver here." Houghton lifted the unit and showed Coltrane the ports on the side, similar to the computer input and output ports he was so familiar with.

"How much is this?" Coltrane asked, and prepared for the answer.

"$1500. But you'd be crazy to buy one. Just rent one. The phone company salesman is always on my ass to rent these units. Apparently they are big in Miami. Probably the drug dealers like them because they can't be traced." Houghton smiled.

"Can they be tapped?" Coltrane was surprised at the newfound implication.

"This Motorola 9505 unit is digital, very secure. In fact, the NSA cleared it for top-secret transmissions. I suppose it could be tapped, but it would be extremely difficult to do. But their location can't be traced like a cell phone can. When they want to, the DEA can pinpoint the origin of a cellular phone call to within a twenty foot radius."

"You mean that no one, not even the feds, can locate you through the satellite signal?" Coltrane inquired.

"Absolutely not."

"Too bad. That ability might be useful in the event of an emergency, or a distress call."

"You can interface your GPS with the phone, and that will send out your precise location with the phone calls. I would recommend that highly." Houghton turned the unit to show Coltrane the small input port.

"Amazing." Coltrane looked at the weather-beaten sailor, and smiled in wonder at the piece of sophisticated electronics.

"You want one?"

"How much?"

"About $450 a week plus airtime. Maybe I can get the salesman to give you a special price. He will be peeing himself when he hears I got him a rental. Do you want internet access? High speed data?" Houghton opened a reference manual, and programmed the unit for the Bahamas region.

"Yep."

"Ok, you'll need some accessories." Red turned and pulled two boxes out of the display case. "A RS232 data adapter and a fixed mast marine omni-directional antenna. The standard land antenna has to be perfectly vertical to function. Try keeping anything vertical on a pitching and rolling sloop." He fitted the unit and accessories into the aluminum case and passed it to Coltrane.

"I'm gonna be vertical as often as possible," Coltrane grinned.

"Then why bring this damn thing?" Red laughed.

"Good question." Coltrane hefted the Halliburton case. "Thanks, Red. I appreciate it." Coltrane shook his dry, leathery hand, and turned to leave.

"My pleasure, Doc. Hey, if you can, bring me back some more of that habanero pepper sauce you got last time. That shit was great."

"Yeah, it was, wasn't it? I spent two weeks trying to reverse engineer that recipe, with no luck. I'll try to get a case this time. Thanks again." Coltrane left.

Driving back towards town, Coltrane passed Doctor's Hospital. Remembering that he had medical records to complete there prior to his trip, he swung into the parking lot. He parked by the ER and ran into the hospital by the physicians' entrance. Coltrane never saw the swarthy man in the sedan watching him with interest. One hundred meters away, the Cuban noted the man's stride and wrote down his license plate number. Next to it he wrote "White Expedition". His list now numbered twenty-two prospects, and he was no closer to his quarry than when he began. He cursed and settled back in the car seat. He picked up his cellular phone, and dialed a Miami number. He left a coded message on the answering machine to contact him on a previously arranged payphone that afternoon. Maybe his client could help him find the doctor.

Chapter 38

Coltrane was late arriving at the medical society office, a small building in a run down section of town. The parking lot was gravel, and filled with the cars of the office personnel. He parked, gathered his papers and notebook computer, and went in.

Coltrane and Susan Kerr went into her office, and reviewed the arrangements for the upcoming conference. All was in readiness, and the hotel conference site prepared. The meeting was scheduled to begin the coming Monday, with the entire membership in attendance for that session. Afterwards, the conference would be split into working sessions, the schedule becoming complicated. The number of physicians registered for the program was high, but not as high as Coltrane would have liked. Coltrane asked for a list of the registered doctors, and Susan responded that it was already posted in *Caduceus*. Coltrane turned his computer on and went onto the website. He immediately was greeted on the introduction page with a full list of the physicians involved in the conference. And a second list of all those who were not attending. He turned to Susan and smiled.

"Good idea. Nothing like peer pressure for motivation. Did you get signed onto AOL?" Coltrane opened the AOL application in his computer as he asked.

"I just finished. It was very simple to setup, but I have no idea how to use any of the services."

"I'll show you. I want to set up a secure E-mail and communication system in *Caduceus*, but that will take time. For now we will use the AOL applications for communication and E-mail. One thing to remember always: *assume that anyone can read your E-mail on AOL.* Never put anything sensitive in your E-mails. Never put anything you don't want the world to know."

Susan nodded in assent, obviously concerned.

"Turn on your notebook and plug your modem into your phone." Coltrane helped her set up the modem, and went into another office to hook his notebook computer into a different phone line. Then he returned and taught Susan how to enter the E-mail center at AOL.

"There are many ways to do this, but I will show you the simplest. If you want to send me a message, all you have to do is open your address file, find my name and double-click on it. You will then automatically get a blank screen to write on, and when the message is complete, simply click SEND and it will go electronically straight to me. Amazing, huh?"

Coltrane went through it step by step. He input his name and AOL identification code in her address file, and copied her identification code for his use. He told her to keep copies of his code written elsewhere in the event her computer crashed. Coltrane went into the nearby office, and sent Susan several questions via the E-mail. She responded with answers to the questions, and easily mastered the technique.

"There is one more way of communicating with AOL that I want you to use. The E-mail is similar to a letter, you send it and I may read it hours or days later. If we want to talk in realtime, we can use the Instant Message application. I find you using the address book, join you on an IM private screen, and we can type messages to each other on a split screen." Coltrane went into the application and opened it for Susan.

"Why do this rather than a phone call?" Susan asked the obvious question.

"Several reasons. For one, if I am out of town, we can talk like this essentially free, there are no long distance phone charges because AOL uses a local trunk line. Also, we can send data from your computer to mine and back through this system, as well as faxing letters. It has limited but specific uses." Coltrane did not tell her the real reason he found it so attractive.

"Wait a minute. Don't tell me you have plans to go out of town. Not now."

"I have a meeting that I may have to attend in New York next week. This conference has been on my schedule long before I was elected President, and I'm obligated to attend. I'd cancel, but I have to present a paper at the scientific session. If I go, I'll be back as soon as possible." Coltrane lied, knowing that it was best.

"You'll miss the meeting. How am I going to run a meeting of six hundred doctors all by myself?" Susan cried, on the verge of tears.

"Look, you know only one in five guys will show up, and half of them will leave after twenty minutes, You'll do great, and the meeting will be run by the specialty committees regardless. No problem. It will be much better if I am not here anyway, no one for the media to shit on. They like you." Coltrane smiled at her, calming her. "I will be in contact with you every day, and you can Instant Message me all day long if you want. The meeting will run itself, I promise you."

"There are too many details to leave unanswered like that. I can't answer all the media's questions. They'll demand a physician spokesperson." Susan was obviously very uncomfortable at the sudden and unexpected responsibility placed upon her by Coltrane's absence.

"Susan, listen. Let them demand whatever they want. Smile and ignore them." Coltrane wrestled with whether to tell her the whole truth, then decided that to do so could be an injustice to her. If he ended up named in a federal indictment, he did not want her involved. "The less media exposure the conference gets, the better. If I'm not available, then the interviews will have to wait until I get back. All you have to do is keep them out of the hotel conference area, and delay them until I return. You will do just fine."

"Don't leave me high and dry like this. I need to have a physician to refer the media to. I can't even begin to answer all the questions that are going to arise." Susan was getting upset.

"Listen, the last thing I want is to have some doctor taking over *your* position, and making himself the society's media liaison. All physicians have healthy egos. If we didn't, we could never make the critical decisions we make, day in and day out. The problem with us is that we often deceive ourselves into the delusion that we have powers and skills outside the field of medicine. Why do you think that doctors have the highest private pilot fatality rate? We are so arrogant, we believe we can overpower nature. And there are quite a few of the membership that can't seem to get enough attention. Especially Pennington."

"The psychiatrist?"

"Yep. He's an idiot. The worst kind of idiot. An idiot who doesn't realize that he is an idiot, and thinks he's a genius. There are a few of them in the society, for sure. They will have to be muzzled."

"How? I won't feel comfortable shutting them up. You're going to have to do that."

"Fine. We will do it in a way that all members get the message. Do we have an opening message on *Caduceus*?"

"Yes. Right now it's a request for the assessment, and a list of those who haven't paid their share as yet."

"Good. Keep that on, but add the following message." Coltrane wrote a short paragraph for the membership, and handed it to Susan. It simply stated that no member shall communicate with the media in any form, and in the event that physicians were quoted, a public announcement refuting any such statement, and severing any association with that physician would be made and circulated.

"What are you trying to do, humiliate our members?"

"No, just keep them quiet. All our talking has to be done professionally, and it has to be coherent and consistent. That reminds me. I should have one more, in-depth meeting with Elizabeth Volk before I disappear. Can you arrange that? At my office?"

"I will try."

"Good. Are the position papers ready?"

"The ones you gave me are on *Caduceus*. The papers from the heads of the specialty committees are not all in yet."

"Okay. What I want you to do today is contact *every* chairperson, and get a paper from each one. I don't care if it takes all day, I want to see all our papers, and have them finalized before I leave. And that will be *all* we give to the press, to the public, and to anyone else who is interested. A well worded, consistent and thoughtful presentation of our concerns. It will certainly simplify your life." Coltrane started to gather his equipment and moved toward the door before she could continue her remonstrations. She watched him leave, cursed softly to herself, and got back to work.

Coltrane had several things to do before he could consider leaving the country. He drove to the County Hospital, parked and went into the gray imposing building through the physicians' entrance. He had only three inpatients, and all three were in the County Hospital. He had inherited their care while he was on his weekly rotation for the ER, and they were almost ready for discharge. The first was a teenager who had broken his arm rollerblading and was very happy to be sent home. Coltrane discussed his follow-up care with his attentive mother, and discharged them to be seen in the office.

His second patient was an unemployed bouncer who had injured his heavily tattooed fist in an assault. He had smashed someone in the mouth, suffering fractures of the ring and little fingers with an open, infected wound. He had thus far refused surgery, despite the risk of long term disability. Coltrane had an instinctive distrust of the man, feeling that something was irregular about his behavior. Coltrane was surprised to find that the patient had left the hospital that morning because the nurses would not let him smoke in his room. He cursed, and called the social worker to begin the long process of tracking him down and arranging for his appropriate care. She took the information over the phone, and told him that she would get a letter out today. Coltrane thanked her, wrote a long note in the chart describing the incident and left to find his last patient in the surgical intensive care unit.

His third patient was a young girl involved in a motorcycle accident with her boyfriend. They had been brought into the County ER together, but the boy had died hours later from massive injuries. The girl had once been a beautiful child, her fresh youthful skin now swollen by the bruising and fluids. She was in a coma that the neurosurgeon felt would last for weeks. She had suffered multiple hand fractures that Coltrane had pinned several days ago. Coltrane checked the bandages as the family looked on, and saw that the wounds were clean and dry.

"Which doctor are you?" asked a woman in the room, as she turned a tear-stained face up to him.

"The hand surgeon, Mrs. Gardner. Your daughter is doing well from my standpoint, and I will be seeing her in my office when she leaves the hospital. I understand that she may be here for a while as she wakes up." Coltrane tried to comfort the woman, and gave her his card. He stayed for a moment, then left the family in their grief.

Coltrane went to the medical records department and finished all his current records, signing orders, and checking diagnosis codes for the charts. He knew that if he was delinquent in his records, he would return from vacation in two weeks to discover that he was suspended from medical staff. He had done the other hospitals earlier in the week. He signed the last chart, piled them on the desk, and headed out the door to the parking lot. His digital cellphone chirped, and displayed a message that Ms. Volk would meet him at his office in an hour.

As he drove to the office, he sadly reflected on the tragedy that had befallen the young girl. An irrevocable mistake, a tremendous tragedy, all in the flash of an instant. Coltrane thought of the lost possibilities and dreams that were the result of that motorcycle crash. It was this kind of tragic waste that kept him from buying the black Harley-Davidson Fatboy he had always lusted after.

Chapter 39

June 22

Elizabeth Volk was waiting in the reception area when Coltrane returned to his office. He led her down the hall, and into his private office. She seated herself, and waited patiently as he opened his briefcase and arranged a stack of documents before him on the huge desk.

"Ms. Volk, thank you for coming on such short notice. I will be leaving town in the next few days, and want to fully brief you on some of the events that will transpire during my absence." Coltrane started to explain.

"Shouldn't we wait for Barbara Farrell?" Elizabeth interrupted.

"She was not invited." Coltrane answered bluntly.

"May I ask why not?" Ms. Volk persisted.

"I view the local news as purely entertainment, with no educational value whatsoever. They will not devote the necessary time to presenting the issues in any meaningful form, and will only cheapen and sensationalize whatever is presented to maximize shock value. Let them concentrate on car accidents and murders."

"You are losing a great deal of exposure by shunning the television audience." Elizabeth warned.

"I prefer to present the issues to a jury of literate citizens. A newspaper can devote pages to these issues. Hopefully, you will get a section in the Sunday paper devoted to healthcare issues. But even in that form, too much will be lost and condensed. The newspaper is the only forum for thoughtful discourse of weighty matters."

"I am sure the paper would like everyone to have that opinion."

"Listen, if it was up to me, reading a daily newspaper would be a prerequisite for voting."

"I don't know about the constitutionality of that idea, but let's get back on record about the Society's agenda, please."

"Right. I have prepared a series of position papers for you, and Susan Kerr will be getting several more to you in the very near future. The purpose of the papers is to present, in layman's terms, the concerns of the society, and our vision of how to improve the current state of healthcare delivery in the Tampa-St. Pete area. Each paper outlines the problem, gives a short history of how the situation developed, and our solutions. Often, there are a number of options, and it will be up to all of us to determine the direction we travel as a city."

"Are these papers your personal agenda, or the agenda of the society?"

"All the papers are consensus opinions, not mine. I am really just a figurehead. My opinion has no greater weight or value than any other society member's. Later Susan will be getting you the papers from each specialty committee. Those papers will present the views of the individual specialties."

"Do you give me permission to republish these papers if I wish to?"

"Absolutely. I only ask that they be presented in complete form, no editing or abridging."

"If they are brief, that's not a problem."

"Frankly, one thing I am concerned about is that, during my absence, individual physicians will be tempted to voice their own unique ideologies, on behalf of the society. Hence the position papers."

"If you could put the goals of the Medical Society in one sentence, what would you say?"

"Our primary goal is to take medical decisions out of the hands of insurance plans, bureaucrats and attorneys and put control back into the hands of physicians."

"What about the patients? Where do their rights fit in your picture?"

"Ahhhhh, yes. The Patient's Bill of Rights. I agree with the concept. But I think many patients don't fulfill the responsibilities. Maybe I should draft a Patient's Bill of Responsibilities."

"Are you serious?" Elizabeth was puzzled by the turn of thought.

"Half-serious. Let me be the devil's advocate for a moment. What percentage of Emergency Room visits are true emergencies? Take a guess."

"Seventy-five or eighty." Elizabeth answered after some thought.

"Not even close. Ten to fifteen percent, depending upon the criteria that is used. Fifteen percent at the most. The rest are colds, flu, nausea, vomiting, diarrhea, stomach pains, grandpa is disoriented, boils, falls, aches and muscle pains, sprains, headaches and so on. And every time a case of meningitis in Orlando makes the evening news, our ERs get packed with people who have headaches and self-diagnosis of an exploding brain. Add the many minor injuries of drunks and drug abusers to the equation, and there is a huge cost to the system, and a huge waste of manpower and resources."

"Unbelievable. Why is that?" Elizabeth was skeptical.

"Many reasons, I suppose. Maybe they don't want to take a day off work to go to their family doctor. For many patients, the services are free, or require only a minimal co-payment. ERs, by law, cannot turn anyone away."

"You would deny a patient's right to healthcare?" Elizabeth was now incredulous.

"Yes. But let me clarify what I mean by that. I have never refused to treat a patient on the basis of their ability to pay. And I have never seen a true instance of that occurring by any other physician in my lifetime. I have no qualms refusing to treat difficult, or troublesome patients. But I have never refused to treat non-paying patients. And nine times out of ten, I know when I am not going to be paid. Or paid very little, like Medicaid which pays about one tenth of standard fees. But I take issue with the common assumption that every American has a right to healthcare. I imagine that sometime, somewhere, some politician told people that healthcare is a right. Absolutely false. Where in the Constitution does it say that?"

"I don't know. Are you saying that only the wealthy should be given treatment?"

"No. I am saying there is no *right to healthcare*. There exists a right to *access to healthcare*. No one can be denied the medical attention on a basis of color, race, religion, existing medical condition, AIDS, HIV, or hepatitis, or whatever. That is the distinction that I am trying to make here."

"Back to my question. Who will take care of the poor, the sick, the elderly, or children who can't fend for themselves?"

"That is an entirely different question, and we will get to my ideas on that later. But my point is that there is no *right* to healthcare. That, by definition and practice, confers a *right* to the *labor* of another human being. No one has the right to the uncompensated labor or services of the hospital or clinic involved, the secretary that processes the patient, the nurses and technicians that care for the patient, and the physician that delivers the definitive care to the patient. It's not just. It is a form of slavery, or indentured servitude. Unique to healthcare. What other profession is forced to provide free service? Did you know that lawyers went to the Supreme Court in 1989 to obtain a ruling that they may *not* be forced to provide free service to the indigent? Despite the fact that there are many references to legal rights in the Constitution?"

"Interesting. Physicians as slaves. That will be a hard sell to my readers." Elizabeth smiled.

"Of course. I know. And the public will not have any great sympathy for us; they are sure that we all have good lives, and are overpaid. The same guy that will defend some illiterate baseball player's right to make 200 million dollars will expect me to give him a complete physical exam for his five dollar co-pay. And then bitch that he has to pay anything at all. I'm not expecting a great deal of sympathy from the public, simply because they don't know all the facts. No one knows that I performed two hundred thousand dollars of free surgery last year. Or that every single physician in this country writes off huge amounts of free services each year. American physicians performed over 25 *billion* dollars of charity care last year. I don't know of any other profession that does that kind of community service. Understand that the hospitals are businesses, and always make a profit. And the nurses and other personnel are salaried. Physicians are bearing the burden alone. And unlike a retail business, which can claim their losses as tax deductions, physicians just have to eat it."

"I think that the public expects that their doctors do a certain amount of charity work. Isn't that in the Hippocratic Oath?"

"There are many different versions of the Hippocratic Oath, but as far as I know, nothing is mentioned about money or payment. It does specify that only men shall be taught the healing arts, so perhaps the Oath is outdated for our modern use." Coltrane smiled at his female interviewer.

"I would think so."

"Please don't misunderstand me. There is no greater satisfaction for me than to help someone, especially if they cannot help themselves. Traditionally, the medical community has borne the costs of indigent care without complaint or expectation of recognition. But the situation has changed dramatically in the past decade. Our costs have become suffocating, and our reimbursement has been decreasing at the same time. We can't continue. Something has to change, something has to give."

"What do you see happening?"

"What is happening, and has happened, is that the older physicians are leaving the profession in droves. While twenty years ago, we were practicing into our sixties and seventies. Now these seasoned and extremely wise clinicians are retiring. The stress is too much, the aggravation is too high."

"Shouldn't those older guys be put out to graze, anyway?" Elizabeth couldn't see an eighty year old surgeon operating on her.

"Certainly there comes a time to retire. But medicine is a cerebral pursuit, and experience bestows wisdom. The clinician who has seen five hundred cases of gallbladder disease will always be better at diagnosing an unusual presentation than someone who has seen fifty cases. These physicians, in the prime productive years of their lives, are leaving practice. We will never get their skills back. Everyone suffers."

"All I have heard thus far is complaints. What are your solutions? What can the society do to improve the situation?"

"That is why I prepared the position papers. If you take the time to read through all of them, you will get a very good feel for the consensus view of the society. But remember, these are just starting points, and very preliminary. This is a crisis of immense proportion. It will take years of gradual change to overcome all the obstacles. And require some very hard choices by the American public."

"What kind of choices do you mean?"

"Now we are getting into philosophical issues, and I can only give my opinion, not the position of the society."

"Fine. I'll listen to your opinions. That's why I am here."

"Then we will have to go off the record. Would you turn off the recorder, please?" Coltrane looked at the tiny digital recorder she had on her lap.

"You don't want these comments reported?" Elizabeth smiled knowingly.

"No. I will give you my thoughts because I want you to know the whole picture, and see my viewpoint. But please don't attribute these radical ideas to me. I'll deny it."

"Fine." She turned the recorder off.

"What are the hard choices?"

"First, Americans have to accept responsibility for their own health. I hear these talking heads whining about *empowerment* of personal healthcare. If I hear one more imbecile whining about empowerment of their healthcare, I'm going to choke them. Forget that. Patients don't make healthcare decisions, physicians do. When you get on an airplane, do you tell the pilots how to fly the thing? Do you question them about the flight plan, or the weather, or the maintenance schedule on the jet engines? No. You trust that they are professionals, and you either take a seat, or go get a bus ticket. Same with healthcare. Patients make choices. What people need to do is become empowered by assuming the responsibility for their *own health.* Americans are still smoking cigarettes at an alarming rate. Alcohol abuse is at an all time high. Americans are now over sixty percent obese. Obese people take a hugely inordinate proportion of the healthcare dollar. Diabetes. Heart disease. Stroke. Arthritis. Americans need to exercise. But why should they exercise when there is a little pill to replace their pancreas. Or a little pill to give them an erection?"

"On that topic, what is the stand of the medical community with regard to prescription drug coverage?"

"Excellent question. Ever wonder why the evening news on all four major networks runs ad after ad for *Nexium?* Or *Ambien?* Or *Lipitor?* Or *DitropanXL?* Or *Viagra?* No one in the television audience can go and buy them; they are all prescription drugs. For very specific medical conditions. But these are multimillion dollar ad campaigns aimed at getting patients to diagnose themselves, and then go and ask their internist to give them the *perfect pink pill,* or whatever else is the top seller for that company. Ever wonder why?"

"Now that you mention it,..."

"Just another example of more bureaucratic interference from the government, effectively blocking marketing of pharmaceuticals to physicians. Too much red tape, too much interference with the drug companies' research and development. Too much politicization of the FDA. That having been said, not everyone needs the most expensive drug available."

"You would restrict the sale of pharmaceuticals?"

"No, but if walking a mile every night is better than a pill, and free, then everyone should be out there walking. And if you smoke, be prepared for the health problems that will inevitable result. And I want the federal government to tax cigarettes five dollars a pack to pay the health bills. You and I shouldn't have to carry that burden. Look, I'm just like everyone else. I would love to sit in front of the television and eat Whoppers and drink wine all night, every night. But I don't. If I can get off my ass and walk around the block every evening, so can others."

"People aren't going to like your plan, Doctor."

"Of course not. The American people want the best possible healthcare in the world, and they want someone else to pay for it. That's the theory behind HMOs. John Q Public doesn't want AIDS patients to have costly medications at his expense, but when he has back pain, he's going to demand a MRI to rule out the one in ten million chance of a tumor, or herniated disc. It's just human nature."

"And we all want our personal physician to be like Marcus Welby, MD. Not Dr. Jack Kevorkian," she added.

"Right. Speaking of Dr. Jack, modern medicine has the ability to keep us alive almost indefinitely. Transplants. Artificial hearts. And so on. But the cold fact is that the resources are finite. Someone has to decide whether to immunize five thousand children, or transplant one liver. Should Mickey Mantle have had a liver transplant? He was an alcoholic, and very ill. Should old men, who have smoked all their lives and now cannot get an erection, should they get Viagra? Or penile implants? I remember during my training at the Veterans Administration Hospital, I put a penile implant in a smoker who was impotent. He continued smoking. When he and his wife came for their yearly check up, I asked them how it was working for them. She said he had only used it once, but it seemed to work fine. That was the most expensive lovemaking the VA has paid for, I bet."

"The VA paid for that?"

"Sure. The VA provides everything any hospital provides. And more. But the entire system needs revamping. My personal opinion is that we must have a universal plan, funded by the federal government, and administrated by Medicare. Covering everyone, from the cradle to the grave. No more malpractice claims, and one hospital system. Look, now we have this bizarre, redundant system of hospitals and clinics and teaching institutions. Veterans Administration Hospitals. County Hospitals. University Hospitals. Cancer Hospitals. Heart Hospitals. Private Non-Profit Hospitals. Private Not-For-Profit Hospitals. And Private Hospitals. If some cosmic jester tried to design a more screwed up and confusing system, he couldn't. We have to take the VA, the county hospitals, the university hospitals, the Catholic, Baptist, Presbyterian, all the private hospitals, and make one system."

"Eliminate all thc privatc hospitals?"

"I don't know. Maybe keep them, and have private insurance plans for those who want a private room, with a color television, and gourmet food. But the primary delivery system has to be one centralized system. Australia has a good system. We can pattern ours after the Australian system. We don't have to re-invent the wheel."

"Why do you prefer the Australian system, Dr. Coltrane?"

"It's a logical, no frills system. America has the resources to provide high quality, free healthcare to every one of our citizens. The technology is spectacular. There are retinal implants that give sight to the blind. There may be breakthroughs in Parkinson's Disease within the next years that reverse all the symptoms and degeneration. Spinal cord research is promising. We can improve the quality of the lives of millions and millions of people. We can expand healthcare coverage so that it benefits all Americans. Everything is in place, everything is ready. We have to be strong and eliminate the waste, the fraud, the red tape and the bureaucracies that absorb fifty cents of the healthcare dollar."

"I'll explain the advantages of their centralized system next time we talk. I am sure you've had enough of my insanity for one evening. And I think if you read all those position papers, it will give you the background information to better appreciate our perspective. Please feel free to contact me any time via E-mail." Coltrane wrote his E-mail address on a business card, and slid it across the oaken desk to her.

Chapter 40

June 22

Britt had been frantically busy all day, preparing for the unexpectedly early trip to the Bahamas. She scheduled and picked up the plane tickets without difficulty. American Airlines flew directly to the Abacos from Miami twice weekly, and seats were available. She used a different travel agent than they usually used, and paid for the tickets in cash. Coltrane had told her to take those precautions. Britt thought it was melodramatic, but followed directions. She also picked up $1000 in traveler's checks at her bank. She had spent the rest of the day organizing the sailing gear, and reviewing the checklist they prepared for sailing trips. They had learned early that thoughtful and thorough planning was essential to safe and comfortable blue water sailing. There were no second chances on the open ocean.

All the gear was laid out on the living room floor, Britt knowing that Bill would want to pack the sea bags himself. Their scuba gear, masks and snorkels, regulators, fins and booties were lined up along with Bill's spear gun and the dive knives. They could get tanks and buoyancy vests in the islands. Sterile medical supplies, wrapped and sealed in a waterproof nylon bag, sat by the scuba gear. Laid out next to the dive gear, she arrayed the sail gear. Heavy sailing gloves, handheld VHF radios, a night vision monoscope, a Lexan 1 million candlepower Q-Beam, Coltrane's treasured pair of Steiner binoculars, brass shackles and numerous specialty tools and pieces of equipment that they have come to prize as essential. She had selected and packed all the usual decongestants, antibiotics and headache medicines they might need, along with her cosmetics. And the two newest books by Dave Barry and Jimmy Buffet for Coltrane, hoping that he would lose himself in them, and forget the stress and tension he was living with.

She had everything packed into soft-sided luggage when Coltrane returned home, walking in with an excited smile and a large silver aluminum case at his side. He was beaming as he demonstrated the satellite phone to his suspicious wife. What she understood was that the addition of two large carry-on cases for the phone and computer meant that she had to abandon one bag full of clothes. She cursed him and went back into the bedroom to select what she could leave behind.

Coltrane contemplated pursuing the argument as he followed her into the bedroom, then thought better of it. He quietly selected the cotton clothes he wanted packed and piled them on the bed. He went out into the living room and viewed with satisfaction his gear, arranged in neat rows on the carpet. He carefully packed the equipment into a heavy ballistic nylon duffel bag, arranging the heavy sturdy items around the outer edges, and packing the scuba gear in plastic cases and bundling them inside the sleeping bags. He carefully placed his speargun and shotstick in special pouches and hid them in the recesses of the sleeping bags. He took the cartridge out of the shotstick and placed it in a separate bullet wallet, then slipped it into the sleeping bag.

In a heavy-duty plastic storage container, Coltrane packed all his basic sailing gear. Sailing gloves, compass, charts, books, shock cords, brass shackles and other indispensable items were lovingly packed away, and checked off the list. Coltrane found that mountaineering fasteners and military gear was very adaptable to sailing use. Over the years, he had assembled equipment that simplified the serious task of small craft seamanship. Few feelings were worse than trying to untie an old, knotted rope in the middle of a black night with ice cold, driving rain slamming into your face.

He went to the kitchen, and pulled open the cabinet doors where the spices were. He selected a variety of spices, red pepper, Italian seasoning, curry powder, Hungarian paprika, garlic powder. He intended to enjoy some cooking in the two weeks they would be gone.

Coltrane went to his study and found his handheld GPS unit. He turned it on, and ran the instrument's self-test. It functioned perfectly. He got two spare sets of batteries for the unit from his desk, and packed it into his computer's protective case. He checked the computer battery, and made sure that he had all the cables and adapters for the modem and the satellite phone. Assured that all was in order, he spun the combination locks on the cases, and set them by the front door.

He went to the small bar in the living room, and cut a fresh lime in half, squeezing the juice into two glasses. He opened the bottle of Myers's, savoring the sweet heavy aroma of the rum. He swirled the rum with the lime juice and made two rum and cokes. Coltrane sat in the half-darkened living room, and watched as his wife came down the hallway, dropping the luggage in the foyer with his cases.

"A Myers's and Coke, my love? In celebration of our upcoming escape?" Coltrane raised his eyebrows and smiled.

Her irritation spent, and having finished the task of packing, Britt's mood was improving. Her husband could never comprehend how difficult it is for a woman to make do for two weeks on a boat with the barest of necessities. Despite all the many inconveniences, she truly enjoyed the seclusion and exotic settings that only yachting provided. The smell of the

Myers's brought back memories, and she drifted towards the living room sofa. She took the drink, touched glasses with him, and draped a long, bare, suntanned leg over his lap. Coltrane kissed her and idly stroked her silky leg, as they both drifted in thought and sipped their drinks.

Chapter 41

June 22

The Cuban left his hotel, and walked down the alley between the hotel and an empty parking garage. He turned left onto the street and walked through a gas station to a twenty-four hour convenience store. Around the side of the store was a bank of payphones, painted with gang graffiti and smelling of urine and vomit. He found the payphone that he wanted, and stood by it lighting his cigarette. Five minutes later, the phone rang.

"Hello, is that you?" The electronically scrambled voice on the other end of the line was cautious. The chief of security for AthenaHMO had enjoyed a long and successful career. He meant to keep it that way.

"*Si*, it is I. I have found and destroyed one of the discs that you wanted, but the other is very difficult to locate. Perhaps you can give me some direction." The Cuban replied.

"We have very little on our end. Hendricks has no family contacts, or close relatives according to the personnel file. No girlfriends either. He's a dead end. His secretary is clean, and has cooperated with our internal investigation completely. After Hendricks' death, she showed no change in attitude or behavior. I don't think she is involved. Examination of the computer terminal in Hendricks' office shows that he copied data onto only two 650MB discs. The third disc was still in the CD-R drive."

"No telephone contacts the day he quit?"

"None of significance."

"Let me decide that." The Cuban disliked the supercilious arrogance of the man.

"He talked to the attorney about the case that he fucked up, that is all I know," the man snapped back.

"The case that he fucked up, that was the reason that he was fired?" The Cuban demanded.

"Yeah." his tone was sullen.

"Tell me about this case."

The insurance security man related the story to the Cuban. Hendricks had made a serious error in judgment that resulted in the death of a young man insured by the company. Subsequently, the security man had found in his internal investigation that Hendricks may have spoken at length with both the family and a physician involved in the case. This had been verified both by Hendricks' secretary and electronic phone logs. The corporate attorney handling the case felt that Hendricks had disclosed damaging information to the family or the physician, but could not obtain hard evidence to verify his suspicions. Hendricks had become rapidly unstable during this time, and was discovered stealing confidential corporate data and fired immediately.

"Tell me about the doctor." The Cuban cursed silently at the man's blindness.

"I don't know much beyond his name. Coltrane. And there exists a taped conversation between him and Hendricks, but we're dealing with that."

"Find out everything you can and call me back in thirty minutes. Find out his license plate numbers first. And ask that lawyer what he knows. Coltrane is tied to this somehow."

"I have got a meeting that I have to go to."

"*Fuck your meeting.* Unless you want to read about your disc in the newspaper, you get me that fucking information now. The trail is gone cold down here. You *understand* me?" The Cuban snarled into the phone, his back to the street to shield his conversation.

"I'll try." The phone went dead.

The Cuban slammed the receiver down on the cradle, and walked into the store. He bought a pack of cigarettes, and a cup of coffee. He watched the customers shuffle in and out. Some glanced at him briefly, feeling his tension and avoiding him. He resisted the temptation to buy a beer, and read the girlie magazines instead. When twenty-five minutes had passed, he returned to the payphone. Again the phone rang and he picked it up.

"Is that you?" the voice began again.

"*Si*. What about Coltrane?"

"I have your information. Coltrane is a trauma surgeon who is also the president of the local medical society. He was asked to consult on the case by the kid's father, but the kid died before Coltrane ever saw him. But our lead attorney feels that his interference was responsible for the delays in appropriate treatment. We're going to depose him this week."

"Depose him? What do you mean?"

"A deposition is an informal interrogation of a witness before the trial, in order to get an idea of what the other side will present. It is conducted usually in the doctor's office, but is recorded by the court reporter, and is sworn testimony. We will find out what he and Hendricks talked about by that deposition."

"What does he drive?" The Cuban got out his notebook, and looked down the list as he listened.

"He has only one car registered with our hospital security, a white Expedition. It has current Florida plates. I have his address too. Got a pen?"

The Cuban smiled as he wrote down the license plate number and house address. He knew Coltrane was the one. He had been in the business too long to believe in coincidences. "Thanks. How did you get all this so quick?" he asked the security man.

"He's on our insurance plan, a participating provider. Everything is on his application for hospital privileges. And for his parking lot decal and gate cards. Need a photograph?"

"No, I know what he looks like. You are going to owe me big when this is over, amigo."

"You know our agreement. Call me when you are done."

"*Adios*."

Chapter 42

June 23

Coltrane was always anxious and irritable going to the airport. He was usually late and worried about missing his flight, something he had done twice before. Today, they were on time and halfway to the Tampa-St. Pete airport when his cell went off.

"Why don't you turn that damned thing off?" Britt asked as he cursed viciously and reached for the cellphone.

"I can't until I check out with the office at 8AM." Coltrane looked at the number, and called his office. "What is it, Cindy?" Coltrane asked his office manager.

"Sorry to bother you, Dr. Coltrane. You had two calls that I think you should know about. Davis Clark called, asking to arrange a time for a deposition. I told him that you would be gone for two weeks, but he wants to speak with you. And Scott Lynwood from the FBI called. He wanted to talk to you, he said it was urgent." She gave him both phone numbers.

Coltrane called Davis Clark at his office, and waited as his secretary put him through. Clark came on, unruffled as usual.

"Morning, Bill. I have just gotten a subpoena from the insurance company attorney to depose you next week. What does your schedule look like?"

"Next week? They can't do that with such short notice, can they? I'm going to be out of town next week." Coltrane felt his anger rising. He could not ignore a subpoena. He knew that a very effective tactic of lawyers was to utterly disrupt and destroy the schedules of their opponents.

"Calm down, Bill. It is just a harassment tactic. I'll deal with them. When will be a convenient time to meet with them? I imagine that the deposition will take two or three hours."

"What will they ask? Do they know about the discussion that Hendricks and I had?"

"They will certainly ask you about details of the case from a medical viewpoint. I think that they are suspicious about your transformation from a defendant to an expert witness, and will concentrate on that area of testimony. They have no way of knowing the substance of your conversation with Hendricks, do they?"

"No, I suppose not. The only way they could know about that is through Hendricks himself or his secretary. I doubt that Hendricks would have admitted to having revealed that information. His secretary knew that we spoke on several occasions, but not what we spoke about. I don't think she knows much."

"Good."

"Do I have to tell them about the tape?"

"You have to be truthful at all times, you will be under oath. You only have to answer with a yes or no, however. Don't get too talkative. If they ask about the tape specifically, you must answer truthfully. But I doubt they will have any idea about the tape yet. Alistair will eventually have to list the tape as evidence during the discovery phase, if we are going to use it in the trial. But I think he will delay that move as long as possible. I think he will use it as a trump card, and hope to force the insurance company to settle out of court. One thing, though. He placed a condition that, if he doesn't use your testimony, the deal is null and void. That was the only way I could finesse the deal without actually playing the tape for him."

"Good. I will need to spend some time with you preparing for the deposition. I will be back in about two weeks. Can I call you then?"

"Sure. No problem. We will do it at your office. I want them to see your diplomas and certificates, your credentials. I'll tell them that your schedule is full, and I will arrange a deposition time at your convenience. Call me when you get back. Have fun, you deserve a break."

Coltrane hung up after thanking Clark. He thought about calling the FBI man, but decided that the less that he interacted with him, the better. He called Cindy back, and told her that he was checking out for the week, and that all medical calls were to go to Dr. Hernandez, who was covering for him. He told her that he would be in New York, and that she could reach him via E-mail on the Internet. He told her not to tell anyone where he was, and not to call him unless it was urgent. He hung up, and turned his cellphone off. As Britt watched, he symbolically placed it in the glovebox. He smiled at his wife, and turned into the airport exit off the freeway. He didn't see the white sedan three cars behind him make the same turn.

Chapter 43

The Cuban had been following Coltrane himself that morning, not trusting his partner. He was very grateful that he had. He watched the couple park their car in the cavernous lot, and carry their baggage into the passenger terminal. Interesting that they didn't drop the bags off at the curb, or have the porters take them. He contemplated attacking the defenseless Coltrane as the physician hefted two heavy bags and carried them toward the terminal. The arrival of another car made the decision for him.

He easily tailed them into the American Airlines corridor, and observed them check in. From his vantage point, fifty yards away, he could not make out where they were headed. He looked up at the television screens announcing the flight arrivals and departures. There were six AA flights leaving in the next hour, and any one may be Coltrane's flight. And even if he found the first leg of their journey, there was no guarantee that they had a non-stop flight. A change of planes in Miami or Dallas would lose him completely. He couldn't follow them to the gate, security would allow only ticketed passengers past the final checkpoint. He did not want to be seen by Coltrane or his wife, any recognition could have dire consequences at a later date.

He edged forward, hoping to catch a glimpse of something. Coltrane turned, looking around the terminal with a sweeping gaze. The Cuban turned his head, looking out the glass face of the building as to spot an arriving relative or friend. He moved closer, keeping his back to the line of people waiting at the counter, watching Coltrane in the reflection on the glass. When he turned back, Coltrane was again facing the counter agent. The Cuban backed to within two yards of Coltrane, behind the velvet rope forming the queue. A middle aged woman scowled at him, thinking he was butting in line. He ignored her.

The Cuban was catching bits of the conversation. Coltrane's wife was doing all the talking, asking about customs in Miami. The agent confirmed that they would have to claim and re-check their luggage in Miami, and that they would not pass US Customs then, only upon their return from the Bahamas. He told them that they would check their baggage through to Marsh Harbor from Miami. The Cuban smiled at the scowling woman in line, and strode away, still keeping his back to Coltrane.

Luck favors the prepared, he thought.

Chapter 44

Unburdened by the shackles of his practice, and having checked into the gate for the flight to Miami, Coltrane began to relax. They boarded the plane, and were again amazed at the stupidity of the flying public. People rushed to get onboard, ignoring the attendant's instructions for orderly boarding, then blocking the aisles talking or adjusting their luggage as others tried to reach their seats. Coltrane pitied the flight crew for having to deal continually with these assholes as he guided Britt to their seats.

The flight to Miami was very short, the jet ascending to altitude, then descending to land. Miami International Airport was, as always, a mass of frantic travelers. Europeans mingled with huge crowds of Latin Americans, all lost in the corridors of the terminal, all looking for food, drink, relatives, and flights. The jabber of foreign tongues mixed with the smell of bodies, sweat and the dank humidity. The long deserted rows of counter space under the Continental Airlines banner mutely testified to the changing fortunes in the airline industry.

Coltrane and Britt found their bags, and took them from the domestic terminal to the international terminal. They took a huge diesel bus from one concrete building to the small outlying section for Caribbean flights. They rechecked their bags, and sat in the crowded waiting area. The flights to all points in the Caribbean originated in Miami, and all passengers flew out of this area. The scene was always the same when they passed through. Couples sitting close together, dressed in tropical attire, aglow in the anticipation of an exotic escape. Large knots of coal black Bahamian women with huge shopping bags full of toys, hats, and cheap stuffed animals. Loud middle aged white vacationers with their fat wives, wearing cheap imitation safari wear bought in New Jersey, lecturing each other on how to beat the casinos at blackjack. The noise and humidity was oppressive. When their flight was finally called, even the heavy oily smell of the jet fuel was welcome.

The turboprop aircraft seemed tiny by comparison to the enormous jetliners that they usually flew, but they were on board and wedged into their seats before any thoughts of retreating could take hold. The flight crew went through the safety instructions dully. Coltrane wondered why these crewmembers were stuck on these backwater Caribbean routes, and hoped it was a matter of low seniority, not a form of punishment for prior ineptitude.

The flight took them over the infamous Bermuda Triangle, and Nassau and Freeport. The waters of the North Atlantic Ocean were dark blue, heavy and rolling with swells that had white caps visible from the plane. As they neared the islands, Coltrane could see the water transformed from dark ominous hues into the inviting emerald and turquoise waters he loved so much. Ever since his parents had first brought him to the islands years ago, he had been drawn back again and again. The spectacular beauty of the crystal clear water, the white sand beaches with their knee deep shallows and the lush tropical vegetation entranced him. And the unmistakable, intense aura of sex, of passion, of lust. Things were different here, always would be. It all came back to him as the plane banked sharply, jolted hard on a rising thermal, and turned for final approach. Coltrane saw the long stretches of empty beaches, the tidal pools of salty water, and the mangrove swamps as they hurtled over the tip of the small island. He saw the many tiny islands that formed the outer barrier of the Sea of Abaco, and recognized them all. From his vantage point high in the air, he spotted the submerged wreck of a two seater plane that he and Britt had scuba dived around during the last trip. With that thought in mind, he grasped Britt's hand and settled back in his seat for landing. In the back of his mind, he wondered how the conference had gotten off.

The small plane landed hard, and bounced sideways as it careened to a halt. As he deplaned onto the broken concrete runway, Coltrane was hit with a blast of humid, hot tropical air. His light cotton shirt immediately stuck to the sweat rising from his chest and back. The passengers made their way towards the Customs line, and the baggage inspection area. Coltrane showed their passports to an unsmiling black woman in dark blue uniform of the Bahamian government. She stamped entry visas on each, and curtly directed him to the luggage inspection area.

Guns and drugs were the primary concerns of the customs officials in the outlying Bahamian islands. Both came from not only the main islands, but with vacationers as well. The Bahamian Parliament had recently passed strict firearm controls, with severe mandatory penalties for weapon possession. The long legacy of domestic peace, a result of gentle British rule over three hundred years, had recently been shattered by a series of brutal murders. The criminals were found to be local toughs who had traveled to New York City, and adopted the style and methods of American gangs. In an immediate backlash, handguns were outlawed, and gun control was enacted.

Coltrane had always carried a pistol with him on his sailing trips in the past, declaring it to US and Bahamian Customs. Yachtsmen were a preferred target for drug smugglers and pirates, especially in Caribbean waters. Remote, isolated surroundings without communication and no effective law enforcement presence made sailors ideal targets for armed robbery, rape or murder. This vulnerability had always been a concern for Coltrane.

This time, he had no gun. Instead, he brought with him a powerful speargun and a sharkstick. The sharkstick was a primitive firearm, a four inch steel tube at the end of a handlegrip which fired a .357 Magnum pistol cartridge, meant for use underwater. The diver carried it lashed by a cord to his wrist, like a magic wand. If threatened, he could pull a safety pin then slam the nose of the barrel against the fish, firing the bullet and the explosive gasses into the body of the shark. It would instantly kill sharks up to 15 feet long. Coltrane was not thinking of sharks when he packed the sharkstick and the speargun. Both were illegal for use in Bahamian waters. If discovered by customs, he would argue that he was traveling into international waters, and might need them there.

Thc Customs agent examined the visas and asked Britt where they were staying, and the purpose of their visit. Coltrane moved the heavy bags of gear and luggage behind her, as the man's handsome smooth skinned face followed him. Coltrane met his all-knowing gaze and smiled amiably, hoping that his nervousness didn't show. He wondered how the agents all managed to keep their uniforms starched and razor sharp in the oppressive muggy heat. The man beamed a toothy smile, and waved them through.

Coltrane found a cab quickly, before the Customs official changed his mind. They loaded the gear and took a forty-five minute terror-filled ride down sandy gravel roads to the marina, nestled up high in Marsh Harbor. The town was clustered around a calm little bay, protected on three sides by low-lying hills and scrub. Coltrane had been coming back to the Sea of Abaco for over ten years now, and despaired as he watched the area grow and become despoiled with time. He shook the sad feeling off, and headed for the office of the base manager.

They found Dennis conducting a charter briefing with a young American couple, an arrogant preppie kid and his sullen, stunning girlfriend. Dennis went through the motions, knowing that neither was listening. They were anticipating five days of fucking in paradise before returning to the tedious business of their shallow lives. He was finished and headed for his office when he looked up and recognized Coltrane and Britt. Smiling, he beckoned them to follow into the relative cool of the shaded verandah.

Dennis liked the Coltranes. He had known them for many seasons now, and appreciated the care that they gave his boats and equipment. The Coltranes had made three passages from Abaco to the Exumas by now, and were seasoned blue water sailors by his estimation. They never got lost, never damaged his boats or gear, never made unrealistic demands of him and his crew. Dennis himself was an accomplished sailor, having ferried a

Beneteau sloop from France to the Abacos five years ago, and then staying on as a dock hand. Like many of the European ex-pats that worked in the islands, Dennis had developed a distaste for the ugly Americans, with their loud boorish scenes and ridiculous behavior. Like the black native Bahamians, he slowly learned to tolerate and ignore their presence, understanding that his job and the economy of the town was entirely dependent upon American tourist dollars. The Coltranes were an exception to the rule, and he respected them for it.

They sat under the verandha, drinking ice cold Amstel and going over the charts and the weather reports. Coltrane proposed an itinerary, and Dennis agreed to his plan. The only problem left was to select a boat. The last charter they had taken was a Beneteau 38, a beautiful sleek sloop that slept four people in two staterooms. Because of the sudden change in arrival dates, Dennis had not been able to give them the same boat again. He had promised them something equivalent, but would not know until they arrived which boat they could charter.

"What boat can you give me, Dennis?" Coltrane looked out down the dock, at the rows of sailboats moored in slips. Clearly some of the boats were in far better condition than others. Charter yachts get rough treatment at the hands of unskilled and drunken captains.

"Wait until this yuppie prick casts off, Doc." Dennis grinned and pointed to the couple as they hurriedly loaded their gear and prepared to leave the dock. "I gave you his boat. You'll love it, it's brand new, just arrived three weeks ago. His mind's not on sailing anyway."

After the couple had motored out of the harbor, Dennis took them down the dock to a sparkling white Hunter 426, a forty-two foot sloop so new that the gelcoat on the fiberglass shell was sparkling and translucent. The teak was oiled and fragrant, the stainless steel fittings and rails bright and polished. The craft had been brilliantly designed and outfitted, with a roller furled main mast and roller furled jib. The winches were two speed, self-tailing and positioned for easy access. All the lines and sheets were curled and secured neatly in their places, and the cockpit electronics glowed with blue-green LCD readouts. The boat was gorgeous, and virgin. Even the deck cushions were still in their plastic factory wrapping. And this boat had the feature that Coltrane valued the most, a walk-through transom set into the sloping aft of the boat. The transom was a series of steps that descended from the cockpit down into the water, and made entry and exit from the sea effortless. It was priceless to a tired diver, loaded with heavy, cumbersome scuba gear and awkward fins. Tied to the stern was a brand new Zodiac dinghy with a Mercury outboard.

Dennis looked at Coltrane with a knowing smile. "I knew you would love this boat, Doc. It's not a part of our regular fleet; the owner is an American Airlines pilot who is down here frequently, and put her into the charter fleet just to defray some of the expenses. This boat is far better equipped than any bareboat you will find anywhere else. He even gives you a CD of Pink Floyd. *Learning to Fly*. Great sailing tune."

Coltrane was impressed. When he and Britt had started bareboat chartering fifteen years ago, it had been a much more primitive adventure.

The boats had been older and unpopular models, brutishly ugly and usually abused by inexperienced and indifferent skippers. But as the bareboat chartering industry expanded, sailboat manufacturers like Beneteau and Hunter began to design and produce craft specifically for that market.

Sailboat design is an exercise in compromise. All sailors want a fast, sleek boat; one that will perform well at all points of sail, and is responsive and quick. Those boats, exemplified by the 12 Metre America's Cup racing monohulls, were extremely fast and able to sail into the wind and carve turns into the seas with aggressive agility. But belowdecks, a racing hull had no room. They were meant solely for racing, not living aboard. And if you were going to live on a boat, even for a short period of time, you needed room. Cramped, humid quarters invariably led to cabin fever and a miserable, quarrelsome experience. So gradually, over the years, the French and American and Scandinavian designers had adapted and refined offshore racing formulas, and produced sloops that were roomy belowdecks, yet still maintained a responsive feel under sail. The Hunter 426 was the pinnacle of this evolution, benefiting from a racing heritage and the extensive use of Kevlar and high tech composite materials.

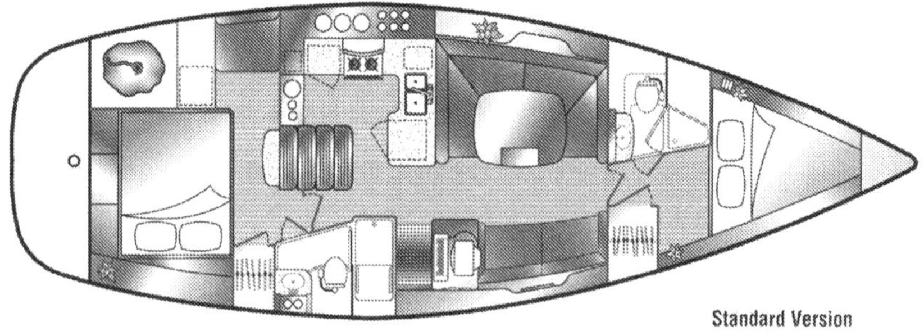

Reproduced with the kind permission of Hunter Marine
www.huntermarine.com

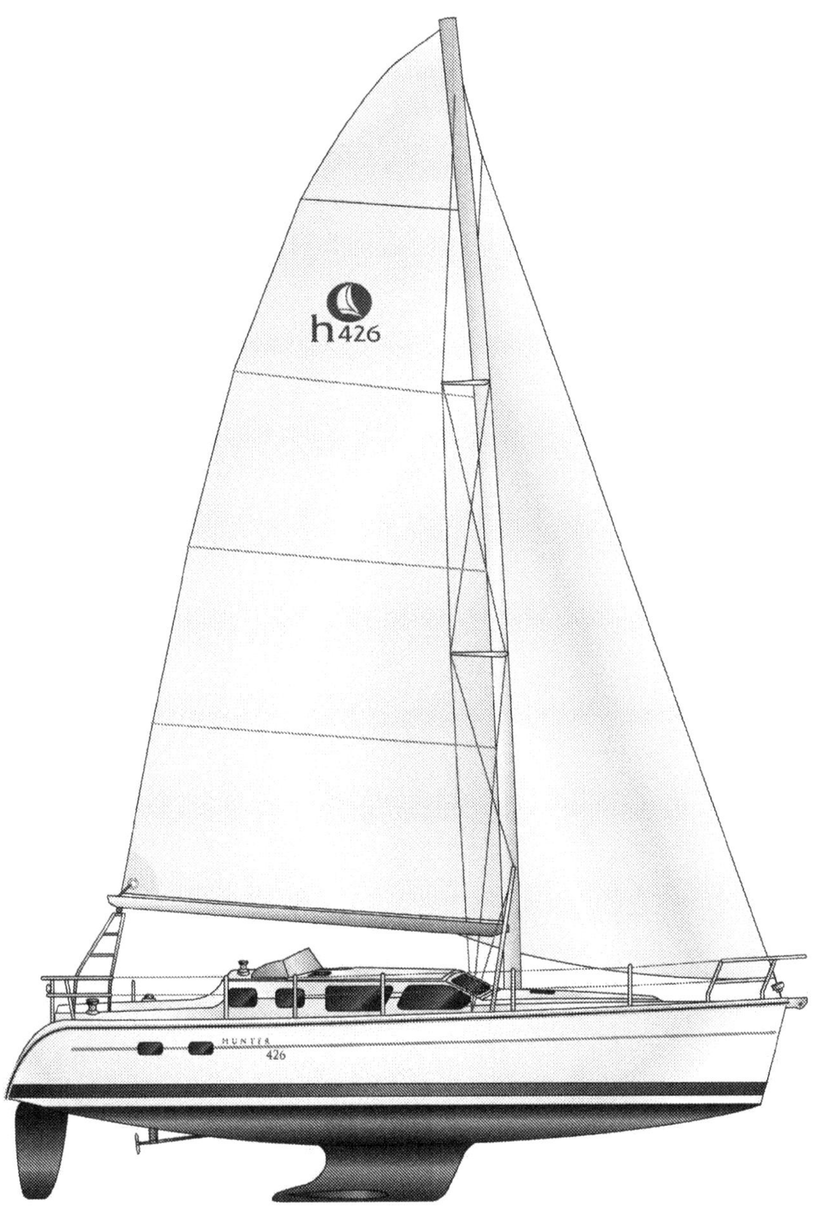

Reproduced with the kind permission of Hunter Marine
www.huntermarine.com

Coltrane looked admiringly over the sloop. Both the mainsail and the jib were roller furled, and the main boom was raised and anchored to a stainless steel arch above the cockpit. No more fears of being smashed by a wildly flying main boom and killed or thrown from the boat in heavy weather. In offshore racing, more than one skull had been crushed when the wind shifted suddenly, and sent the five hundred pound boom swinging violently across the cockpit, catching a crew member unawares.

The anchor windlass was electric, and there were even two electric halyard winches. Rare for charter boats, the cockpit was equipped with an AutoHelm autopilot, GPS and full electronics. A digital knotmeter, depthmeter and alarm and VHF radio were integrated into the pedestal console.

While Dennis gave Coltrane the briefing, Britt went below to check the living quarters.

"Ohhh, baby. Look at this," she purred from below.

"What?" Coltrane peered down through the companionway.

"This boat has *air conditioning?* Is that possible? Am I dreaming?" She asked in disbelief.

"Yes, yes, and no," Dennis replied. "And a 110 volt inverter, and a dehumidifier, and a ten speaker, 100 watt stereo system, and a microwave, and Corian countertops. But no TV."

"Damn, Dennis. We may not bring it back," Britt beamed.

"Don't blame ya. It's better than my apartment, by a long shot," he smiled.

Coltrane went over the mechanical and electrical details of the sailboat with Dennis while Britt checked out the refrigerator, cooler and the gas stove. Both Coltranes knew the drill well. Radio protocols and the times of the local news weather reports were noted, and emergency procedures discussed. Dennis opened the engine cover, and showed Coltrane how to purge and clean water from the diesel's fuel filter, and how to change the oil. They checked the huge array of batteries and the battery charging system. They checked the fuel tank and the fresh water tanks, then topped them all off.

When Coltrane was satisfied that he was familiar with the boat, Dennis left them to stow their gear. Coltrane hefted the heavy bags off the dock, and carried them below to the aft stateroom. As he quickly stowed the gear and clothing, Britt went to the marina store and provisioned the boat, buying fresh Bahamian bread, eggs, vegetables and fruit. She found their favorite local hot sauce, a blend of Bahamian serrano peppers and spices, and bought several jars. Most of the other staples were imported. Meats, pasta, sauces, cheeses and, most important of all, wine, beer and rum, all came from outside the islands. She provisioned the boat for two weeks, then added an extra margin for safety. There were no grocery stores where they were headed.

Their gear secure, Coltrane helped Britt put the food into the small electric refrigerator and pack the pantry. He didn't want to stay in the still, humid air of the harbor for any longer than necessary. Below deck, the salon of the sloop became like a sauna in the afternoon heat. They stowed the fourteen plastic one gallon containers of deionized water below the floorboards of the yacht, and closed all the hatches. Britt went through the checklist as Coltrane started the diesel. Dennis came down the dock, and wished them Godspeed as he slipped the dock lines. They drifted backward before the prop caught, and spun the heavy boat slowly away from the wooden piers and into the main channel of the harbor. Coltrane stood steady behind the large stainless steel wheel of the sailboat as he guided it out through the maze of anchored yachts, sailboats and fishing vessels. He was glad to be alive, glad to be a man.

The sun was already dropping into the sea, the light on the water making it difficult to read the depth of the shallows. In the Bahamas, the challenge for the captain was not in the art of setting sails, but in the skill and judgment of navigation. The Bahamas was a long chain of small limestone islands, lying in a shallow sea. More than once, Coltrane had misjudged the color and depth of the many coral heads and sand bars in the shoal waters. Running aground was part of sailing, but damaging the boat or becoming stranded was not.

After clearing the harbor entrance, Coltrane lay a course directly for a small sandy barrier island seven nautical miles away. It was their favorite spot in the world, a strip of pristine beach with a small tidal pool that filled and emptied with crystal clear water each tide change. Hundreds of brightly colored marine creatures would find themselves swept into the three foot deep pool for hours before the rising tide released them, and Coltrane and Britt loved to swim and play in their little world. They could overnight there before attempting the long ocean voyage the next day.

Coltrane was tired, sore from the long day's travel in the cramped airline seats, and the jolting cab ride. He stood mesmerized behind the wheel of the yacht, numb to the beauty around him. He piloted the sailboat straight to his favorite anchorage, a little depression in the shoreline with a perfect sandy bottom and clear turquoise waters ten feet deep. They were the only boat within sight, and the sun was setting. Coltrane slowed the diesel, and shifted the prop into neutral. He gave control of the boat to Britt, and moved to the fore of the sleek craft as it gently nosed into the cove. He watched the sandy bottom carefully, through the perfectly clear, brilliant waters. He could see the starfish nestled in the white sand. A school of small yellowjack darted away from the keel, the sun glinting on each shimmering iridescent scale and fin. The visibility and clarity was startling.

When he was happy with the depth, he hand signaled to Britt from the pulpit to point the boat into the breeze, and give a burst of reverse. The boat stopped dead in the tranquil bay, and he played out the heavy main anchor with its iron chain. It settled lazily onto the rippled sea bottom. Coltrane walked along the side of the boat back to the cockpit, and Britt shut off the diesel. It was a nightly ritual that they had performed countless times before. The heavy boat, pushed by the slight breeze and pulled by the tidal flows, settled back on its anchor. In the space of fifteen minutes, it would dig its anchor blades deep into the soft sand bed. They sat and relaxed in the comfortable silence. When the slight backward motion of the boat had ceased, Britt turned the diesel on momentarily, and steered the sloop gently off in a sixty degree angle to the anchor line. Coltrane dropped the smaller, secondary anchor into the bay, and let the line slack. She cut the motor, and again they drifted back.

Satisfied that the primary anchor had bitten the sand, Coltrane stripped off his clothes, and dove into the warm Caribbean water. He allowed the effusing warmth to bathe over his tired muscles, and circled like a dolphin around the boat. Rejuvenated, he returned to the walk-through transom, and pulled up to the submerged staircase. Britt handed him his mask and snorkel, admiring his wet body from above. He smiled up at her, loving her, marveling in her affection.

He swam slowly along the sleek, clean side of the Hunter to the anchor line, then followed it down into the sparkling waters. He cautiously scanned around him, ever aware that Caribbean seas were home to sharks, and that swimmers were often taken here. He had seen an enormous eleven foot bull shark on their last trip, cruising in just six feet of water, right off a popular swimming beach. The shark had lazily swum directly under his boat, with the diesel at full bore. It was as if it was saying this was its world, and dared you to enter. Coltrane never forgot the look in the shark's dead eyes.

He found the main anchor, and dove down to handset the flukes deep into the sandy bottom. Confident that it was solid, he repeated the procedure on the smaller secondary anchor, then swam slowly back to the boat. He pulled himself out of the salty water, and sat on the transom steps. Britt rinsed him off with the freshwater shower that was built into the back of the boat, and handed him a towel. He toweled off, and stepped up into the cockpit to an awaiting Myers's and Coke, complete with fresh cut Caribbean lime.

"*Alles klar.*" Coltrane scanned the sailboat appreciatively.

"What, you speak French now that we are in the islands?" Britt laughed.

"That was German. Can't you tell German from French?"

"Maybe it is your Southern accent. What's it mean?"

"*All is well. All clear.* Remember 'Das Boot'? It is a submariner's term for everything on the boat is functioning, and right. I like it. A good practice for us sailors."

Britt lifted her drink, and they touched glasses. Long ago, they had decided never to drink while sailing until the anchors had been set for the evening. Errors made at sea were more than inconvenient, they could be fatal. Alcohol increased errors exponentially, as Coltrane saw frequently in the ER. Fortunately, he learned from others' mistakes.

They watched the sun set into a blaze of red, orange, rose and peach, gradually fading into blues and purples. Calm beset them, hypnotized by the gentle rhythmic lapping of the waves against the smooth sides of the boat. Only the final drop of the dying sun brought them out of their reverie.

Britt went below to begin a quick supper. There was not enough room in the tiny galley for two, so traditionally they alternated cooking honors. Both were creative and avid cooks, and they found that something about the islands made cooking and eating even more enjoyable. The cabin was fitted with a small propane oven and a four burner gas stovetop, and all the necessary pots and pans. Coltrane preferred to cook on the small stainless steel barbecue that could be attached to the rear of the transom, hanging out over the water. Tonight, Britt boiled pasta and made a seafood marinara with fresh shrimp, squid and conch she had just picked from the marina store.

Coltrane folded the leaves of the teak salon table upward, locking them into position. He went back into the aft stateroom which would be used as a storage area, getting his satellite phone and computer. He opened the aluminum phone case, and arranged the components. He ran the antenna cable to the back of the transceiver, and fed it through the closest open hatch. He secured the cable with a short bungee cord, selected the marine antenna, and climbed up through the companionway onto the deck of the sloop.

The boat had settled into a stable position, swinging slightly on the taut anchor lines. He fixed the antenna in front of the mainmast, and angled it toward the darkening sky. He screwed the cable tightly into the antenna coupling, and returned below.

Opening his computer case, he removed and turned on the powerful Pentium IV notebook. He connected the computer to the RS232 input terminal of the satellite telephone, and verified that the interface was functioning. Then by double-clicking on the AOL icon, he opened the main menu to the Internet service. The AOL set-up program went through its steps, and asked him for the local trunk line number. He checked his directory for AOL, and selected the number for New York City. Coltrane input the New York City phone number, then sat back as the program completed itself. It would now automatically dial the New York phone number, and anyone trying to trace the origin of his computer transmissions would be led in that direction.

Coltrane leaned back on the thick cushions of the salon lounge. He opened AOL again and went through the process of going online. The computer clicked and buzzed, and then dialed the area code and the New York number, Coltrane hearing the rapid series of tones emanating from his computer's speaker. The system functioned perfectly, with the AOL service coming online quickly. The connection status rating, a measure of how good the telephone line contact was, showed ninety six percent. Coltrane sighed with relief, and was astounded yet again at the sophistication of the technology.

He double-clicked on the mailbox icon for the E-mail function. The service paused as it searched the main frame computer for E-mail. A message box flashed in the corner of his screen saying that two messages were waiting for retrieval. He clicked twice to retrieve.

E-mail
June 23
5:23:46 PM
From: SKerr
To: WmColtraneMD

Have had a call from a FBI lawyer.
He claims that he is investigating this conference for anti-trust violations. He wants to speak with you urgently. I told him that you are in New York.
He wants to know where? What is this about? What should I do?
Please respond ASAP.

Coltrane cursed outloud, startling Britt as she stirred the pasta by the stove. He had known that Agent Lynwood would not be easily avoided, but he hadn't anticipated that he would be so aggressive this early. The conference had not even started yet.

E-mail
June 23
7:33:12 PM
From: WmColtraneMD
To: SKerr

I am in New York City, at a conference and cannot call him during the day. I will call his office tomorrow at 4:30pm.
Please relay message. I have the number.
Keep up the strong work. I will be back soon. Think about someone who may make a good interim media spokesperson if necessary.
wc

Coltrane sent the message, and then turned off the computer and the satellite phone. He mixed another drink for both of them, and helped Britt finish cooking dinner. He outlined the news from Susan as they seasoned the marinara with the incredible Bahamian hot sauce. They ate quietly, contemplating the alternatives available to them. She could see that a sense of dread hung over him, and she wondered how far they had to go to escape the stress and pressure of his practice.

Chapter 45

June 24
5:18AM

Coltrane rose early, having slept well. The fore cabin was the master stateroom, larger than the aft cabin, with a roomy bathroom and shower, meant for the captain of the boat. A queen bed sat in the center of the suite, and teak racks swept forward along the sides of the room as it narrowed toward the bow of the sailboat. There were ample lockers for stowing clothes, luggage and gear built into the beautiful, teak paneled walls. A large, screened hatch opened directly over the center of the bed, allowing cross-ventilation of the cabin. Britt slept peacefully in the bed, her naked body draped in the white linens. He let her rest, closing the teak cabin door softly.

The boat rocked gently, and the lapping sound of the waves soothed him. He pulled on a pair of shorts and slid open the companionway lid, stepping out and into the cockpit. The sun was just rising, and the waters of the Sea of Abaco were flat as glass. Across the small island, past the reef and shoals that protected the Sea of Abaco, lay the North Atlantic Ocean. The tranquil, pale green and turquoise water changed abruptly into dark blue rollers, white capped and powerful, two meters high. Coltrane had profound respect for the immense power of the ocean, a primeval fear mixed with admiration. Today he would again venture out into the trackless desolation.

Coltrane pulled on his swim goggles, preferring the triathlon equipment to the heavier scuba mask. He dove off the end of the transom, and swam lazily around the sailboat, then dove under the keel. He checked the prop for damage or obstruction, and removed a small piece of fishing line from the rudder blade. He checked the winged keel, and saw that it was smooth and undamaged. The gelcoat of the sides of the hull was slick and polished like glass. The boat is virgin, he thought as he surfaced. Confident in the seaworthiness of the sloop, he hoisted himself onto the transom, and went below to prepare breakfast.

Britt was up, and had made fresh coffee. They went over the charts and the local charterguide, planning the passage from the Abacos to Eleuthera. It was an eight to ten hour trip, depending upon the strength of the winds and the direction and speed of the ocean currents. The entry channel into Eleuthera was treacherous, littered with hulks of ships dating from the pirate days to modern iron freighters. The channel would be hard enough to find in the daylight, and Coltrane feared arriving in Eleuthera after dark. They would have to weigh anchor and sail as soon as possible.

Moving to the bank of electrical switches mounted above the small navigation desk in the salon, Coltrane turned on the power to the cockpit gauges. He climbed through the companionway, and started the motor. As the powerful diesel warmed up, he went forward, and prepared to weigh the anchors. The smaller secondary anchor he pulled up by hand as Britt motored the boat directly over its position in the sand. The main anchor was broken free by powering the sailboat over and beyond it, jerking the blades loose with the mass of the sloop. Coltrane hauled the heavy Bruce anchor and chain up using the electric windlass. He stored the anchors in the triangular forepeak, and latched the lid. Using hand signals, he directed Britt out of the anchorage, watching the bottom carefully for shoals and coral heads. Once he was satisfied that they were clear of danger and into deeper water, he walked back and took the helm.

There were only three passages from the shallow, protected Sea of Abaco into the North Atlantic Ocean. Coltrane was forced by time and tides to use the closest one, a thirty foot wide gap in the treacherous ring of coral and rocks that encircled the islands. The cut was passable only in a falling tide, when the razor sharp coral could be seen, partially submerged in the dark blue water. At a high tide, the rocky shoals were completely submerged, and the cut impassable even by experienced local sailors.

Coltrane checked the proper heading, and re-checked a bearing on the prominent lighthouse directly at his stern. He began the passage towards the cut, with Britt at the bow guiding him. He could clearly see the waves boiling over the jagged, exposed rocks as the boat was drawn inexorably toward the gap in the reef. The withdrawing tide, and the millions of tons of water flowing outward into the ocean, gripped the sailboat and angled it sideways. Coltrane felt the tide and current pulling him, and corrected the rudder and accelerated the diesel. The sloop shot through the cut, missing the coral heads by ten feet on the starboard side.

The Atlantic Ocean was dramatically different from the tranquil Sea of Abaco. The colors changed from emerald to deep azure blue, from crystal clear to endless depth and darkness. The ocean was quiet, with gentle rollers of six to eight feet, moving the heavy yacht with ease. Coltrane motioned Britt to come back from the bow. She took the helm as he went below to check the charts and take a GPS reading. The voyage to Eleuthera was eight to ten hours, and an error of two or three degrees in their heading would translate into lost daylight, or worse. He called a bearing out to her from below, and she brought the boat about. He stood up straight in the companionway, felt the wind on his face and the salt spray on his body. He heard and felt the vibrant, rhythmic humming of the big diesel, driving the boat through the swells. He tilted his head back and howled like a madman, raising his voice to the heavens, exulting in the freedom and the adventure.

The wind was steady at seven knots from the south. Coltrane knew that they would not be able to sail the passage with the wind coming from that quarter. Sailing into the wind, they would have to tack back and forth, losing valuable time and light. Disappointed, he increased the throttle on the diesel, and maintained the engine revolutions at 2500 rpm. They motored southeast for three hours, allowing the diesel to grind out the distance. Both watched with mild apprehension as the low-lying Bahamian islands slowly disappeared behind them, leaving them in a vast, empty ocean.

Coltrane kept them on a straight course to the mouth of the inlet at Elcuthcra, and used the GPS data to calculate the speed of the ocean current. As he held the GPS unit in his hand, he marveled again at the leaps in technology that had occurred in the space of months. After the end of the first Gulf War, the Department of Defense granted limited use of its vast satellite array for civilian application. Using the same technology that guided the MIAI Abrams tank and the F-16 fighters to exact locations in the desolate, featureless Iraqi desert, marine electronics companies produced handheld Global Positioning Satellite units that could pinpoint its longitude and latitude accurately to within ten feet. Coltrane had bought the GPS unit for their last sailing trip, and it had brought them safely back through the Abacos cut in the middle of a blinding rain. Now he would never sail without it.

Blue water sailing and navigation was one of the few surviving domains of the adventurer and explorer. It combined the key elements of manly joys: freedom, isolation, danger and expensive, technologically sophisticated equipment. Coltrane reveled in the challenge, and the vast distance that sailing placed between his practice and his daily existence. The dangers, remote but very real, only heightened his pleasure.

Coltrane had experience in navigation beginning with training for a private pilot's license in medical school. The fundamentals of sailing and flight were the same, motion through the air using a wing to provide lift. In the case of a sloop, the wing was the jib foresail and the mainsail working together to pull the boat forward. The angle of the sails to the boat and the boat's heading determined speed and efficient use of the wind. And the relationship between the origin of the wind and the desired course of travel was critical. A modern rigged sloop could sail into the wind, but progress was slowed by the necessity of tacking back and forth toward the destination. On the ocean, navigation was further complicated by the effects of tides and swift ocean currents upon the path of the yacht. Coltrane stood in awe of the bravery of the ancient mariners, sailing limitless unknown oceans, guided only by celestial navigation and crude wooden floats to measure subtle ocean currents.

When they had motored for four hours, Coltrane handed the helm to Britt, and went below to check the charts. He verified the GPS coordinates, and plotted their progress. Sure that they were ahead of schedule, he asked Britt if she wanted to sail. In answer, she cut the diesel to idle, and pointed the nose into the wind as Coltrane pulled on his thick leather gloves and checked the jib sheets. He secured the lines and jumped up onto the center of the boat, clearing the lines that ran to the mainsail. Coltrane stepped back down into the cockpit, and awaited Britt's command. When the boat was directly into the breeze, she told him to raise the mainsail. Coltrane had never used a self-furling mainsail before, and was delighted with the simplicity it provided. By using a hand winch in the cockpit, he was able to quickly and effortlessly wind out the huge sail from its housing within the mainmast. The sail was wound around a stout aluminum shaft, much like a window shade, and could be rolled out or retracted back in by twisting the shaft within a protective mast housing. All the other boats that he had sailed required that the crew balance on the top of the pitching deck and hoist up the sail as it snapped and fluttered in the wind. In a gale, on a rolling and yawing boat, it was a miserable and dangerous job. He smiled as he cranked out the sail, felt it crack sharply as the wind buffeted it side to side.

Coltrane turned to Britt, and gave her the heading and point of sail. She nodded, and waited for him to prepare to unfurl the jib. The jib was the larger of the two sails, and was on a roller furling like the mainsail. Coltrane took the heavy winch handle and whipped the line around the winch, pulling and drawing the sail out. The wind immediately grabbed the white sail, and it shot out across the sloop, and flapped in the air as Coltrane tightened the line on the winch. As the jib was cranked down, the wind caught the sloop, heeling it over and pulling it forward with a surge. Britt cut the motor, and it died, leaving a silence. Coltrane checked the lines and sheets, and secured the precious winch handle. He made a complete circuit of the yacht, checking running gear and lines. When he was satisfied that all was right, he moved aft, and dropped into the cockpit by Britt.

She stood balanced on her right foot as the boat heeled to starboard. She held the three foot diameter, leather wrapped steel wheel in both hands, holding a perfect heading as the boat rose and fell into the rolling waves. The air was filled only with the rush of the wind and the sound of the water slicing off the bow as it knifed through the dark blue water. The breeze blew the soft, strawberry blonde hair off her neck, and Coltrane bent down and nuzzled her, biting the muscle of her neck, tasting her flesh, smelling her hair. Her beauty intoxicated him. He stood silently behind her watching the sea over her shoulder.

The sloop made eight knots under sail, faster than under power. But the heading was not perfect, so after four hours of sailing and tacking, they were obliged to drop the sails and resume motoring. The passage was smooth, uneventful. Coltrane slid his rod and spinning reel into a sleeve holder on the stern rail, and ran out one hundred yards of light line and an artificial lure. He loved trolling off the back of a sailboat, and almost always caught something. Usually it was catch and release, because some species of Bahamian reef fish had a fatal neurotoxin in their flesh, and Coltrane always forgot which species were affected. So he usually released everything.

He had frequent hits on the line, and caught and released several small snapper and a brightly colored dolphin. A two foot barracuda hit the line once, and it took Coltrane an exhilarating twenty minutes to bring him in on the eight pound test line. The barracuda jumped off the line at the last second. With blinding speed, he twisted and disappeared into the depths.

Britt was relieved as the low scrubby outline of Eleuthera came into view over the bow, the sun still above the water to the west. They stayed in the deep water as long as possible, finally turning to angle into the channel that wound through the coral and wrecks that dotted the shoals. The water changed rapidly from the deep blue to aqua, to emerald. The sandy bottom was barely visible, with the brown coral heads everywhere. The angle of the setting sun behind them made it difficult to discern the channel, but Coltrane had done this many times before. They headed for the small anchorage they always used, and anchored just after four o'clock.

Coltrane dropped the main anchor, and Britt cut the diesel. As the boat settled, he went below and set up the satellite phone, hurrying not to miss the scheduled time of his call to Lynwood. He pulled the FBI agent's business card from his wallet, set up the antenna, and dialed the number. It rang for a long time.

"Agent Lynwood." The voice was tired.

"Mr. Lynwood, this is Dr. Coltrane. I got a message that you wanted to speak with me?" Coltrane started calmly.

"Yes, thank you for calling. This pertains to the conference that is scheduled for next week. As we discussed in your office, there have been formal complaints filed with the regional FBI office alleging that this conference is simply a sham, a front for an illegal labor action by the physicians in the society. As the investigating attorney assigned to the case, I have been asked to obtain a preliminary written statement from a representative of the society. I assume that you are the appropriate person for that statement?"

"Yes, I am the president of the society."

"When can we meet?"

"I'm in New York, and I don't know exactly when I will be back. I can call you when I return."

"I'm sorry, but that will not work. I require some form of response within forty-eight hours or I will have to issue a subpoena for your appearance. I would like to avoid that if possible."

Coltrane cursed to himself. He thought feverishly, seeking a solution that would buy him time without revealing his location or plans for the conference.

"I will be in New York for some time. Can I meet someone in your New York office for a brief statement?" Coltrane gambled that a show of good faith would buy him time. He was wrong.

"Fine. I will give you the address and the name of the chief investigator there. He'll be expecting you. Please bear in mind that this statement will be taken under oath, and carries with it the penalty of perjury for false or misleading statements. Do you understand?" Lynwood was very curt in the demand.

"Yes." Coltrane saw his ploy dissolve, and felt a gnawing pain in his gut. But the die had been cast. He took the number for the FBI office in New York, and hung up.

"I'm fucked," Coltrane swore. Britt had come below and was looking at him with concern. He told her about the conversation with Lynwood and the tactic he had tried to use.

"You lied to the FBI?" Britt asked. "Was that wise?"

"Probably not. But I was not under oath, and they can't prove that I was not in New York."

"Alright, but now what do we do?" Britt sat down across from her husband on the settee.

"Stall. I have forty-eight hours before they get pissed. I'll call the FBI office tomorrow late, and make an appointment for the next day. That will give me some time. Hopefully, by then I will have an idea what to do." Coltrane wondered whether leaving Tampa had been opportune. Too late for regrets now, he reflected.

The main anchor was set, and Britt helped him drop the second anchor and they rested together as the sailboat dug the hooks into the soft sandy bottom. The evening was quiet, and a soft breeze cooled and refreshed them. After awhile, Coltrane stripped and dove into the clear water to hand set the anchors. They were well dug in, and he surfaced and climbed onto the transom platform. He lay back, half in and half out of the warm water, watching the sun settle into the ocean. He wished he could stay there forever, away from the demands and pressures of humanity, alone with his beautiful bride in paradise.

He rose and climbed the steps into the cockpit, accepting the glass of Merlot that Britt offered him. Her eyes wandered over his wet body, the drops of saltwater glistening on his chest and belly. She reached down and caressed him gently, sipping on her wine. He stiffened in her hand, and they went below, bathed in a spectacular sunset.

Chapter 46

Marsh Harbor
June 24

It had taken the Cuban just ten hours to get to Marsh Harbor. After overhearing the Coltranes' destination at the Tampa airport, he went directly to the phone and tried to schedule a flight for himself and his associate. He found to his dismay that American Airlines flew to Marsh Harbor and Treasure Cay in the Abacos only twice weekly. The next flight he could book would be next Tuesday. He couldn't wait that long. He called Johnny and arranged to meet him back at the hotel. They packed quickly, and hopped a commuter flight to Miami before noon.

Once in Miami, it was an easy matter to charter a plane for the hour flight to the Bahamas. There were seven outfits based in the Miami-Fort Lauderdale area that specialized in running gamblers, fishermen and lovers out to the islands, and picking them up at pre-arranged times. The Cuban chose the largest company, and paid the charter fee up front. By the time a flight plan had been filed, and the plane fueled, it was early evening. The flight over the azure waters of the Atlantic calmed the Cuban, and he slept most of the way. They landed in the dark, and went straight to the hotel that the cabdriver said was the best on the island.

The resort was set on a half-moon bay, brand new, with a modern concrete and steel marina sheltering rows of gleaming sailboats and sixty foot Bertrams. Sport fishermen rocked gently next to beamy fifty foot Pearson sloops. They ate quickly down by the boats, then started their search for the Coltranes. They walked the grounds, checked the resort bars, the beach and the pool for hours without luck. They went into town, and scoured the small, sweaty beach bars filled with tanned young Americans and Europeans, dancing to reggae and drinking rum and Heinekens. But Coltrane and his young wife were nowhere to be found. At three in the morning, when the drunks poured out of the bars, and paired off to wander down by the palm lined beach, they gave up and went to their hotel room.

They split up the next morning, and the Cuban went into town while Johnny played the Yankee tourist at the resort. The only clue they had to work on was the heavy bags of gear that Coltrane had been carrying. The Cuban reasoned that Coltrane had scuba gear, boating equipment or camping gear. He doubted that Coltrane would be camping in the Bahamas. Even the backpacking kids who floated around the Caribbean stayed in the youth hostels, rather than be brutalized by the flies and mosquitoes in the brush. Most likely, the Coltranes were on the water somewhere. It would take time to sift through the many fishing charter and scuba diving operators on the island. But the Cuban had all the time in the world.

Chapter 47

Eleuthera
June 25
3:11AM

The wind shifted at three in the morning, clocking around to the southwest. Coltrane stirred as the boat swung gently on the anchors, moving like a weathervane to point nose into the freshening breeze. Coltrane went topside to check the anchors. He saw the main anchor line running taut into the clear water, saw it disappear below the shimmering surface. The sailboat had moved ninety degrees from her original position, but the anchors were holding her well. Coltrane sat on the deck of the boat, and looked up at the stars above. The cloudless Caribbean sky was dazzling, the stars bright and clear, unobscured by city lights or smog. Coltrane found Orion, Polaris, and traced the Milky Way. He breathed deep, leaned back against the shiny steel mainmast, and let the magnificence of the sky bathe over him. Even at night, the water was crystal clear, the depths visible. At first glance it seemed blue, featureless. As Coltrane watched, he saw past the reflections on the surface, and fathomed deeper, saw light penetrate into the emerald water, saw tiny fish, gars, shadows and motions in the crystalline pools of light. The rhythmic swaying of the sloop and the sound of the waves lapping lulled him into a trance.

The boat was gently rocking, the waves lapping at the sides of the craft. He sat in the cockpit, laying back and looking at the night sky. Pliedes was overhead, first five stars, then six, ever elusive. Orion descended in the night sky, moving towards the horizon. To the west, he could see the lights of Nassau, bright against the darkness of the ocean.

It was a full strawberry moon, and the tides were high. The flow off the sound would be strong tonight, and he had prepared for the tidal surges by laying two anchors in a Bahamian Moor. He walked along the side of the sloop, hunched over to keep his balance as the boat rocked back and forth. He checked the anchor rodes as they angled off into the dark water, one taut as a rod of steel, the other lying slack in the sparkling water.

The Hunter was a beautiful boat, designed for speed, but easily adapted to cruising. It was a sloop, narrow and fast, with a racing heritage. The single mast held a self-furling, Kevlar reinforced mainsail. Providing the driving force for the sloop was the huge foresail, also self-furling. The running gear was all placed in the aft cockpit, easily reached by the crew. Two people could easily sail this boat without difficulty. Four large self-tailing winches were set into the forward cockpit, and the console with the electronics was set slightly behind the sail controls. GPS, AutoHelm and the VHF radio were arranged under a plexiglas protective shield at the wheel.

He sat back in the sculpted fiberglass cockpit, admiring the design and beauty of the sailboat. No experiences in his life equaled the wonder and thrill of ocean sailing. Few people would ever know the pleasure of mooring alone in a remote, pristine anchorage. The dangers involved in getting there and the beauty of the unspoiled wilderness were exhilarating. The soft glow of the cockpit light cast a halo on the surroundings; the gently swaying mast rising into the night sky, the well oiled teak benches and the sparkling stainless steel wheel. He could hear the wind whistling through the guy wires and stays. He could have stayed in that moment for the rest of eternity.

The sense of rapid motion startled him out of his dreams. He felt, rather than saw, the sleek gray shadow move past his vision. Startled, he pulled back from the edge of the boat as the dolphin came up from under the keel, and rolled over, looking at Coltrane with a curious eye. Then it was gone. Coltrane stood up, and opened his hands, holding his arms above his head to show the dolphin that he was harmless, a friend. He wanted to dive into the water, to somehow communicate with this beautiful, intelligent creature. He heard the dolphin surface just out of sight, heard him exhale heavily, blowing into the air. He went to the stern of the boat, and sat in the transom by the faintly glowing stern light, hoping the dolphin would return. For a long time he waited, listening to the dolphin's intermittent surfacing and exhaling, the soft puffs of air blowing through the warm water. Then it was gone.

Chapter 48

Eleuthera
June 25
7:55AM

The rising sun heated the stateroom, and Coltrane and Britt allowed the warmth to permeate their bodies. They luxuriated in the soft sheets, and resisted the urge to rise. Coltrane encircled his wife in his arms, and rocked her in time with the boat's slow motion. They made love tenderly, and drifted back to sleep.

By the time they eventually got up and ate breakfast, cleared their heads, it was almost eleven o'clock. Coltrane knew that it was far too late to attempt the crossing to the Exumas that day, and Britt enjoyed the excuse to stay another day in the perfect little bay. Coltrane swam down the anchor lines and checked both the main and secondary hooks, setting them well into the soft sand. He drifted in the salty water, face up, gazing up the steel cables that secured the sixty-foot mast. The boat was gorgeous, clean and sparkling new. The brilliant white of the fiberglass body shone in the sun, reflecting onto the blue rippled water.

Britt emerged from the belowdecks wearing nothing but black thong panties. Coltrane watched her move, with feline grace, out along the narrow gunnel and fore to lay topless on the sundeck. Coltrane had known women before he met her, but none had her natural sensuality. Few women had it and it couldn't be taught, he thought. He could never define or describe the essence of her, he just knew the instant he had first laid eyes on her that she was fine and rare.

The moves she made. The way she arched her back as she lay on the deck, one coltish leg flexed, arms over her head. The sinuous way she moved. The way she would look at him over a dropped shoulder.

Her body caught the light and beads of sweat glittered in the hollows of her flat belly, along her lean muscular thighs. She had a swimmer's body, sleek and athletic, well defined. Even from the water, he could see the cuts on her thigh and calves, the delicate arch of her foot. He knew the feel of her, the taut stretch of her skin over young muscle, the velvet smoothness of her body. Coltrane watched her for several minutes, drank in her beautiful, lithe body and then rolled on his back and thanked God for his life, and his hard won dreams.

They decided to play the day and night away, but before the rum lamp was lit, Coltrane had to contact Tampa. He set up the computer and the satellite phone, running the antenna up onto the deck. He dialed into the New York trunk line for AOL. The service came on, and Coltrane found his mailbox empty. He composed a message for Susan.

E-mail
June 25
3:55:27 PM
From: WmColtraneMD
To: SKerr

> Would you arrange a media interview? There are some points that I want to express to Elizabeth. I will be available to talk via phone for the next several hours. Send me an update on the schedule for the conference.
> wc

Coltrane sent the E-mail message, and leaned back on the built-in settee in the salon, contemplating his next step with the FBI. He had already deliberately misled them, so he doubted that another fabrication would matter. Picking up the sat phone, he dialed the number for the New York FBI office, and felt the knot in his gut tighten as it rang. A female voice answered. Coltrane introduced himself, and the woman replied that they had been awaiting his call. As he had hoped, the chief investigator was out of the office for lunch, and would return in twenty minutes. Coltrane explained the situation, and asked for an appointment the following afternoon. She gave him his choice of times, and scheduled the meeting. Before she could ask for a contact number, Coltrane thanked her and hung up. He had given himself another twenty-four hours. Coltrane turned off the computer and the phone, and prepared a picnic lunch for the beach. It would be some time before he could do anything further.

Coltrane dragged in the heavy inflatable dinghy and threw their snorkel gear into the bow. Britt handed him the food and drinks, and they stepped in. When he had the outboard motor running strong, he released the slip line, and headed for shore. They cruised in lazy circles over the gardens of coral and sea grass, seeing a profusion of marine life. Coltrane dropped the dinghy anchor near a trio of coral heads that formed a tiny protected cave, teeming with tiny brightly colored fish. They snorkeled in the warm water for hours, playing with the curious angelfish. Tired from the swimming and diving, they rowed to the beach, ate and lay in the sand, relaxed and peaceful. Twice, they made love in the powdery soft sand. Spent and exhausted, Coltrane slept deeply.

Britt woke him as the tide came in and the sun began to set. They got into the Zodiac and made their way back to the boat, and washed off in the transom shower. Coltrane set up the computer and satellite phone. He dialed the New York access number and checked his E-mail. He had one message.

E-mail
June 25
7:43:21 PM
From: SKerr
To: WmColtraneMD

> Things heating up here in anticipation of the conference.
> Hospitals are angry that elective admissions have dropped off sharply. No one is admitting patients because they are planning to attend the conference all week. Insurance companies have increased the pressure, calling this a strike in the media. ERs are full with routine problems, colds, flu, back pain, etc. Pressure on the physicians, threats of losing hospital privileges or being dumped from HMO lists.
> Some members are quitting the society.
> Need media support. Call Elizabeth.
> She is in her office all afternoon.
> Good luck.
> sk

Coltrane closed the AOL program and sat still on the settee for several minutes. He calmed himself with a series of deep breathing exercises, taught him years ago by his martial arts master. Breathing slowly and from the belly, he gradually obliterated the unrelenting, distracting thoughts from his consciousness. He concentrated upon the task at hand. At peace and focused, he dialed the main switchboard of the newspaper.

Elizabeth Volk had been awaiting Coltrane's call. She had been assigned to the newspaper's medical desk just two months ago. Hardly a sought after appointment, she had accepted that it was part of paying her dues in the long climb up the ladder. The recent controversy involving the city-wide medical conference and the interview with Dr. Coltrane in his office had pushed her into immediate prominence in the newsroom. As the situation intensified, the veteran newspaper columnists and reporters were coming to her for reference and background information on the personalities and issues at hand. She reveled in the attention. And if she could pull off an exclusive interview with Coltrane, maybe she would find her way out of the hemorrhoid and acne department sooner rather than later.

She took the call that had been directed to her by the operator, and switched on a small recording device attached to her phone. She leaned back and looked at the prepared list of questions her editor had given her, and introduced herself to Coltrane.

"Dr. Coltrane, this is Elizabeth Volk. Susan Kerr asked me if I would present the society's positions. I would like to record this interview, if that is acceptable?"

"I have no objections as long as you provide me with a copy."

"Certainly. I understand that you are out of town, Dr. Coltrane?"

"Yes, unfortunately I had prior commitments. The conference will proceed very well without me, I'm sure. As president, I am really just a figurehead and spokesperson for the society. Physicians are, and have always been, very independent."

"In our previous interviews, you delineated very well the issues that physicians face in modern healthcare, and the solutions that you feel are needed. But now this conference has developed a life of its own. The HMO insurance entities claim that you are using financial blackmail to achieve your goals, and that you are extorting them with the blood and suffering of the patients of Tampa-St. Pete. They claim that your membership has violated the terms of their contracts, and that they intend to bring suit against each and every doctor refusing to see patients. Additionally, they claim that there are provisions in the provider agreements that allow for this, and even specify that fines and damages may be recouped by the HMO in the event of breach of contract by the participating physicians. How do you respond?"

"The charges of blackmail and extortion are ridiculous, and do not merit comment. As far as breach of contract, do they expect that the physician will never attend a conference? Or take a vacation? Again, that is ridiculous. We are trying to improve healthcare for everyone. This is our goal."

"Your only goal?" she persisted.

"The society has many long range goals to improve the delivery of healthcare in the Bay area, but the most pressing problem at this time is to limit the influence and interference of third parties in the practice of medicine. In our first conference weeks ago, the membership voiced a very strong and unanimous opinion that critical decision making has been taken out of the hands of the physician and the patient. Our primary goal is to return the control of medical decisions to physicians and patients."

"I think the real question here is what means you will use to achieve these goals."

"Absolutely nothing illegal. We have retained legal counsel to advise us; a very established and reputable firm specializing in labor law. Our meetings are now in the stage where we are in specialty planning groups. It is my hope that each group will draw up and present a list of problems and immediate solutions for these problems. I will present them to the state insurance board, and hope that they will be acted upon quickly. I should mention that I have personally requested meetings with the insurance executives and their representatives, and repeatedly they have refused to meet with us. If nothing significant arises from the state insurance board, I plan to go to Tallahassee to the Florida state legislature with the proposals."

"How do you respond to the allegations that this is an illegal strike, a tactic to increase doctors' fees at the expense of the public? Along those lines, is an increase in your fees on your agenda?"

"First of all, this is not a strike or a labor action. I stress again that the physicians' offices are providing continuity of care, even if a different physician may attend the patient. You probably know that is the norm in most other countries. Americans are used to the luxury of a personal physician, a luxury unknown elsewhere in the Western world, especially in countries with socialized medicine. The public may be inconvenienced for the short term, but the gains in the long term will justify the minor inconvenience. Secondly, the current fee structure is unfair and confusing and we will try to make it more equitable."

"How can you complain about physician incomes with any clear conscience? Physicians are one of the best paid groups in the country?"

"Actually, we are behind lawyers and entertainers, by a long, long way. But income is not the issue here. Reasonable reimbursement is the issue. How can our society justify 55 million dollars to someone for playing on a football field thirteen times a year, but pay a physician fifteen dollars for the physical examination of a sick human being. Bear in mind that physicians are our most highly trained and educated professionals, in some cases spending ten years of intense study after college to even qualify to treat patients. These are important and valuable skills, and need to be viewed as such."

"Still, there is common feeling that this is an illegal strike. Can you comment on the status of the FBI anti-trust investigation?"

"There were complaints filed with the federal court, and that is all I know."

"Have you spoken with the FBI?"

"Yes, and I told them just what I told you."

"Dr. Coltrane, I have what I need for the column today. May I contact you as things progress?"

"You can contact me through Susan Kerr, or via the Internet. Susan has my E-mail address. I will be glad to answer any questions you may have."

"Thank you for your time." Elizabeth finished, hung up and disconnected the recorder from the line. She frowned, disappointed that nothing significant had surfaced in the interview. Next time she would have to press him harder. No more kid gloves for the doctor.

Coltrane hung up the phone, thinking of the things he should have said as he turned off the transceiver. The interview had been too short, too abbreviated. There was so much more that he had wanted to get across to her, to her readers. Maybe next time.

He got up and made two Myers's Rum and Cokes, slicing a fresh lime in quarters. He climbed out of the salon, into the cockpit. Britt sat watching the sunset, a loose cotton sundress draping over her body, clinging to her tanned, lithe legs, revealing her taut form. Coltrane sat close to her, gave her the drink. The ice tinkled in her glass as she touched his. They drank in a comfortable silence, watching the sun's spectacular descent into a sapphire sea.

Chapter 49

June 26
5:56 AM

Coltrane was up with the sun, and had the coffee brewing after he did a preliminary survey of the sloop and the anchor lines. He ate a quick breakfast, and allowed Britt to sleep late. While he sipped the dark, aromatic coffee he plotted the day's sail. The Exuma Cays were still nine hours sail away, and this passage was difficult in a different way. To sail from the big island of Eleuthera to the Exumas meant passing through a vast garden of coral heads, some reaching to the surface of the shallow sea. The coral grew on a sandbar that ran the full length of Eleuthera, then tapered over the miles to form a narrow fingerlike projection upon which the tiny Exuma Cays lay.

The Exuma Cays are felt to be the most pristine, most spectacular group of tropical islands in the world. The Exumas are an archipelago of low lying, sandy cays that have the finest white powder sand and clearest turquoise water known to man. All dreams of paradise must have originated here. The first time that Coltrane had sailed here, he had not wanted to leave. Ever.

Coltrane checked the charts and compared them to the aerial photographs that his charterguide provided. He mapped a course for Beacon Cay, the northernmost of the Exumas. He finished his coffee, and took his time stowing loose gear and securing supplies in the cabin. By this time, Britt was up, moving sleepily about the cabin. He cranked up the diesel, and prepared to weigh anchor.

The passage was slow and nerve-racking. Coltrane guided Britt from the bow, leaning out over the pulpit and hanging onto the metal spine of the jib, searching the shallow water for a path through the coral heads. He preferred to motor this leg of the trip, because sailing did not allow for rapid turns. They started slow, as he gained confidence in reading the depths. The underwater panorama was frighteningly beautiful. The water was so crystal clear that he could easily see the ripples in the white sand bottom, smooth irregular wave patterns, perfectly spaced and perfectly parallel. The coral heads were large, some eight or ten feet in diameter, rising off the sandy bottom. Their mushroom shaped domes ascended to within inches of the surface in areas, and Coltrane intensely scanned the water in their path as they motored along.

The shoreline had vanished from view long ago, and they found themselves in the center of an ocean of varied colors, the white sand visible between the dark brown and black of the coral and rocks. Coltrane knew that the sailboat drew nearly five feet of water, and Britt had been reading out the depthmeter at a constant ten feet. That gave him less than a five foot safety factor; five feet between the top of the winged keel and the sandy bottom. Judging the size of the coral heads to be at least six feet, he knew that he would never be able to clear one of them. Further complicating the task of determining the amount of water under the keel was the scattered clouds, reflecting shadows on the surface of the water. As Coltrane scanned the water and checked shadows on the surface against the small cumulus clouds above, he watched a single engine plane far in the distance as it made a slow turn towards them. Britt waved as it passed overhead and continued flying towards Eleuthera. Coltrane thought once again about his dream of starting a small charter flight service in the out islands, then Britt's shriek brought him back to reality as they narrowly missed a huge coral head. He concentrated once again, his head hurting from the sun, his eyes squinting against the dazzling glare.

Seven hours later, they emerged from the maze of coral and rocks to glide into deep water east of the Exuma Cays. The cays were the boundary between a large shallow body of water on the west and the much deeper Exuma Sound on the east. Over thousands of years, the coral and limestone deposits from the shallow sea had gradually formed the tiny islands, and the small reef that protected them.

Coltrane brought the sloop even with the first of the many small cays, and then took a heading parallel with the line of islands. He needed to refuel, and get some more block ice and cold beer. He headed for the small marina at Highburn Cay that served the northern half of the Exumas. He knew the owner there; he had removed a deep fishhook from his wife three years ago. Coltrane hoped that Calvin would be there. He went below and called the marina on the radio, requesting fuel and water. Calvin answered and told him to come right in, there were no other boats at the dock at the time.

Coltrane turned off the radio and went topside to the two large gear lockers in the cockpit. He selected three large oblong bumpers to protect the sides of the boat, and hung them on the starboard side of the sloop. He shortened the line to the dinghy to prevent it from being caught in the prop as the boat slowed. Then he swung into the cockpit, taking the helm from Britt. She laid out the bow and stern lines as he piloted the large sailboat through the small channel cut into the little bay. The small marina and fuel dock lay to the north, with a beautiful little cove opening to the south. In the cove were anchored several sailboats of varying size and age. On a chartered thirty-six foot Beneteau, a middle aged couple sat in the cockpit, and waved cheerily at Coltrane. Nodding back, he slowed the boat to a crawl, barely making headway as they prepared for docking. The inertia of a cruising yacht was tremendous, and Coltrane had seen boats and pilings destroyed by inexperienced skippers who underestimated the mass of their craft.

He got the sloop nearly dead in the water, and gave the helm to Britt as he went forward to handle the lines. As the boat inched up to the wooden dock, a huge black man came out onto the rickety structure, flashing a toothy smile. Calvin welcomed them back to the islands, and took the stern line Coltrane handed him. He expertly flipped a loop around one of the oil-stained pilings and the boat swung gently to the pier and stopped. Coltrane stepped off the bow with the bow line and secured it to the cleat on the dock.

Calvin and Coltrane adjusted the bumpers between the sailboat and the dock, then turned to each other and warmly shook hands. Calvin Persons was six foot six, and close to three hundred pounds. A lifetime of hard labor in the islands and on the New Orleans docks had given him strong, calloused hands. He was not losing his strength with age, Coltrane noticed, even if he was carrying some excess weight. His warm smile was studded with a gold capped incisor that flashed in the bright Caribbean sun.

"How's Shirley?" Coltrane asked about Calvin's wife.

"Fine. Her hand is just fine, Doc. Maybe you should open a practice down here when you retire, eh?" Calvin grinned.

"Maybe I should, Cal. What's the weather look like for the next week?" Coltrane asked as he opened the fuel cap and began to pump the diesel into the boat.

"Weather looks good for the next few days, low pressure over ESE. I got a message from Dennis for you, too. I wrote it inside, in the office. What else you need?"

"Amstel Light and some block ice. And some fresh water. How much for the water?" Coltrane knew that fresh water for boats was sometimes more expensive than fuel. He shot a sideways glance at Britt as he asked. The issue of her long, hot showers always came up when they had to refill the fresh water tanks.

"Screw you." Britt laughed at him. "You want me to skip showering, Captain? Fill it up and take it out of my allowance."

"Seventy cents a gallon, Doc. Better keep the lady happy, my advice." Calvin left them to tend to the boat, and went to get the beer and ice.

Coltrane finished and walked up the dock to meet him in the office, a small aluminum shed with a drink cooler and photos of trophy fish and local guides taped on the walls. Fishing tackle and boating supplies were displayed, attached to the ceiling by wire. Calvin could do most marine repairs, and was a decent diesel mechanic. He was limited only in his access to parts. Everything in the Bahamas was imported, and freight and taxes were expensive. Twice Coltrane had sent Calvin parcels full of specialty items that he needed and couldn't find here. Things could get boring on a remote island, even if it was paradise.

"Need anything from the States, Cal?"

"No, we're fine. Thanks for the Florida Gators hat. My nephew loves it."

"No problem."

"Let me find your message. Here it is…Dennis spoke to two friends of yours but did not give them your itinerary. He will if you want him to. That's it."

"Friends of mine? Here, in the Bahamas? Or on the phone?" Coltrane was confused.

"I think he meant in Marsh Harbor." Calvin had not given the message much thought.

"Can I use your phone, Cal?" Coltrane asked quickly, hoping to catch Dennis before he left for the day.

Calvin nodded, and turned the dial phone around on the countertop for Coltrane to use. Coltrane dialed the number, finding it in the tattered Yellow Pages. The phone rang for a full minute before it was answered.

"Hello, this is Bill Coltrane. Is Dennis there?"

"One moment."

"This is Dennis." He sounded winded.

"Dennis, this is Bill Coltrane. You have a message for me?" Coltrane sounded perplexed.

"Yeah, Doc. Are you planning to meet two guys here? They say that they missed hooking up with you."

"They came to the charter base? Looking for me?" Coltrane felt his heart racing.

"Yeah, two days ago. I don't ever release information about our clients without their consent, but one of the guys talked to a dock hand who checked the charter sheet and told them which boat you had taken out. I didn't give them your plans, but I can if you want me to. They were friends of yours."

"Describe them."

"One was from the States, he did all the talking. Tall, skinny, maybe twenty-five years old. The other guy was Latin, older, shorter and stocky. He didn't say anything."

"Did they leave you any names?"

"No."

"If you see them again, don't give them any information about our plans. We don't want any guests, and I don't know who they are. Alright?"

"Absolutely. I wouldn't have said anything, but that dock hand loves to talk, and the cat's out of the bag. They didn't look like friends of yours, anyway."

"What do you mean?"

"Well, not to insult your friends, but they were sort of sleazy, like they wanted to sell you something. One had a tattoo on his knuckles, real amateur job."

"No, thanks for your honesty, Dennis. I don't know anyone that fits your description. Just don't tell anyone anything about our trip, please."

"No, sir. Sorry about this." Dennis finished, and hung up.

Coltrane slowly replaced the receiver, and looked up at Calvin, who had been listening to the entire exchange. No one knew that they were in the Bahamas, not even their parents or family. Britt had protested going without telling her mother and father, but Coltrane had insisted on absolute secrecy. And he hadn't told anyone. The airline tickets were purchased with cash, leaving no credit card trail to follow. Coltrane was puzzled and concerned.

"Not friends of yours?" Calvin asked, frowning.

"No one I recognize by Dennis' description."

"Well, watch yourself, *mon.* We had two yacht hijackings last year. Three people killed. Vicious."

"Fuck. The one time I travel without a gun, I get trouble."

"Guns are outlawed in the Bahamas now, Doc. Don't you get caught with one now. You don't want to go to Fox Hill Prison, that the worst hellhole in the world."

Coltrane walked out to the office door and looked around the dock. The area was empty, no one to be seen. He returned to the counter, and leaned close to Calvin looking him level in the eyes. "You sure that there are no guns at all on this island? I want one if you can find one for me. Cash, no records of the sale."

"Doc, if there was a gun here, I would try to get it for you, believe me. But there just plain ain't no guns here. We don't need guns here. Only four people on the island. No lions, tigers or bears." He flashed a big toothy smile and laughed aloud.

Coltrane laughed with him, and shook his hand after paying for the supplies and the fuel. Calvin cracked a beer, and they walked out along the dock to the sleek sloop. The tide was rising. It was late, and the sun was setting. Calvin helped Coltrane cast off. The marina was too small and cramped to spend the night, and Coltrane preferred the peace of an open water anchorage. They waved goodbye, and Britt piloted the sailboat out of the cove, and to a sheltered half-moon bay on the leeward side of the island. Coltrane dropped the small secondary anchor as he surveyed the tide and current before selecting a place to anchor for the night.

Just as he was savoring the idea of a night alone with his bride in this spectacular anchorage, he saw the thirty-six foot Beneteau come motoring around the point, headed directly for their position. Coltrane cursed outloud.

"What's the matter?" asked Britt.

"We've got company. Fuck."

Tropical vacations mean many things to many people, and yacht charters were no different. Some people take their kids on the dream trip, hoping that it will be a lifetime memory. Some couples come for romance, during the intense infatuation phase of courtship. Some couples go purely for the adventure. Still others savor the companionship of fellow travelers, and seek interaction with new friends. The Coltranes went purely to get away from the rat race, away from all contact with strangers, away from the stress and rigors of dealing with people. Coltrane got plenty of that in his practice, he needed to escape it in his vacations. During the course of a day at the office, he might insert his finger in the rectum of two or three strangers. You just don't get much more personal than that. And that is why Coltrane preferred the solitude and peace of yachting to any other form of vacation. Over the years, Britt had come to understand and respect that.

As he watched the yacht bearing directly for them, Coltrane realized that this couple was looking for some friendly companionship. Any other time, and he would have been glad to see them. Often the long passages made sailors crave human contact. But not tonight.

The middle-aged sailor waved, and pointed toward an area to the lee of *Blue Pearl*. Coltrane acknowledged his courtesy request to anchor near his yacht, and the man slowly and cautiously circled, yelling orders to his flustered wife, and dropped anchor. Midway through the process, the wife cursed loudly at the man, and went below. By himself, he struggled to set the two anchors.

Britt and Coltrane sat in the cockpit of *Blue Pearl* and watched the farce with amusement.

"That looks like the way we did it the first ten times," Coltrane laughed.

"Until you learned not to yell at me."

"Sometimes you screw up, and I have to yell. You don't get second chances on a boat at sea. I take our safety very seriously."

"You don't have to yell orders at me like I'm one of your lackeys."

"*One* of my lackeys? I wish I had a few lackeys. You are my only lackey, babe," Coltrane laughed.

As they were talking, the VHF Radio crackled and came to life.

"*Blue Pearl, Blue Pearl*, this is *Nautique*. Come in please."

"*Nautique*, this is *Blue Pearl*." Coltrane replied.

"Would you care to join us for a cocktail? I'm buying."

Coltrane took his thumb off the handset and looked at Britt for an answer. She had been a very shy girl when Coltrane met her years ago, and despite his gradual attempts to immerse her in the whirlwind of medical society, she still avoided most social interactions. She was starting to shake her head no, when the woman came above decks and waved a huge bottle of Pusser's rum.

"Who can refuse a Pusser's and Coke?" she grinned, her spirits momentarily lifted.

"Sure, *Nautique*, we will be right over." Coltrane responded.

They grabbed a nice bottle of merlot from the provisions, and stepped down through the transom and into the Zodiac. Within seconds, they were tying up to the stern of the *Nautique*, and being helped aboard by their hosts.

"You're Americans, right? Where from?" the man asked immediately.

"Bill and Britt Coltrane, from Tampa," Coltrane replied, as he shook the man's hand.

I'm Dr. Judith Berkin-Tayler, and this is my husband, Stephen. We're from Boston."

"Steve," the yachtsman said, somewhat apologetic for his wife's formal bearing. "Would you like a Painkiller?" He referred to the local favorite, a mixture of two types of rum, pineapple juice, mango juice, coconut milk and pureed papaya.

The Coltranes agreed and sat on the port settee, and Judith sat on the starboard settee, as Steve poured two drinks for his guests. They all sat back and watched the sun set.

"Bill is a physician also, what is your specialty." Britt asked Judith.

"Really?" Judith looked at Coltrane, clearly unimpressed. "I have a doctorate from Vassar in the history of the romance languages. But I really specialize in poetry, mostly sixteenth to eighteenth century."

Steve sat quietly, as if he had been through this before.

"The poets and the poetry of that era are divine, unbelievably pure and deep. Are you familiar with Joachim Du Bellay and Pierre de Ronsard?"

"No, I never got into poetry in any depth. Just what we learned in high school," Britt was beginning to feel stupid.

"There are no poets anymore," Judith declared, and leaned back to sip her rum.

"No poets?" Coltrane laughed, and looked at Steve. "Ever heard of Bob Dylan? John Lennon? Don Henley? Tom Waits? Tom Petty? Jagger and Richards? B.B. King? Muddy Waters? Iggy Pop? Janis Jop…"

"Jesus Christ! You think Iggy Pop is a poet? That's laughable," Judith interrupted.

"Okay," Coltrane laughed. "Maybe he has been guilty of some weak lyrics, but they all are poets by any definition. Better than poets. They write the lyrical poetry and then put it to music as well. How can that not be poetry?"

"Poetry is about the questions of life, the meaning of the universe and our eternal soul. Mick Jagger is a misogynist who sings about sex and rock and roll. And drugs. Our society has been destroyed by drugs. I detest people who glorify drug abuse."

"I agree with that," Coltrane answered calmly. Holding his glass of rum high up in the air, he continued. "This is a very destructive drug, the demon alcohol. More deaths, more disease, more lost days of work, more decreased productivity, and disability than any drug known to man, except perhaps cigarettes. But I have to admit, this is my favorite drug."

Judith glared at him, momentarily ceasing to sip her drink.

Coltrane smiled at her pause. "Don't stop drinking, now. As the Irish proverb goes, 'Take the drink for the thirst yet to come'."

"And the Scottish proverb, 'He who decries my drinking, never thinks of my thirst'." Steve replied.

The two men grinned, and touched glasses.

"Now that is true poetry. And just because Mick Jagger sings about chasing tail doesn't make him any less of a poet. I based my adolescence on the Rolling Stones… "Under my Thumb", "Satisfaction", …those songs had much more meaning to me than Walt Whitman or a twenty page poem about trees."

"Bill, shut up. What the hell do you know about poetry?" Britt glared at him.

"Steve, you know the story of Pusser's Rum?" Coltrane laughed and changed the subject.

"No, tell me," Steve leaned forward, glad that the topic had been changed before he would be forced to enter the discussion on his wife's side.

"Pusser's rum was the official royal purveyor of rum to the Royal Navy for years, since before Lord Nelson. That's what they made grog from."

"Grog?" Judith asked.

"Grog was a mixture of one part rum, three parts water, plus some lime juice to combat scurvy and maybe brown sugar. The recipe varied from ship to ship, but the intent was the same. Life on a seventeenth century warship was very hard, and discipline was brutal. The sailors needed something to keep them happy, and the officers needed something to numb the crew enough for them to brave the horrors of naval warfare. So every afternoon and before any battle, the crew got their daily ration of grog. That's where the word *groggy* comes from. The practice continued into the Second World War, I think."

"Very interesting. I'd heard of grog, but I thought it was just slang for hard liquor," Steve sat back, and swirled his drink and sipped it.

"Actually, it's slang for *grogham,* a kind of cloak that Admiral Vernon, the inventor of the recipe, used to wear. And *Pusser* is corrupted from the ship's *purser*, the sailor responsible for the ship's stores."

"Where in the hell did you learn all this useful trivia?" Judith asked sarcastically.

"Off a Pusser's bottle, I think." Coltrane laughed.

"Perfect." Steve laughed with him.

"How do you like the boat?" Coltrane asked, looking around the vessel. It showed signs of hard use, and misuse.

"Beneteaus are great. I picked this one up in Georgetown, they ferried it over from Eleuthera for us. No one is allowed to sail down here in a chartered boat. Did you sail from Tampa?" Steve turned his head and admired *Blue Pearl.*

"No, we chartered in the Abacos. We have sailed over here a couple of times, and they are beginning to trust us. It's not a fun passage."

"Damn, you two must be good sailors. That is a long, difficult trip. Two, three days?"

"It's two days, and more tedious than physically hard." Coltrane put his arm around Britt, suddenly proud of her nautical skills.

"Stephen, when you are finished kissing the doctor's ring, pour me another drink," Judith said, clearly annoyed.

"We will finish ours, and then we'd better get going. I've got to move the boat and I want to leave early in the morning."

"Did I park too close to you?" Steve looked at the distance between the two yachts, afraid that he had committed an error choosing his anchorage.

"No, no, you did fine. It's just that Britt makes a lot of noise when I spank her, and I don't want to keep you guys up." Coltrane smiled a huge grin, and lifted Britt up from the settee, guiding her to the Zodiac before she could castigate him.

"Nice meeting you," Judith said, half rolling her eyes and not getting up from the cockpit.

"Same here," Coltrane got into the Zodiac, and made momentary eye contact with the man, as if to apologize for debating with the guy's wife.

"Safe trip." Steve flipped the line to Britt as they pushed off the stern of the *Nautique*.

As they whipped the quick little dinghy around and shot toward *Blue Pearl*, Britt gave Coltrane a dirty look. He said nothing until they were back on the boat.

"Sorry, honey, but that woman just aggravated the fuck out of me. She calls herself 'Doctor' right out of the gate, and demands respect for that? I'll bet you that she's one of those patients that refer to their physician by his first name, too. Doctor of fucking poetry? Her poor parents probably paid over $200,000 for that degree, and I would bet you a hummer that she has never made a single cent on her own. Plus a hyphenated last name. What happens when two people with hyphenated last names get married? Will it be like Spanish royalty, with twenty last names? No more poets, she says. What a cunt."

"Don't use that word around me." Britt snapped.

"Sorry. She just irritated me. That is the beauty of America, everybody is free to voice their opinion, regardless of how little they know about the topic. I saw some washed up old crone British actress on the national news last night, giving her views on the American Presidency. Who the hell cares what an actress thinks about politics and world history? And a foreign actress as well. Jesus."

"You can't stand it when a woman speaks her mind."

"If she has a mind. But it's not just women. Look at that Irish rock star, whatever his name is, Bozo or Bobo or some shit, running all over the world like he is some UN diplomat, pressuring the US to increase foreign aid. Why doesn't he just tour again, and donate the $200 million to AIDS research? That would actually be helpful. Or solve the problems in his Northern Ireland?"

"You done?" Britt had learned to tolerate his occasional tirades, and let them run their course.

"Almost. Did you see the outfit she had on? Two inch heels and diamond jewelry on a sailboat? And a huge skirt to hide her fat ass? The uglier and older the woman, the more jewelry you see." Coltrane took a deep breath, looked once toward *Nautique,* and went below.

Coltrane fired up the diesel, and turned on the mast light. As Britt manned the helm, he went fore and pulled the small Danforth anchor up easily. With him watching the water depth, she made a long sweeping curve and they dropped anchor a mile away from the original site. He had Britt position the boat in the center of the small bay, and threw out the secondary anchor only. He needed time and space to think. Something was bothering him, and he didn't know exactly what it was.

Coltrane had felt uneasy since the conversation with Calvin. Initially, the news from Dennis had not registered as danger. He knew that the FBI would eventually query the airlines and a ticket check would show that they were in the Abacos. Or check with the Customs and Immigration Service who would have record of their passage through Miami Customs. He had anticipated that eventually their whereabouts would become known. But he had hoped that the process would give them enough time to achieve the conference goals. They had tracked him too quickly.

Then, as he sat in the dark cockpit alone, it hit him. The plane! The single engine aircraft that he had noticed this afternoon had flown over the boat, in a wide arc. He plotted the position of the boat and the plane in his mind, and realized that it could only have come from the Abacos. But it flew over them, and then circled back to Eleuthera. His mind was racing, searching for an explanation. Whoever had been in that plane had spotted them, and flew to the nearest airport to touch down. Who had followed them here? He thought frantically. Why?

He went below, and pulled his charts of the Bahamas out onto the teak dining table. The nearest airport was on Eleuthera, at Deep Creek. He plotted his previous position at the time of the flyover, and calculated the bearing to the airport from that spot. The direction coincided with the plane's path. They had flown to Deep Creek at about two that afternoon.

Coltrane paced the cabin nervously deciding if he should alarm Britt with his suspicions. She came below after shutting off the diesel and checking the anchor line. She could tell something was very wrong, and concern lined her loving face. Coltrane related the discussion with Dennis and his conclusions about the plane flyover. He showed her the location of the airport on Eleuthera. The nearest harbor was Powell Point.

"How far is that from here?" Britt asked, looking for their little bay on the chart.

"Twenty-five nautical miles to Powell Point."

"Well, we're a day ahead of them, if they want to follow us. We can get easily lost in the cays, can't we?"

"They know that we are at the north end of the Exumas. There aren't enough places to hide that I could guarantee they won't find us. My guess is that they will charter a fishing boat, maybe a fast sportfisherman. Our sailboat will motor at eight knots. Even a shitty little twenty foot center console fishing boat will do twenty, thirty, maybe forty knots. They can just cruise through the Exumas and run us down. We can't escape." Coltrane slumped into the settee, and cradled his head in his hands. In two short hours, their carefree vacation had become a nightmare.

"Who are they? What do they want?" Britt asked.

"FBI probably. They may want to serve me a subpoena. Who knows what's happening in the anti-trust action the Feds are bringing against me and the society?"

"How many FBI men have jailhouse tattoos on their hands?" Britt looked straight into Coltrane's eyes. She had seen many similar tattoos in his office, relics of someone's past that they regretted, wanted removed.

"Maybe they hired a local Bahamian process server. Maybe a private investigator from Miami. Who knows?"

"What if it's the insurance goons, the guys who killed Hendricks?" Britt was up, pacing back and forth in the small cabin. "They would have the cash to get here fast, and to hire a plane, and to hire a boat. And they have several very good reasons to want you dead. The tape of your conversation, and the compact disc."

Coltrane stiffened as he followed her logic to the obvious conclusion. She was right. Certainly the highest probability lay in her conclusion. Any number of people knew about the disc. Resendez could have been found and picked up by the killers. Or more likely, greed overcame wisdom and he simply tried to sell a copy of the disc back to the insurance company. Either way, his name would have come up in conversation. His stomach knotted with a sickening, hollow cramp. He looked up into the expectant eyes of his wife, anguished that he had delivered her into mortal danger.

"Let's go back to Marsh Harbor, or sail to Nassau. They will never find us in the city," Britt said.

"If you are right, and they are the insurance company's hired killers, then they're professionals. They killed Hendricks, and everyone still thinks it was an accident. They'll find us, and it will be easier to kill us in a city. I can't watch our backs constantly, and I don't even know what these guys look like."

"But there would be people around, they wouldn't be able to kill us in the open and get away. We can tell the police. They will track them down." Britt believed the system would protect them.

"And what do I tell the Bahamian police? That someone is after me? I don't have a description of them, or how many of them there are. The authorities here will check with the States, and who knows what the FBI will want with me. There may be a subpoena or warrant for my arrest for all we know. Even if we get back to the States without a problem, they will have months to kill us before the trial. We're fucked."

"Have you called the FBI today?"

"No. It's too late, eight o'clock in the evening in New York. By now they will know that I had no intention to meet with them and give a statement in New York. Lynwood will be looking for me. I guess I had better check *Caduceus*."

Coltrane set up the satellite phone, his practiced hands working swiftly. He entered *Caduceus* and checked his mailbox. In it was one message.

E-mail
June 26
2:35:42 PM
From: SKerr
To: WmColtraneMD

Dr. Coltrane
The meeting started today without a hitch.
The attendance was excellent, with 68% of the membership attending either the morning or the afternoon sessions. Groups are established with the specialties evaluating the possible courses of action. Media interested in the conference, and wanting to speak with you. They will run an interview with the insurance lobby this evening.
The lobby is calling this a strike, a work slowdown. We need to respond soon. When will you be back?

Your interview must have had a positive effect on Elizabeth, she wrote a nice article in today's paper about the need to change the healthcare system, and the problems that we face daily. I gave her all our position papers and have been talking with her frequently.
Otherwise, everything was status quo over the weekend. The FBI agent, Lynwood, called yesterday, big time pissed at you. He told me to tell you to call him immediately. If the FTC does not get our response to the complaint, they will file an injunction and close the conference. I think he wants to put you in jail.
Please call him.
When are you returning from New York?
sk

Coltrane sat and thought about his answer. The New York farce was wearing thin, and soon it would be obvious to Lynwood that they were not in the city. He would have to change the charade somehow. It had to be believable, because if Lynwood could show that he was evading contact, his suspicions that the conference was truly a labor action would be strengthened. Racking his brain for a foolproof story, Coltrane sent another E-mail.

E-mail
June 26
8:31:36 PM
From: WmColtraneMD
To: SKerr

> I have finished at the meeting here, and plan to take a short trip with Britt to Vermont. A friend of ours has a cabin in the mountains. I will keep in touch via *Caduceus*.
> I will call Lynwood.
> Thanks.
> wc

Coltrane opened his wallet, and found Lynwood's business card. Dialing the after hours number, he waited as the phone rang. He heard clicking as the call was routed to another line. Abruptly, Lynwood picked up the phone.

"Agent Lynwood."

"Lynwood, this is Coltrane. I'm sorry to call so late, but I missed the meeting with your New York office. I'm at a conference, and got tied up in a meeting." Coltrane paused to see where Lynwood would take the conversation.

"Dr. Coltrane, I need something substantial in the form of a statement from you immediately. Allegations have been made that your society is staging an illegal work slowdown. The only way that I can stop a judge from ordering an injunction against you and the entire society's membership is for you to show to me that what you are doing is legitimate. Do you understand?" Lynwood sounded conciliatory.

"Yes, I do. But what I don't understand is why so much attention is being directed to this conference. What makes it any different from the annual meetings of any other society? For example, the AMA meets for week long conferences every year, year in and year out. How is our conference different?" Coltrane asked politely.

"The complaint that has been filed alleges that you and your membership are conspiring to restrict availability of medical services to the public in order to negotiate higher fees with insurance carriers. This is illegal on several levels, violating both anti-trust laws and Medicare guidelines. Listen, Doctor Coltrane. I am not accusing you of any wrongdoing. My uncle is a family doctor in Chicago, and I empathize with your position. But I have to have your response to these accusations." Lynwood sounded almost friendly.

"I don't know what to tell you other than what I stated before. We are *not* orchestrating any type of labor action *whatsoever*. All specialties have provided complete coverage for patients and the local emergency rooms. The quality of patient care has not been, nor will it ever be, compromised. I will be glad to have Susan Kerr provide you with the society's position papers if you desire. Like I said before, the society is more like a social club than a labor union. As president, I don't make policy. I am a spokesperson only. All decisions are voted upon by the membership." Coltrane finished, hoping Lynwood would be appeased.

"Does your society have a secretary who records the minutes of each meeting?" Lynwood inquired.

"Yes." Coltrane was startled by the question. He knew minutes were taken, but was not sure what they said. Nor was he sure who was responsible for recording the minutes. But he was sure that he had followed the letter of the law in all his addresses to the membership. Every move had been cleared with the St. Petersburg law firm they had retained.

"If you will allow me to review those minutes, I may be able to clear you of these charges. Otherwise, I will be forced to subpoena you and the records in the morning. Help yourself out here, Doctor." Lynwood waited for a response.

"Alright. I will direct Susan Kerr to give you full access to the society minutes in the morning. You understand that some of the transcript may be censored if any patient names are mentioned during case presentations. Otherwise you will have unrestricted access to the record." Coltrane hoped that he would be cleared by Lynwood's review. Either way, Lynwood could easily get legal access to the transcripts.

"Good. I hope I can resolve this quickly." Lynwood concluded the discussion.

"Listen. One last question. And do me the honor of an honest answer." Coltrane asked quickly before Lynwood could hang up. "I think that I am being followed. I have had messages that two men are looking for me. Do you have agents trailing me for any reason?"

"No. Absolutely not. This is still a preliminary investigation, not a criminal prosecution. No one from the FBI is observing you. You have my word on that. Probably some old colleagues from medical school are trying to track you down. I will contact you after I have reviewed the minutes of your meetings. Goodnight, Doctor Coltrane." Lynwood hung up.

A chill went down Coltrane's spine despite the Caribbean heat surrounding him. The men searching for him were not FBI agents or officers of the court as he had hoped. They must be Hendricks' killers. He would have to stay far ahead of them to survive. Setting that thought aside, he sent another E-mail to Susan.

E-mail
June 26
9:55 PM
From: WmColtraneMD
To: SKerr

> Susan, please check with legal counsel if we can or should allow the FBI to review the minutes of the society meetings over which I presided. I think it will be OK. If possible, I want to let Lynwood examine them, but you must delete any patient names for confidentiality reasons.
>
> Thanks
> wc

Coltrane shut off the computer and satphone and sat on the settee, rocking back and forth, thinking. He computed the distance from the island of Eleuthera to their present position, and added additional time for transit from the airport and time to hire and provision a small boat. He realized that it was possible, if the timing was right, for them to arrive here tonight. There were only three islands of any interest to sailors in the northern end of the cays, and any idiot would check those three first. And Coltrane was anchored in the first of the three islands.

The sun had set, and the night was calm, clear. The breeze was from the east, and the moon was waxing, half full, and bright. Coltrane let the small anchor out, and decided not to drop the main anchor. If they had to run, weighing the main would take too much time. He would have to watch the water closely thorough the night. Coltrane didn't think he would sleep anyway.

Coltrane went belowdecks. The main cabin of the yacht was spacious, and in the manner of all sailing craft, incorporated function and utility in a compact and efficient design. The small galley kitchen area was located near the steps of the companionway, and all the cabinets storing food, water, spices, pots and pans lined the sides of the cabin at chest height. Above the teak cabinets, a row of watertight high-tech oval portholes allowed light in and enabled the crew below decks to observe the full 360 degree arc outside the cabin. Opposite the galley, a teak desk and swiveling stool sat below the banks of electrical switches and communications gear that was the heart of the boat's mechanical system. Two huge red switches controlled the batteries, and the radio and fresh water pumps and bilge pumps were operated from this station. The desk was illuminated by a tiny red map light and all the navigation equipment and charts were stored under the lift top of the teak desk.

Further forward of the galley and the nav desk, the salon grew wider near the beam of the sailboat. A huge aluminum shaft came from the center of the floor of the boat, and exited through the center of the ceiling of the salon. The shaft was the housing of the main mast, reaching from its position on the upper deck, down through the cabin, to sink its base into the lead counterweight of the keel. It was the massive five ton lead weight in the keel that kept the huge sailboat from heeling over in strong winds, and prevented the craft from being tossed about in heavy seas. When the portholes and hatches were sealed, and the companionway closed and sealed, the boat was virtually unsinkable. Unlike motor yachts, it would not rollover or founder, rather it would bob like a cork in the waves and weather the most vicious seas. Theoretically, at least.

In the center of the salon, astride the mainmast housing, was a large teak dining table, with folding leaves and an upholstered circular settee encircling the table on three sides. It was open on the stern end, near the nav desk. At night, the table could be lowered and custom fitted cushions placed between the edges of the seating area, forming a large queen sized bed. The sailboat was designed to sleep six in comfort, two in each of the two main cabins, and two on the salon bed. Fore and aft of the large salon were two staterooms, each with its own bathroom and freshwater shower. Coltrane always preferred to sleep in the larger fore cabin, opening the large hatch above the bed for ventilation. But tonight he would sleep on the deck.

Coltrane set up the main salon bed for Britt, and considered his options. Sailing at night in these waters was suicide, with no way to read the depths of the channels and see the coral heads. The boat drew five feet with its keel, and would certainly run aground or rip its belly open on a reef or coral head. They would have to stay in the bay, at least for tonight. Beyond tomorrow, he had no plan. Coltrane was getting very tired, the stress of the passage to the Exumas having taken its toll on his mind. He considered how he could keep a watch from the boat, and decided that the only way was to sleep out in the cockpit. He could easily throw some cushions on the bench seats in the cockpit, and keep vigil from there. Britt would have to sleep in the salon in order for him to awaken her quickly if necessary. And he would leave only the small anchor out, he could leave it if necessary. If pushed, he could try to get to the deep water of the Exuma Sound and sail south in the safe water of the channel. But the weather out there could rapidly get brutal, with twenty knot winds and ten to fifteen foot seas. He was not ready to attempt that now.

Coltrane regretted that he had left his PPK\S at home. He cursed outloud, then resigned himself to using whatever weapons he could find. He went to the aft stateroom, and opened the seabag containing his scuba gear. He pulled out the speargun, and checked and oiled the stainless steel shaft. He visually checked the thick rubber cords that fired the shaft, and pulled on their metal connections to the trigger mechanism. Coltrane considered removing the steel trailing wire that attached the shaft to the speargun, then decided against it. The wire would allow him to retrieve the shaft if he missed his shot, even if it would shorten the effective range of the speargun. Coltrane figured that beyond about ten paces, a hit would be pure luck. He released the safety and pulled the trigger of the gun, easing the shaft from the gun. Carefully, he removed the plastic protective tip used for packing and examined the threaded tip of the spear. He oiled the threads, and then opened a small plastic pouch containing the spearheads.

There were eight spearpoints that he carried with him on dive trips, different sizes and shapes for various types and sizes of game fish. The tip had to penetrate the fish, and hopefully kill it instantly, then resist being torn out by the inevitable rapid and vigorous thrashing in the water that the speared fish would make in its death throes. Each point had a hinged metal barb, some had a pair of barbs, that held the shaft in the flesh of the fish. After spearing the fish, the diver could swim to the surface, with the fish impaled on the end of the spear which was connected to the gun in his hand by the wire cable. But it did not always go that way. More than once, Coltrane had scored an off-center hit on a big fish and fought in panic as it pulled him deeper and deeper into the depths, until finally he had to let go of the impaled fish, speargun and all.

Coltrane selected a medium sized point, brand new and razor sharp. He turned it over in his hand, and measured it against the shaft of the speargun. It would have to be small enough to pass between and through someone's ribcage. Satisfied, he screwed the point onto the threaded end of the speargun, and laid the gun on the bed. He found his dive knife, and pushing the quick release button, removed it from the plastic sheath. Coltrane had special ordered the Japanese knife because of the combat design, rather than the clumsy, thick blades of typical dive knives. The seven inch Wenoka blade was double edged, with one edge serrated along the entire length. He hefted the heavily ribbed rubber grip, and turned the weapon in his hand.

The edges were razor sharp, unusual in a dive knife. Coltrane never did have any use for dull knives. He lightly oiled the knife, and slid it in and out of the sheath, checking the release button before he oiled it as well. He laid the knife on the bed next to the speargun.

Gently, Coltrane lifted a small hard plastic box out of the sea bag. He opened it, and examined the shotstick fastened securely within the case. The device was designed to protect divers from shark attack, and could kill large sharks by firing a handgun bullet directly into the body of the fish. It was a simple design, a handle with a wrist cord to allow underwater carry, a screw-on firing head and short barrel, and a safety pin. Coltrane unscrewed the three inch barrel, and selected a .357 Magnum cartridge from the case. He inserted the shell into the base of the barrel, and then checked to see that the safety pin was in place. The pin was very similar to the pin in a grenade, a large stainless steel cotter pin that mechanically blocked the firing pin. Coltrane oiled the moving parts, and placed extra lubricant on the safety pin. Positive that the mechanism was safe, Coltrane screwed the barrel and cartridge onto the end of the handle, snugging it down tight. He checked the ease of motion of the safety pin. By pulling the pin, and slamming the muzzle of the stick against the fish, the barrel and cartridge assembly were forced backward and down onto the firing pin, and the weapon fired. At point blank range, the effect would be lethal. Out of arm's reach, it would be useless. Satisfied, he laid the shotstick on the bed.

Coltrane picked up his binoculars, and stepped up into the cockpit. The moon was rising behind the island in the clear sky, and a few small, scattered clouds drifted high above. The water of the small bay was smooth, gently rippled by the wind. The boat pointed nose first into a light breeze coming offshore. With the moon to his back, Coltrane could see the entrance to the bay, and the small cut between Allen's Cay and the next island to the north. Any boat coming from Eleuthera would have to enter via the cut, or come around the island to the north. From Coltrane's position in the cockpit, he commanded the high ground. No one would be able to surprise him. As long as the weather held.

Coltrane went below, and finished cleaning the dinner dishes. He pumped up seawater into the small steel sink, and washed and rinsed the plates. He took the pots and pans out to the stern of the boat, and washed them in the bay, watching the hundreds of tiny fish feast on the leftover food. Years of boating had taught him the precious value of fresh water, a lesson lost on much of the civilized world. On a sailboat, there were two storage tanks, one for diesel and one for fresh water. The water tank held 550 liters, and that supply had to provide not only for drinking but also for showers, cooking, washing and cleaning. The profligate waste of water normally practiced by Americans would be disastrous for the sailor. Coltrane limited his showers by wetting his body, then soaping with the shower turned off. Only when he was finished did he rinse. He never let the water run as he shaved or brushed his teeth. And he only used fresh water to rinse the dishes, never to clean them. In that fashion, he had always had enough water to last the trip. Fresh water was hard to find in the Exumas, and almost as expensive as gasoline was in the States.

Britt finished preparing for bed, and came into the salon from the fore stateroom. Coltrane made the bed for her in the salon, and explained the unusual sleeping arrangements. She nodded, too tired to argue. He gave her the speargun, but did not draw the rubber tubes to cock the gun. He also gave her the shotstick, with the safety pin in. Britt was capable of using both weapons, having spent time spearfishing with her brothers and father as a teen. She laid them on the bed beside her, thinking the scene melodramatic. Coltrane told her to get some sleep, for he would be dead tired by morning. He gently kissed her, and went above to stand watch.

Coltrane went topside and surveyed the situation again. The wind was gentle, from the east, five knots. The boat pointed toward land, giving him a view of the open mouth of the bay. He walked to the bow of the sloop, and checked the single anchor line. It felt tight, and he could appreciate no change in the boat's position since he dropped anchor one hour earlier. They were in seven feet of crystal clear, luminous water, and he could see conch and sea stars on the ocean floor. The beauty of the Bahamas never ceased to amaze and delight him.

Shaking himself back to reality, he moved to the aft cockpit. He lay the thick cushions on the bench, and propped himself up into a comfortable position from which he could see the water before him. He strapped the dive knife onto his right calf, and checked the catch. He calculated that even with a boat capable of twenty knots, it would be hours before they could arrive here. He set his Timex Triathlon watch alarm for two hours, and settled himself for a short nap. He was asleep instantly.

It was the chirping of the watch's alarm that woke him from his deep and luxurious sleep. Resetting the alarm, he straightened up from a sitting position, feeling the muscles in his neck tighten as he did. He rubbed the cramps from his shoulders and looked around the bay. Nothing moved but the water, rippling as the waves rolled out on a receding tide. He stood and walked forward to check the anchor. It was holding well, and he scanned the shore for anything unusual. The long white sand beach had no motion, no activity. Satisfied, he returned to his lookout position, and settled in.

He had no idea how long he had been watching when he sensed something. He frantically searched the water for movement, straining his ears for sound. Nothing. A feeling of unease crept over him, a primal fear, a sense of danger. He forced himself to relax, and scanned again the horizon and the bay using his peripheral vision, knowing it was sharper for night vision. Still nothing. Then it came to his conscious mind, the sound that his ears had been hearing for minutes. The low rumble of a powerful motor, intermittently coming to him from across the water. He looked at his watch. 2:55AM.

He jumped up and bolted below, awaking Britt roughly. He looked around the cabin for protection as she shook the sleep from her mind. The sink and refrigerator were set into a waist high countertop that formed the foot of the salon bed, and would be a protective wall from which Britt could hide. He took a soft cloth cushion, and laid it onto the counter top. He grabbed the speargun, laid it on the cushion, and sighted toward the companionway. Satisfied, he turned to Britt.

"Someone is coming. I can hear a boat, maybe five hundred yards away. I can't see it yet. I am going to hide in the starboard locker. If they board us, you wait until one is framed in the light of the companionway, then shoot him with the speargun. You'll be safe behind the bulwark of the counter, he can't see you. Aim for the navel. If you miss, lock yourself in the fore cabin. You still have the shotstick to protect yourself. I'll try to knife one or throw him overboard. That's our only hope."

"What if they are FBI?"

"FBI will not board a vessel in the night, in foreign waters. That would be a violation of international law, and they have no jurisdiction here anyway. Anyone coming aboard will be doing so illegally, and we are perfectly within our rights to defend ourselves. Don't waver. If you see someone in the door, shoot him. Don't worry, I will know not to step into your sights. You see a target, fire."

Britt nodded. Coltrane took the speargun, and cocked the three rubber tubes, engaging them in the notches in the spear. Checking that the safety was on, he laid the gun on the cushion.

"Once I am through the companionway and in the locker, release the safety. Aim the gun for the center of the stairs and the companionway. I'll be able to watch from the locker, and hopefully this is just a fisherman coming in late."

Coltrane jumped through the companionway, and looked out into the bay. He could see the low black outline of a powerboat rounding the heads of the cay. As he watched in horror, the boat nosed around and headed directly for the yacht. The low long silhouette changed to a narrow V, and Coltrane could only see the froth from the ship's bow wake. As the boat slowed, the prow gradually dropped down, and the sound diminished.

"This is it. They are headed straight for us. Britt, can you hear me?" he whispered.

"Yes," her voice shaking with tension.

"Take the safety off. Take it off."

"No. What if I hit you?"

"Goddamn it, I know where you are and where the gun is pointed. You can't possibly hit me. If you wait til the last minute, he'll hear the sound and it will throw off your shot. Take the fucking safety off. Please."

He heard the raspy metallic click as she thumbed the lever.

"Alright, the safety is off."

"I am going to get into the locker, I can still watch from there. Deep breathe. Finger off the trigger until you are ready to fire. *Concentrate*."

Coltrane watched the boat as it came towards them. They could not make rapid progress due to the outgoing tide, and their slow motoring. Still, it was hard to estimate distance when viewing the boat dead on. He crouched, and gently lowered himself into the deep rope locker built into the cockpit deck. The locker was four feet deep, and three feet wide, designed to hold the large bumpers that protect the sides of the sloop when it was tied up at a dock. There was ample room for Coltrane to stand, crouched over. He wedged a coil of rope in the lid of the locker, propping it open enough so that he could see out. He could still hear the motor's drone, but could not see the boat. He guessed that they were still fifty yards away.

He shifted the ropes and bumpers around in the locker, and arranged a solid stance among the gear. He hefted the heavy lid of the locker onto the nape of his neck, so that he could throw it up when he stood up. As an afterthought, he removed two of the large bumpers and lay them on the floor of the cockpit opposite his position, blocking off that pathway to the companionway. This would force them to pass directly in front of his locker, within arm's reach.

"They are here. I will wait to charge until after you shoot. Hold your shot until you are sure that you will hit his midsection. You hear me?" Coltrane whispered rapidly to Britt.

"Yes. I am shaking like a leaf. I don't think I can hit shit." Britt pleaded.

"Detach yourself from the fear. These fucks are coming to kill us. They will not be expecting resistance. Wait and choose your shot. Deep breathe, my love." Coltrane calmed her, gave her confidence.

"Good luck, sweetheart, I love you."

"I love you. No more talk until it is all over."

As Coltrane spoke, the thrum of the motor abruptly ended. They cut the engine at thirty yards out, and were drifting towards the anchored yacht on the current. Coltrane could no longer see the boat, or hear it. He tensed, every muscle in his body feeling the weight of the heavy locker door, the skin of his neck bleeding under the shear and weight of the heavy deck lid. Nothing. He imagined he could hear the boat slice through the dark water.

A gentle tug told him that they had hooked his dinghy, and were pulling themselves forward on the dinghy line. A subtle, imperceptible bump told him that they had come alongside the sloop. They had to be good, experienced seamen to be able to quietly board an anchored yacht in a strong current like tonight. Coltrane hoped that they would underestimate their quarry.

Coltrane eased down in his hiding place, leaving a two inch crack in the deck lid to see out. Dim illumination came from the anchor light, a white light on the tip of the mast, sixty feet above the yacht. It threw enough light onto the boat to easily make out the layout of the cockpit, and to silhouette anyone moving into the relative darkness of the cabin below. Coltrane knew that the darkness would protect Britt, at least initially. If all went according to plan.

The stern of the boat dropped under the weight of a man as the first intruder came aboard. Immediately after, a second man boarded, smoothly and easily. The first man hesitated, and turned toward the shorter man behind him. The shorter man whispered harshly, and pushed him forward. He grabbed the wheel of the boat, and swung around it, moving directly forward, hunched over. The stocky man followed closely behind him, intent on the open companionway. They passed directly in front of Coltrane as he crouched in the locker.

As Johnny looked into the cabin through the companionway, he could see nothing. The pitch darkness, combined with the rolling of the yacht in the waves, disoriented the killer as he crept forward. He had never been on a boat like this before, and had no idea of what to expect. He saw the stairs that led below into the cabin. Grabbing the edge of the companionway, he lowered himself into the salon. He knew that there was a woman aboard, and his groin tingled in anticipation of the sport he would have with her.

Coltrane now was looking at the back of the lead man. He was tall and gangly, his clothes ill-fitting. His right arm and hand was held behind his back, gripping a small pistol shoved into the waistband of his pants. Opposite Coltrane moved the other man, visible only from the knees down. Coltrane's brain screamed, the events moving far faster than he had anticipated or hoped. He was watching the skinny man and questioning his plan when all hell broke loose.

Britt had felt the boat rock as both men come aboard. She had spent many nights on sailboats, and had never completely become at ease with the noises and pitching of the yachts. She settled back and centered the speargun on the rectangle of light that poured through the companionway. Within seconds, the frame of the hatch was filled with the head and shoulders of the skinny man. He paused, squinting and straining to see in the blackness below. She breathed deeply, exhaled slowly and waited for him to move just a foot forward. He hesitated, then grabbed the handrails in the stairway and bent forward.

Britt centered the speargun on his scrawny waist, and squeezed the trigger. The gun jerked violently in her hands, and the four foot spear shot straight out. As the spear left the gun, the cable that connected the end of the spear to foreguard of the gun twisted and caught on the cushion, sending the spear wild. Instead of hitting Johnny in the navel, it hit him high in the chest, impaling him through rib and lung, through muscle and bone, embedding its barbed tip in his scapula. He screamed a high pitched cry, and fell backwards to his knees in the cockpit.

The sound of the speargun was very different transmitted through air than through water. It had a high pitched metallic shrill that shocked Coltrane into action. He stood upright in a great lunge, slamming his head and ripping his skin on the raw fiberglass undersurface of the deck lid. His leap pushed him directly into the center of the cockpit, and the blinding pain of the blow to his skull sent him into a mindless, animal rage. He looked up and saw the startled face of the stocky man as he spun to meet him, his pistol in his right hand. Coltrane struck with the knife, sweeping upward from his right to left. The Cuban was pinned between Coltrane's attack from the right and behind, the cockpit console to his left, and his partner to his front. He tried to back up, but was blocked by his partner, who was howling in pain and terror.

Coltrane missed completely on his first stab, and the arc of the swing carried him up into the cockpit and almost to the level of the Cuban. He twisted his torso, and slashed downward toward the short man's belly as he pivoted into him. The Cuban backed up, tucking his chin to his chest, pulling his head back away from the attack, grunting. He moved easily, gracefully, like a dancer. The knife slashed by his belly, cutting his shirt and flesh. He tried to bring the pistol in his right hand to bear, but slammed it into the console before he could get a shot off at Coltrane. Coltrane closed the gap between them, bringing the knife low for a final upwards thrust at his enemy. The Cuban cursed in Spanish, and jumped up onto the cockpit bench, then dove off the side into the water.

Coltrane watched the body of the Cuban disappear over the side of the boat, then turned back to the cockpit. The scene before him was nightmarish. Johnny lay writhing on his back in a pool of dark blood in the companionway, the stainless steel shaft sticking out of his chest at an absurd angle. Pink frothy bubbles flew out of his mouth, along with obscenities and an incomprehensible babble. At his side lay a small pistol, with an elongated shrouded barrel. Coltrane jumped forward and grabbed the gun with both hands. He spun to look over the side for the Cuban, but could see nothing.

"Britt! Are you OK?" Coltrane shouted down the companionway.

"I'm fine. I'm fine," She replied quickly.

"Get me the searchlight. And the night vision scope. Quick. And kill all our lights," Coltrane snapped.

"Where are they?" Britt asked as she stepped to the electrical panel and turned off the anchor and running lights.

"Above the nav desk."

By the time that Britt had located the hand held Q-Beam and the night scope, the sound of the Cuban's swimming was faint. Coltrane shot the bright spotlight in the direction of the splashing, but saw nothing. He swept the water to the starboard of the yacht slowly and methodically, but found nothing. He kept low, knowing that the man probably still had a pistol. The insane screams of the wounded man distracted and angered him. He reached up and grabbed a stainless steel winch handle from the holster near the Lewmar winch. He brought it up three feet, and struck the skinny killer straight in the center of his forehead. He collapsed in a loose pile on the cockpit floor.

Coltrane returned his concentration to the water. No sound could be heard in the direction that he thought the Cuban had gone. The boat had swung slightly in the wind, and Coltrane was now unsure exactly in what direction the man had gone. He only knew that he now was an easy target, illuminated and silhouetted on the deck of the boat, bright light in hand. Finding the man in the water with the small night scope would be difficult, he realized. Coltrane wanted to be gone, fast.

"Britt, come on up here and give me a hand. We gotta get out of here."

"What about him?" Britt asked as she stepped over Johnny's crumpled body.

"He can wait. Start the diesel and I'll pull the anchor. But don't put it in gear yet."

Coltrane ran forward while Britt cranked up the diesel. The boat coughed to life on the second attempt. He found the anchor line and began to pull it in, straining at the effort, pulling with his back. Fortunately, the small Danforth was in soft sand, and broke free easily as Britt moved the boat gently forward. Coltrane pulled the iron chain and anchor up and hastily secured them to the bow. He raced back to the cockpit.

"Turn her north and head out to sea. I am going to check the dinghy and their boat."

"What bearing?" Britt demanded.

"I don't know. Just get the fuck away from the beach. The other guy still has a gun and could hit us from there if we stay here. The water is plenty deep. Just head out to sea. Full speed. And duck down."

Coltrane climbed down into the transom, and checked the line running to their dinghy. He tried to pull the small inflatable boat closer to the yacht before realizing that the intruders had slip-tied their boat to the dinghy line. The tension on the line snapped it from his grip, tearing his fingers. He debated slowing the yacht to secure the line tethering the powerboat, but decided against risking any further exposure to fire from shore. He stepped up into the cockpit, and took the wheel from Britt.

"Go below and check the depth. My bearing is 020." Coltrane wanted her safely below the waterline. He knew that a .22 could travel over a mile, and today had not been lucky for them. He sat on the floor of the cockpit, trying to gain as much cover as possible in his exposed position. Only when the yacht was safely offshore, and the depthmeter reading 25 meters did he begin to relax.

Chapter 50

Atlantic Ocean
Exuma Sound
June 27
4:30AM

It had taken Coltrane forty-five minutes to move the unconscious man from the cockpit into the powerboat, and secure the craft to the yacht via a separate line. He left the speargun and cable still attached to the embedded shaft, fearing that any attempt to remove it would cause fatal internal injury. Coltrane had lashed him securely to the steel post of the captain's chair as they drifted offshore.

After a short survey of the charts and discussion of their options, they had put out to sea through a wide channel between the islands. They could think of nothing to do but run, as far and as fast as they could. That meant the ocean, where they could race offshore without worry of running aground. Within thirty minutes, they were in the deep blue-black swells of the Exuma Sound. Coltrane took the helm, and Britt tried to get some rest below deck.

Coltrane plotted a course that ran in the deep water, just off the wall that dropped off from two fathoms to eight hundred fathoms. Their path paralleled the island chain, and would get them far from the Cuban by daybreak. Coltrane was still high from the fight, his heart and mind racing too fast to stop or even control. His mind jumped from thought to thought, crystal clear, but out of control. He had experienced this exhilaration before, in Vietnam after combat. He savored the rush, knowing that soon it would pass.

The screams of the wounded man brought him back to reality. Britt was awakened from her fitful sleep by the sounds that drifted to them over the waves and the drone of the diesel. Coltrane cut the power, and turned the yacht into the light breeze. He gave Britt a heading, and then ducked below to grab a small nylon bag. Pulling the motorboat to the yacht by its towline, Coltrane stepped aboard.

For the first time, he examined the craft. It was a sturdy center cockpit sportfisherman, maybe twenty-two or twenty-five feet long. The fiberglass boat had seen much use, but was well maintained. The deck had two beaten captain's chairs, fish lockers and a companionway hatch with stairs leading to a small cuddy cabin in the bow. The big single outboard could easily have gotten the two killers across the sound in two or three hours. The lack of any sophisticated navigational equipment told Coltrane that the men were experienced sailors, and brave to have made that crossing alone and at night. Or very determined.

Johnny lay twisted on his left side, the shaft sticking out of his bloody shirt. His face rested on the deck in a pool of frothy pink blood, and he cursed and screamed to himself as the boat rocked back and forth. He was surprised when Coltrane grabbed him and jerked him upright. Immediately, he lashed out with a vicious kick, striking Coltrane in the flank. The combination of the force of the kick and the pitching deck sent Coltrane spinning on the deck, slick with blood and seawater. He smashed his back and head hard against the bulkhead as his feet flew out from beneath him. Johnny kicked again, but was out of range.

Coltrane clawed back on all fours, blind with pain and anger. On the deck before him lay the speargun. Insane with rage and frustration, Coltrane grabbed the gun with both hands and jerked it as hard as he could. Only the slack in the six foot of cable saved Johnny. Still, the cable snapped the embedded spear down and back, setting the barbs on the spearhead deeper into flesh and bone. Johnny screamed and thrashed on the deck for minutes as Coltrane collapsed in the stern of the boat and watched grimly.

When his captive had weakened sufficiently, Coltrane bound his legs with cord from the nylon bag. Then he untied his hands from the captain's chair, and dragged him down into the cuddy cabin. He pushed him back up against the open wooden ladder that led down into the cabin, and hog-tied him there. He slipped a loop of rope around the man's ankles, and pulled his feet up behind his back, balancing his weight on his kneecaps. Working swiftly and using nautical and surgical knots, Coltrane had him immobilized and in exquisite pain before the man knew what was occurring. Exhausted, Coltrane slumped onto the small cushioned platform that served as a bed.

As his eyes fully adjusted to the gloom of the small cabin, Coltrane looked around. The cuddy was dank, dark. It was six feet long and five feet wide at the entrance, then narrowed as it ran forward to the bow. Along the port side ran a small galley, with an ancient gas burner and a small sink. The starboard side had several cabinets housing spare parts, equipment and oil-stained life jackets. Coltrane lay back and tried to formulate a plan in his aching head.

Johnny was regaining full consciousness, aided by the intense pain building in his knees. "What the fuck are you doing to me, chump? Why did you shoot me like a fucking fish? Get me to a hospital," he yelled at Coltrane.

"We are headed to Eleuthera now. There is a clinic there that can stabilize you, but then you will have to be flown somewhere for surgery.

Without surgery, you are going to die. Soon." Coltrane sat up on the damp cushions and watched the man tied up across from him. From the position, angle and exposed length of the shaft he knew that the spearhead penetrated the right lung and possibly the abdominal cavity as well. The man was doomed.

"This thing is killing me. You're a doctor. Get it out of me."

"How do you know I am a surgeon?" Coltrane snapped back.

"What? That don't matter. Get this thing outta me. If I die, you're going to fry for it, cocksucker." Johnny stared contemptuously at Coltrane, defiant and angry.

Coltrane turned away, picking up his small nylon bag. "Let me look at the wound."

Coltrane held his rage in check, taking a cloth package out of the bag. Unfolding the flaps, he revealed surgical instruments, scalpels and hemostats. From a second case, he removed a syringe and needle, drawing up fluid from a sterile vial. Carefully arranging the equipment on a towel on the cushions, he turned to the bound criminal.

"Hold still." Coltrane bent over, and taking a long bladed fillet knife from his bag, cut through Johnny's bloody shirt and removed it. He could see the entry wound five inches below the nipple and the upward direction of the spear's travel. The spearpoint had buried itself in the muscle and bone of the back, just under the shoulder. Coltrane could feel the tip of the spearhead through the mottled skin. He needed the speargun back. He would have to get the spear out. Sooner or later.

"If I try to remove that spear, it will kill you here and now. Your only chance is if I can get you to a hospital within the next six hours." Coltrane looked at his watch. It read 0445 hrs. Two, maybe three hours until sunrise. The seas had calmed, and the breeze was light. Coltrane climbed over the bound man, and scanned the ocean. No vessels, no lights, no land, just endless rolling, black water. He waved at Britt, and gave her a series of hand signals. Britt cut the power of the diesel, faced it to the wind, then cut the motor. The boats drifted quietly in the predawn darkness.

Coltrane climbed back into the cramped cuddy and huddled over the galley. He fired up the gas burner and tried to run the sink. No water flowed. The smoke of the stove billowed up, and slowly filled the cabin. Johnny watched with growing impatience.

"What the fuck are you doing? Why are we stopped? Get on the radio and call the Coast Guard to come get me. They got choppers that can move me faster than your fucking sailboat." Johnny continued to glare at Coltrane, staring straight into his eyes with unconcealed contempt.

"I'll take you to a hospital, but not before you tell me who you are, and why you are trying to kill us." Coltrane tried reasoning with the man.

"Fuck you." Johnny spat.

"Fuck me? No, fuck you." Coltrane laughed as he pulled his thick neoprene diving glove onto his right hand.

"The Cuban is going to come get me and cut your balls off, asshole. You better get me to land quick. For your lady's sake." Johnny sneered.

"The Cuban? The other guy is a Cuban?" Coltrane asked outloud.

Johnny just stared back, defiant.

"What's his name?"

"Fuck you."

Coltrane lost control. He stood and raised his gloved hand as high as the low ceiling allowed, and in a sweeping arc, slapped Johnny hard on the face. His head bounced on his skinny neck, hit the ladder and dropped forward. Coltrane struck him again, hard on the bridge of the nose, feeling the bones crack. He swung again, this time missing as the head wobbled from side to side. Coltrane beat him until his hand stung with pain from the slapping. Blood poured from Johnny's nose and mouth. Coltrane's heart was racing, fearing that he had done too much damage. He grabbed the man by his hair, and jerked his head upright. The beady eyes gleamed with hate.

"You still don't get it, you stupid fuck. You're tied up, completely at my mercy, and still threatening and playing games with me. I have seen trash like you in ERs forever. Punks. Posers. Drunks. All the same. Tattoos. You think you are so fucking bad. Attacking sleeping unarmed people in the night." Coltrane grabbed Johnny by the throat and pushed his head back, thrusting his own face inches from the struggling man's.

"We are in the Atlantic, miles away from the Cuban. No one could find us, even if they knew where to look. Not for many, many hours. And I can keep you alive, and in the most exquisite pain imaginable, until I'm through with you. We'll see how tough you really are, here and now." Coltrane turned to the stove, and rummaging through the cooking utensils, found an old metal spatula. He straightened the handle, and laid the paddle in the bright flame. Then he took his Leatherman from his pocket, and opened it carefully, selecting the rat toothed pliers function. He turned back to Johnny.

"What is your name?"

"Johnny Davis."

"What were you doing on our boat?"

"We just wanted to rob you, that's all."

Johnny's hands were bound to the stiles of the ladder, at his sides. Coltrane reached down, selected his right index finger, and pulled it free from Johnny's tightening fist. He took the Leatherman, and centered the teeth of the pliers' grip over the first joint of the finger. Then he slowly crushed the joint in the stainless steel jaw, feeling the cartilage and bone splinter in its teeth. Coltrane watched as the tip of the finger turned blue, then purple.

Johnny howled in pain, blood spewing from his mouth and face.

"Don't lie to me again, you miserable fuck. You have nineteen joints left. We can go through them one at a time. Fuck you. Let's do another, just for fun." Coltrane went to the left hand, and twisted his little finger free of Johnny's clammy fist. He crushed the distal joint of the little finger, more slowly this time. As he watched the tissue ooze out from the jaws of the tool, he tried to remember the principle of psychology that he was applying.

Was it intermittent negative reinforcement? Or unscheduled negative reinforcement? All he could remember was that this technique completely destroyed the minds of the lab animals, and in the shortest period of time. The researchers would put the white lab rats in a cage, and then connect electrodes to a paddle in the cage, directly under a brightly colored light. The floor of the cage was electrified as well. In one group, they would train the rat to press the paddle with his forefoot when the light came on, and he would get a food pellet. Positive reinforcement. In a second group, if the rat failed to press the lever when the light came on, they shocked him through the floor electrode. Negative reinforcement. In the third, doomed group, there was no discernable pattern of response to the rats' behavior. The rat got shocked if he pressed the lever, if he didn't press the lever, if the light was on, if the light was off. Never knowing what the result of their response would get them. No correlation between stimulus and response. Even if they gave the correct response, they still got punished. That was it, he thought. That will drive him to madness the fastest.

Johnny panted, his eyes bulging with pain and terror. "You can't do this, you're a doctor. You swore some oath. You can't kill me. You gotta help me. Please."

"I *will* help you. But I want to know *everything* you know. Now. You think that the Cuban would go through this for you?" Coltrane sat back, and paused briefly. He did not want to give Johnny any time to think, to gather his wits. He reached over to the spatula, and grasped it with his rubber dive mitt. It was red hot, glowing in the dark cabin.

Coltrane moved it slowly toward Johnny's face, then lowered it to his left nipple, and pressed it onto the sweating flesh. The skin sizzled and the smell of burning skin and hair filled the room as Johnny screamed in pain. Coltrane turned the flat utensil over, and applied it to the right breast. He ignored the pleas and sobbing of the killer as he repeatedly reheated the spatula and burned the man's chest, hands and face. Finally, Coltrane stopped as Johnny lost control of his bowels. He babbled nonsense at Coltrane, who put the spatula back into the burner's flame.

"You are shitting all over yourself, tough guy. You stinking fuck. Now, for the last time, what are you doing here?"

Johnny couldn't speak. He was sobbing and panting and crying, urinating on Coltrane's feet as his body was racked with pain. He tried to talk, but failed. Coltrane waited quietly, repulsed by the visceral scene and by his own actions.

"We just want that disc. That's all. The Cuban hired me. I don't know who hired him. Somebody real rich, real big. Anything he wants, they get for him. Passports, money, information. Whatever." He panted to catch his breath.

"Where are your passports?" Coltrane looked around the cabin.

"In the shaving kit. Under the sink."

Coltrane opened the cabinet, and pulled out a ragged vinyl shaving kit. Inside were four US passports, two different identities for each man. They were excellent forgeries, complete with the barcodes and watermarks of the US Customs Department. The skinny killer had passports in the name of John Benton and Jason Neville. The Cuban's passports said Miguel Calderone and Javier Reyes. Next to the passports was a thick stack of US dollars and Bahamian currency, and two small unmarked cardboard boxes. The boxes were filled with .22 caliber rimfire ammunition, of a type Coltrane had never seen before. The shells were stamped IMI. Coltrane carefully replaced the contents in the kit.

"Where is the rest of your gear?" Coltrane demanded.

"In the forepeak locker.

"What disc are you talking about?" Coltrane asked.

"Hendricks' disc." Johnny's head hung like a rag doll's as he labored with the answers.

"The tape of our conversation?" Coltrane was confused.

"No. The CD that Hendricks stole," Johnny raised his head with difficulty, looking at Coltrane, realizing that Coltrane may not know what they truly were seeking.

"How did you know I have that disc?" Coltrane was startled at this revelation.

"I saw Ochoa pass it to you."

"Ochoa? You mean Resendez?"

"Whoever you want, man."

"What's on that disc that you will kill my wife and me for it?"

"Don't know."

Coltrane, feeling his dominance slipping, reached down and selected another finger from Johnny's broken left hand, even as the victim began to beg. He crushed another joint very slowly, until Johnny answered.

"Stop! Please! I ain't lying to you. We just wanted the computer discs. The CDs that Hendricks stole from his office."

"You mean the disc?" Coltrane asked.

"No, there were two."

"Why do you think that?"

"We already found the other one."

"Tell me about the other one."

"We got it from Hendricks. The Cuban knew what to look for, something that Hendricks stole from his job before he quit. We found it at his house. The Cuban killed him, not me. I swear, man." Johnny lied, afraid that Coltrane had been close to Hendricks, and would blame him for his death.

Johnny was fading fast, and Coltrane could see the color fading from his wan skin. A thick, dark purple trickle of blood oozed from his chest wound. The veins in his neck were thick and engorged. Coltrane didn't think he would last much longer. He checked his pulse and observed his labored breathing. Coltrane gathered his medical gear, the shaving kit and climbed over the slumped form into a freshening sea breeze. He slowly scanned the dark horizon. Nothing.

Coltrane climbed into the cuddy one last time, and checked Johnny's carotid pulse. The pulse was faint and thready. Coltrane grasped the steel spear shaft and tried to remove it from Johnny's chest. His grip slipped on the bloody steel. Coltrane knew he would never get the shaft out that way. The barbs had set too deeply in the muscle and ribcage. He tried to twist the shaft and unscrew the shaft from the embedded point, but the cable and the attached speargun resisted the effort. Disgusted, he threw his weight against the shaft, and drove it clean through Johnny's dying body, exiting near the shoulderblade. Grabbing a rag from the floor, he removed the gore from the spearpoint and unscrewed it. The shaft slipped easily from the body once the point was removed. He flipped the bent speartip over the side of the boat, and gathered up the speargun.

Using the towline, Coltrane pulled the motorboat up to the transom of the yacht. He tied the boat to the stern cleat, threw the speargun and the men's gear aboard and climbed onto the sailboat. Saying nothing to Britt, he moved below quickly, stowing his gear in the center console. Then he moved to the forecabin. The shotstick lay on the bed where he had placed it the night before. He checked the safety, gathered the ammo box and his flashlight, and went topside.

"Get me a GPS reading, Britt. And a depth reading." Coltrane picked up the charts, and tried to get a feel for their approximate location. He had to sink the motorboat, and it had to be in very deep water where it would never be found.

"What's going on?" Britt asked as she powered up the GPS unit.

"The skinny guy is dead, and we have to sink his boat before dawn."

"Sink it? Why don't we take it? It's faster than this damn sailboat. We can get to Nassau in two hours."

"Then what? There is blood all over that boat, and what do we do with the body? Who knows where the other guy went to? We have to sink the boat, the body, and all the evidence here and now, before sunrise and someone sees us towing it." Coltrane examined the charts closely. "What is our position?" He asked, the debate over.

"24.50.8 by 76.45.2." Britt shot back.

"Depth?" Coltrane demanded.

"Off the meter."

Coltrane plotted their location on the chart, and verified the surface position by cross-checking the depth. They were in eight hundred fathoms of water, almost five thousand feet of water, far enough from the wall drop-off that the sinking boat would be lost forever. There was nothing of any interest to any scuba divers in the area, and no significant fishing that he knew about. The water was very deep, very cold and very rough. The only activity he had ever heard of out here was high speed submarine testing by the US Navy. Hopefully, they weren't running tonight.

"OK. We sink it right here. If it goes down before I can get back on the boat, slip the line fast. And get a knife from the galley in case the line hangs up and you can't free it."

"You mean it could pull our boat down?" Britt's eyes opened with concern.

"I don't think so. But it could tangle on the prop or the rudder. Who knows? Murphy's Law. Get the knife to be on the safe side." Coltrane took his gear and pulling the motorboat alongside, jumped in. He let out ten feet of line, allowing the boat to trail a safe distance from the stern of the much larger yacht.

He grabbed the men's gear bags, and dumped them out onto the bed. Rifling them quickly, he found nothing of interest. He shoved everything back into the lockers, and searched the cabin for any useful nautical gear or equipment. He opened the small port and starboard hatches, and popped up the forward deck hatch. Whichever way the boat sank, there would have to be a way for any trapped air to escape. Reminding himself to take their anchor, he pried up the floor panel that covered the bilge. With the flashlight in his teeth, he looked into the grimy compartment. He selected a spot as far forward as his hand would reach, and wedged the shotstick up against the inside of the hull. He pulled the safety and turning his face, he drove the weapon into the hull. The noise was deafening, and the recoil smashed his hand back and raked it along the sharp fiberglass. Coltrane cursed, but was happy to see black water pour through the rough hole in the boat.

He jumped up, ran to the stern and reached to unscrew the transom drain. The large brass plug was battered and bent, and refused to unscrew. Coltrane's lacerated hand burned from the saltwater as he tore his fingers on the T-handle. Finally, cursing himself for not checking the drain earlier, he reloaded the shotstick. Opening the rear locker cover, he found the lowest point in the boat's hull, and shot another hole through the layered fiberglass. Finding a hammer in a deck locker, he hacked at the small hole until it was the size of his fist. Water shot through, rising in a column and rapidly flowing onto the deck. Alarmed by the speed of the sinking, Coltrane grabbed his shotstick and flashlight, and looked toward the yacht.

"Loosen the line! Loosen the line!" Coltrane yelled frantically to Britt. The boat was capsizing as he scrambled forward, three foot waves slapping over the port side and filling the boat. The stern of the boat went under as Coltrane climbed forward. The bow rose out of the water, and turned slowly as Coltrane tried to balance on the rocking craft.

"*Cut the line. Cut the line.*" Coltrane shouted to Britt, who had come down the transom to help her husband get into the sailboat. Fear shone in her eyes as she watched him teetering on the prow of the sinking boat.

"*No! You jump first! Jump! Jump!*" She screamed.

Coltrane jumped from the side of the bow, slipping as he miss-timed the waves. He landed ten feet short of the transom, and missed the dinghy line by five feet. Holding the shotstick in one hand and the flashlight in the other, he dogpaddled toward the sailboat. The yacht loomed huge and white above him as the seas pitched his body further away with each wave. Britt scrambled down into the transom, her yells barely audible over the ocean. Coltrane dropped his shotstick and flashlight, and swam desperately for the sailboat. The current was barely four knots, but combined with the wave action and Coltrane's tired state, he didn't think he could make it. He steadily lost ground, watching the big yacht drift off in the distance. As the next wave raised him up out of the black water, he saw Britt gesturing wildly to his right. He looked quickly, and spotted the dinghy, trailing thirty meters away. She had let the line out to keep the dinghy from getting caught by the sinking powerboat.

Coltrane knew that it was his last chance. They had practiced man overboard drills before, and Britt knew the maneuvers. Even on a clear day, with calm seas, there were dangers. The sailor remaining on the boat had to make a tight, hard turn back to the man overboard, keeping her eyes on him at all times. It is very easy to lose a human in the vast expanse of the ocean. And she had to remember which side of the keel the prop was positioned. Sailboats never had a centerline prop; the propeller was offset to accommodate the keel design. A hard turn starboard with a port prop would bring the thrashing blades within feet of the surface, shredding the swimmer. You had to turn towards the swimmer, she knew. But it was night, the seas were getting rough, and Coltrane had no life vest. He would be hard to spot and maintain visual contact with during the long circular turn that the slow diesel would need. She could easily lose him. A hard knot formed in her throat, as she stood helpless and watched him struggle.

With strength born of desperation, Coltrane dug into the heaving seas toward the dinghy. Using open water swimming techniques learned from his occasional triathlons, he maintained visual contact with the inflatable boat. It seemed like hours as he closed on the little boat. When he finally hit the soft inflatable dinghy, he held on momentarily, then dragged himself into the little boat. He collapsed on the bottom and vomited seawater. Then he passed out.

When he came around, he was looking up into Britt's smiling face. She had pulled the light dinghy up to the stern of the yacht, and helped him onto the transom. The pain of seawater upon his open hand wounds and his torn fingers brought Coltrane back to reality. He looked for the motorboat, and saw nothing. The towline had been severed at the cleat. He turned to Britt.

"It went down fast. The line got so tight that I couldn't untie it. I had to cut it free." Britt explained.

"Did you see it sink? Are you sure?" Coltrane asked.

"Yes. It went down bow last, with a great gush of air. I didn't watch it too closely, I was watching you try to drown." Britt smiled.

Coltrane looked down at her. There was no doubt in his mind that she would have dove into the water if she felt that he was in danger. He had learned over the years that she knew no fear, nor could pain stop her. She was far tougher than anyone he had ever known, man or woman.

"I love you more than life itself. If I were to live a thousand lives, I would never find another to compare to you. You are my life, my love." Coltrane kissed her gently and held her close as the sun rose in the east.

Chapter 51

June 27
6:25AM

With daylight breaking, Coltrane stripped off his blood-stained clothes and threw them overboard, weighed down with a heavy metal skillet. He showered in the transom, washing the night off his body and mind. Britt piloted the yacht on a southerly bearing, making headway along the eastern edge of the island chain. They were both tired, and needed rest. Coltrane scrutinized the charts, looking for cuts between the cays in the southern chain. They had to get out of the deep water and leeward before the weather came in.

Coltrane looked up the tide charts, and found that high tide was at 0725hrs. They would traverse the cut close to high tide, when there would be very little tidal current. He took a GPS reading and plotted a course for Britt. Taking the binoculars, he scanned the horizon for craft. He saw nothing.

The sun was climbing in the sky behind them as they began the gradual turn to the west. The diesel hummed steadily as the sloop cut through the blue water. Coltrane would have preferred to sail, but the winds were light, and not favorable. He had to be through the cut before the tidal flow reversed and strengthened. He didn't want to run the gauntlet of razor sharp coral battling a ten knot current.

Coltrane searched the low-lying islands for any distinctive rock formation, or man-made landmark to guide him. The Exumas were low, nondescript scrubby islands rising out of the barren ocean, virtually indistinguishable from one another; tiny sand and stone cays clawing an existence against an overwhelming sea. Novice and experienced skippers alike had made errors in identifying the tiny cays. Coltrane checked his GPS against the silhouette of the islands on the horizon, and picked up his Steiner binoculars. With the sun behind him, it reflected pink on the twin engine cargo plane half submerged in Norman Bay, a relic of the prolific cocaine smuggling history of the islands. Sure now that they were abreast of Norman Cay, Coltrane counted down the chain to Hall's Pond Cay and Hog Cay, and calculated a bearing for the small sliver of water that separated the two islands.

As the sun rose behind the sloop, Coltrane made for the passage. The height of the sun and the angle of its rays helped him to read the water, showing the coral and the rocks as they lay in his path. Coltrane went to the pulpit of the sloop, and balanced on the roller furling of the jib. From his height, fifteen feet above the sparkling blue waters, he could see the channel easily. Through a series of hand signals, instinctively understood by each other, he communicated with Britt as she piloted the boat.

The tide was slack, just an hour off high tide, and they traversed the narrow crease through coral heads and rocks easily. Immediately the tension dropped away, as they passed from the six foot swells of the black seas of the Atlantic to the tranquil, pale blue waters of the flats.

This was the beauty that Coltrane sought eternally in his returns to the Bahamas. The spectacular emerald shallows of the banks. White sand shone through the crystal clear waters, warm and inviting. Coltrane could see starfish and branching coral formations resting on the rippled sea floor. So perfectly clear was the water that he could see each tiny grain of sand, each one a perfect little diamond crystal. Tiny silver fish darted by in schools of thousands, and bigger dark blue predators moving lazily in the periphery. Pristine and unspoiled. Dangerous. It was paradise.

Coltrane guided Britt through the confluence of narrow channels that led around the spit between the two cays. They motored slowly, maneuvering between sand bars and shoals as the depth of the channel varied from twelve to six feet. Finally, they entered the tranquil waters of the Great Bahama Bank, and the water turned sapphire blue. The Bank ran from the western edge of the Exumas to Cuba, and was safe water for a cruising yacht, not too deep to inspire fear and generate weather, and not so shallow that running aground was a danger. Coltrane relaxed, and came back to the cockpit, taking the helm from Britt. He turned the sloop south, again paralleling the island chain, now within the sheltered waters of the cays.

"Lay down for a while, sweetheart. We both need rest." Coltrane threw a cushion from the port to the starboard settee to make a bed for Britt. He knew she couldn't stand sleeping below deck on a moving sailboat.

"What about you? You have to sleep too. Just anchor in there." Britt pointed to the next cay in the chain. She wanted to sleep soundly in a quiet cove, the boat at rest.

"We still have a ways to go. I want to get to Saddleback Cay. We can anchor overnight there. I need time to think. I'm too wired to think straight now, anyway. We'll have to sleep in shifts now, and stand watch until we find out what is happening with that other guy."

"Listen, I can't sleep on a moving boat. You sleep for an hour, clear your head. I can get us to Saddleback Cay." Britt reasoned.

Coltrane agreed, collapsing on the settee and immediately falling into a deep but fitful sleep.

Chapter 52

Highburn Cay
11:42AM

Patience is the greatest weapon of the intelligence officer. The Cuban was a patient man, and today had proven that beyond any doubt. His self-control had come perilously close to snapping as he had waited on the sandy spit beyond the marina in Highburn Cay. The transparent stalling of the huge black dock manager infuriated the Cuban, but killing the man would have been a pyrrhic victory. Instead, he sat on the mosquito-ridden sand bar, waiting for the phone. Finally, the arrival at the fuel dock of a cruising yacht with a radiophone afforded him an opportunity to call to Eleuthera.

The Cuban called the Eleuthera marina, and requested a seaplane ferry to the island. He was told by the harbormaster that the plane was busy for the rest of the day, but would be available tomorrow around mid morning. The only other way to get to Hatchet Bay or Powell Point would be to hire a captain to come get him. For that kind of service, cash was the only accepted form of payment. The Cuban didn't have $700US in cash. He thanked the yachtsman whose quizzical gaze was becoming annoying. Giving the man $50US, he climbed out of the yacht and returned to the marina office.

Calvin was busy with another customer, so the Cuban smoothly moved to the phone, and lifted the receiver. He was able to contact his brother in the States, and arrange for a water taxi to Nassau. The rest he would have to deal with on the big island. He bought a cold can of Kalik from Calvin, and set out on a meandering stroll along the strand. He sat and examined his belly wound. He had been very lucky. The knife had hit him flat, inflicting only a long, superficial laceration. He cleaned it with saltwater, then forgot it. Assured that his pistol lay undisturbed where he had hidden it the night before, he returned to the dock to await his ride.

Chapter 53

Exuma Sound
10:23AM

Coltrane woke two hours later, disturbed by a bizarre dream filled with images of horrible knife wounds and medieval torture chambers. He shook the unease from his conscious mind, and went below to check their progress on the nautical charts. The sloop was moving nicely at 7 knots, and he quickly fixed their position. He didn't need a GPS for navigation at this point, he had spent many days piloting this area of the Exumas. He spotted Saddleback Cay in the distance, its prominent twin peaks rising above the low lying scrub of the adjacent islands. To enter the small deep cove where he planned to overnight would require a gently curving approach from the south. He detailed the course to Britt, then went below to contact Calvin. He tried to raise the marina for ten minutes, but got no response. He tried again.

Britt found Saddleback Cay's southern beach, and made for their anchorage in a long, sweeping approach, as they had done many times before. Saddleback Cay was a private island, but uninhabited and pristine. The small southwestern anchorage had been a favorite of theirs for years, protected from the prevailing winds and just large enough for one yacht. A perfect little crescent beach of white sand was nestled among the coral outcroppings. It was paradise on earth.

Coltrane contacted Calvin on the VHF radio, speaking obtusely knowing that their conversation was undoubtedly being monitored. In the islands, without cable television, radio or other forms of entertainment, the locals constantly eavesdropped on radiotelephone conversations. It provided amusement as well as information about the nature of their visitors' intentions. Coltrane didn't want anyone involved in his troubles, but he needed to know if the other killer had come ashore and what action he was taking.

Calvin told Coltrane that a stranger had been found sleeping on the dock at 5 AM that morning, looking soaked and the worse for wear. The man had urgently needed to use the phone, but Calvin had stalled him. Politely but firmly, in the island way, he had asked him to wait on the dock as he conducted supposedly vital morning communications. The Cuban, not willing to attract unwanted attention, had sulked off to the dock while Calvin pretended to use the only phone on the island.

After two hours of delays by Calvin, the Cuban moved over to the fueling dock and struck up a conversation with the crew of a 46 foot sloop. Apparently, he asked to use the cruising yachtsman's radiophone. Playing on the honorable standards of the seafarer and offering the sailor $50US, he was soon talking to someone via radiotelephone. What had transpired during his brief conversation, Calvin did not know. And then somehow, while he wasn't watching, the man had used the marina phone to make a call. Calvin didn't know where the call was placed. But now the Cuban was peacefully sitting on the end of the dock, drinking an ice cold Kalik. Coltrane thanked him for the news, and asked Calvin to hail him when the Cuban was on his way.

Coltrane moved to the salon table, and laid out the nautical maps for the Bahamas. He plotted the distance from Eleuthera to Highburn Cay. Roughly 30 miles, or two or three hours by boat. Nassau was even further. Then from Highburn to their present position was another three hours. If a fast boat set out now from Eleuthera, it would take a minimum of six or seven hours to get to them, assuming that their location was known. But the Cuban would have to check every little cove and bay between Highburn and here. Coltrane figured they had at least ten hours of safety. He sat back against the settee couch and gathered his thoughts.

Coltrane went forward, unpacked the Iridium satphone, and set it up quickly. He picked up the handset and dialed direct to Susan. It was 11AM in Tampa, and she answered on the third ring.

"Susan, this is Coltrane." He was relieved to hear her voice.

"Dr. Coltrane, I'm glad you called. I have been leaving you E-mail all morning." Susan sounded harried.

"Did Agent Lynwood get the minutes?" Coltrane asked immediately.

"I gave them to him this morning. I hope that we're not in trouble with the FBI. If the members find out that the society is under investigation, they will bail like rats from a sinking ship." Susan was rambling excitedly.

"Susan, calm down. Relax. Lynwood is just doing his job. The insurance lobby has filed a grievance in federal court alleging that we are organizing an illegal strike. The FBI is just doing a routine investigation of that claim. Everything we have done so far is completely legal. But keep a lid on it. You're right, the membership will panic if the FBI is mentioned. What else is happening in Tampa?"

"This is the second day of the conference, and I think it is going pretty well. But you were right about the TV news. All four stations ran sensational lead-ins speculating that medical services would be unavailable. Then they devoted only thirty seconds to the story, so Monday was hell. But when it became clear doctors' offices were still open, most of the uproar subsided. The public has calmed down. Many patients are not happy about having to pay the additional fifteen dollar co-pay for office visits, but otherwise all is going well. ER coverage is not a problem, but some trauma patients have been transferred to Orlando. The hospitals are not affected because they are still admitting patients as usual. Hospital bed census is mostly unchanged." Susan was keeping excellent track of the progress of the conference and its impact on the community.

"The physicians' offices are functioning well under the increased loads?" Coltrane asked. He knew that this could be the Achilles' heel of the strategy.

"So far, so good. I think that for the short term, the system will work well. Long term, I can foresee problems. Depending on the number of specialists in each field, the schedule may become too frantic. For instance, take Neurology. There are ten neurologists in town, and that means each is in the office to see patients only one day every two weeks. The offices are getting jammed. It won't work for long." Susan was worried.

"True. It will be busy on the day that the assigned physician is covering the whole city. But look at it this way… then he gets two weeks off. These people are used to grueling schedules. I worked 100, 110 hour weeks when I was a surgical resident. We can handle it. Any response from the insurance plans?" Coltrane was confident.

"Yes. That was what I wanted you to know. The medical director from the PatientsChoice Florida HMO has called twice, asking for a meeting with you and the committee. What should I tell him? This may be a chance to get our demands addressed."

"Outstanding! Now they want to talk. Good. Now listen, Susan. We do not want to talk to any damn medical directors. They are just puppets, they have no real authority or power. Politely respond that we want to arrange a meeting with the HMO plan's regional directors. We will only meet with people who can *change* policy. But when you schedule the proposed meeting, schedule it for late next week. Every day is costing them hundreds of thousands of dollars. Make them sweat for a week or so. Maybe that will bring them to the table." Coltrane was happy to see some progress occurring.

"Yes, doctor. I will E-mail you with any progress. But when are you coming back to Tampa?" Susan pleaded.

"As soon as my business is wrapped up here. Besides, you are doing a spectacular job without me. I wouldn't want to get in your way." Coltrane reassured her and said goodbye.

Coltrane hung up the satphone and climbed up through the companionway to the cockpit where Britt sat watching the sky and horizon.

She was much too tired to relax, much too worried to sleep. She looked at Coltrane, the concern etched in her pretty face.

"We have to get out of here, Bill. We have to let someone know that guy is trying to kill us. How are we going to get help?" Britt was angry and confused.

Coltrane had no answers. He told her that he had questioned Johnny in the hours before his death, and related the little information that he had obtained. They knew only that the men pursuing them were criminals, and that they were after the computer data. While it was obvious to Coltrane that the insurance company had hired the killers, he had no evidence to back his claims. Furthermore, both he and Britt were now involved in the death and disappearance of one of the men. He felt himself slipping deeper and deeper into the mire as the nightmare continued inexorably forward and downward.

"There's no one to help. The nearest police and the Bahamas Defense Force are in Nassau. Even if I convince them that we are in danger, it will take hours, maybe a full day to get a boat here. What are we going to tell them? That this Cuban guy wants to kill us? Why? This is the Bahamas, not the States. They will want some answers to questions that we can't give them. You know the Bahamian authorities. They have a very limited sense of humor." Coltrane was running out of answers.

"Call the FBI. Lynwood knows you. He'll know that you are not making the story up. He can help." Britt was grasping at any solution to save them.

"You want me to tell him that I bought a computer disc from a petty thief, and that I have been withholding evidence in Hendricks' murder, and now we have killed a man here in another country but would like him to help us? Either way we will be in jail, here or in the States." Coltrane could see no way out.

"We can give the disc to the FBI, they can figure out what is on it. Or we can give it back to the insurance company. If they have it back, maybe they'll leave us alone." Britt offered half-heartedly.

Coltrane looked sadly at his young bride. "There is one thing I didn't tell you. The Cuban knows that I saw his face clearly last night. I would be able to identify him and link him to Hendricks' murder. The Cuban will have to kill me, regardless of the contract. We have to deal with him here, now. I will get a seaplane out here to pick you up and take you to Nassau. You will be safe there." Coltrane made his decision.

"No way I will leave you alone. We do this together or not at all." Britt retorted.

"Why risk both our lives? I can move faster alone. I don't want to worry about you." Coltrane was adamant.

"No. I won't even discuss this further. Would you leave me alone here? I will *not* leave you. Now I need sleep, I can't think straight. Wake me in a couple hours." Britt went below to try to sleep.

Coltrane sat quietly in the cockpit for a long time, turning the events of the past days over and over in his head. He could not envision a way out of the quagmire into which they had descended. They had nothing with which to bargain. Coltrane needed to connect the Cuban to the insurance plan and implicate them in the murder of Hendricks. He needed to know what was on the disc. He needed something. He settled back in the cockpit and scanned the horizon. Before he knew it, he was sound asleep.

Chapter 54

Highburn Cay
June 27
4:05 PM

It was four in the afternoon before the small motor launch arrived at Calvin's dock. The man piloting the boat was red-eyed and soaked with sea spray from the trip. The Cuban stepped aboard, gave him $150US and explained that he could put the rest on his MasterCard. The man said nothing, nodded and cast off. He wondered why anyone would be alone in the Exumas, with only a Bible sized bundle wrapped in cloth. But minding his own business was how he stayed healthy. Within minutes they were skimming over the blue water headed for Nassau.

The ride was hard and uncomfortable. The small boat had little in the way of comfort, no cushions or seats. The captain stood, leaning forward into the chop and balancing on the wheel while the Cuban crouched in the stern taking the full force of the spray. The four hour ride was miserable.

Night had fallen by the time Nassau came into view, a crescent of brilliant lights from the distance. They motored slowly into the harbor, a deep protected channel that ran between the city and Paradise Island. He paid the balance of the trip charge, and had the sullen man drop him at the Paradise Island Casino boat dock. Tired, soaked and bone weary from the brutal hammering of the trip, he went straight to the opulent reception area of the hotel. He shook off the disapproving stares as he registered quickly, then headed for the row of high-fashion boutiques by the banks of elevators. He bought swimtrunks, a dark polo shirt, pleated tropical wool slacks and a pair of Sperry Topsiders. He ducked into the newsstand and picked up a copy of USA Today and a razor, toiletries and sterile bandages. Satisfied, he took an elevator to his room.

By the time he had showered and scrubbed the sand and salt from his hair and the dried blood from his body, it was 10 PM. The Cuban ordered a Caesar salad, fried conch, and two Heinekens from room service and ate greedily. He turned the air conditioning to maximum, stripped naked, and climbed into the cool white linens and was asleep in minutes.

Chapter 55

June 27
Saddleback Cay
6:30 PM

Coltrane was awakened by the loud whine of an outboard motor, rapidly approaching the yacht. He leapt out of his sleep and stood in the cockpit, searching for the source of the noise. As he rose, a small wooden skiff shot past, a tall black man standing in the stern, steering the outboard naturally. The lobsterman shot a smile and waved as he flew by, on his way home from a day's diving.

Coltrane vehemently cursed himself as he checked his watch. He had been out for five hours. The Cuban could have gotten there and cut his throat as he slept. He jumped below, and turned on the VHF radio. He hailed Calvin on Channel 16.

"This is Calvin, I read you. Go to Channel 63." Calvin replied.

"Copy, going to 63." Coltrane changed channels on the handset. "Cal, how is my friend?" Coltrane asked.

"Good news, Doc. He was able to contact Eleuthera, but no one could come to get him today. Apparently he is low on cash, so he can't prepay the boat hire. Eleuthera would not come get him. Finally, he got hold of the phone, and he called the States I think. Anyway, a boat picked him up an hour ago and took him back to Nassau. He will not be getting down your way for a day or so, I imagine."

"He could get a boat and meet us tomorrow. That's possible, isn't it?" Coltrane calculated the time and distance to Nassau as he spoke.

"Maybe. But I overhear his phone conversation. He has no cash, no passport. He tried to get some money wired, or get help from the States, but things work slow in the islands, *mon.* No way someone will give him a boat and just let him sail off. A man's boat is his life. We don't got boat insurance down here, Doc. Too many hurricanes. He won't get no boat today. Tomorrow maybe."

"You sure he went to Nassau?" Coltrane was hesitant.

"Yeah. I know the boat he went with, and I watched him leave. No question." Calvin was positive.

"Thanks, Cal. If you hear anything from my friend, please contact me. I will be monitoring all night on 63." Coltrane answered. He knew that if the Cuban returned, he would probably stop at Cal's marina.

"Right, Doc. Out." Calvin signed off.

"Out." Coltrane signed off, leaving the radio on, monitoring channel 63. He cursed himself for his lapse, and by way of penitence, went below to check his gear.

Hours later, thoughts of the conference surfaced in his mind, and he headed into the salon to check *Caduceus*. He plugged the satellite phone into the port on the laptop computer, and booted the program. He used the New York AOL number, and checked his E-mail. There was one message waiting.

E-mail
June 27
3:23:15 PM
From: SKerr
To: WmColtraneMD

Dr Coltrane

All is going well with the conference. The attendance is less today. Many doctors are using *Caduceus* to follow the proceedings from home. Specialist meetings continue. The insurance companies have filed a complaint, and the FBI wants to speak with you. The conference is on autopilot, no problems. It will continue until the doctors or you want it to stop. The delivery of healthcare in Tampa-St. Pete is in continuity. The ERs are somewhat crowded, but the truly sick patients are being seen promptly. The members have devised a system that takes care of the ER overflow by their offices. Thus far, the public and the media have supported us. The media want an interview, and maybe we can arrange this with you by phone?

I await your instructions.

sk

Coltrane read the message and was gratified at the progress of the conference. The first phase in his strategy was to make the public, the insurance providers and the state legislature aware of the problems that physicians faced in the delivery of healthcare. All the previous methods had failed miserably. Now it seemed that he had the media's interest. Clearly he had the insurance industry's interest, as evidenced by the anti-trust action that they had taken. Only through the power of the media would he be able to influence public opinion, or to change the way that healthcare was managed. Coltrane composed an E-mail message to Susan Kerr.

E-mail
June 27
6:39:44 PM
From: WmColtraneMD
To: SKerr

I will be able to have a telephone or IM conference with Elizabeth Volk tomorrow afternoon. She will continue to be our only liaison if she prints accurate unbiased information from our press releases. I want newspaper coverage only, it is much more substantive and complete, the TV news is crap. Let them stick with their car accidents. E-mail me with progress.

Keep up the good work.

wc

Coltrane sent the message, and turned off the computer and the satellite phone. He connected them both to the trickle charger using a cigarette lighter adapter and the power point in the electrical panel of the boat. The green indicators lit up, and glowed in the half darkness of the salon. He flipped a CD into the stereo, and the cabin came alive with The Rolling Stones. Coltrane stood and listened with admiration to Charlie Watts' strong, distinctive snare and cymbal strokes. The high performance titanium speakers reproduced with startling clarity the guitar riffs, and Coltrane smiled as he heard the rasp of Keith Richards' rough fingers on the steel strings. Glancing at the half finished bottle of Merlot, he resisted the urge to pour a glass of deep red wine, and went topside into the sunset.

How had his calm and sweet life become so tortured, so quickly?

Chapter 56

June 27
7:41PM

Coltrane spent the evening methodically enacting rituals of combat preparation as Britt slept in the fore cabin. He carefully disassembled the speargun, and cleaned the blood and bits of tissue from the shaft and cable. Then he cleaned and oiled the mechanism, and test fired the gun into the water. It functioned beautifully. He cleaned and oiled his dive knife. Next he took a clean towel and laid it out on the cockpit cushions. He retrieved Johnny's pistol and examined it closely, turning it slowly in his hand. It was a Beretta .22 caliber automatic, a new design with a fixed barrel. Threaded to the end of the barrel was a thick silencer, four inches long. There were no sights or serial numbers on the weapon. Coltrane checked the clip, and found three shells remained. Coltrane removed a cartridge from the magazine, and compared it to the IMI shells in the boxes. They were identical. He loaded a full magazine, and inserted it into the gun. He knew that a round was already chambered.

Standing up, Coltrane scanned the horizon. They had anchored in the lee of an uninhabited island, and so far had seen no one come or go except the lobsterman. Coltrane saw nothing on the water as far as the eye could see. He rolled another towel into a rest for the pistol barrel, and sighted down the length of the silencer. Coltrane chose a small clump of weeds on the beach, thirty yards away. He gently squeezed the trigger until the gun jumped in his hand. The noise it made was much louder than he had expected, a heavy *thwapp.* He didn't see where the bullet went. He fired again. Still no impact in the sand.

Coltrane went below and picked a piece of orange peel from the trash.

He threw it overboard, and watched it drift on the outgoing tide. As it floated away, he raised the pistol and fired. Now, he could see where the bullets were going. The gun was reasonably accurate out to ten yards, very close range. Beyond that, the rounds went all over. Satisfied, he emptied the magazine at the floating orange peel, hitting it once. Then he disassembled the pistol, and cleaned and oiled it as best he could. He loaded the magazine with seven rounds and pulling the slide back, chambered a round. Then he removed the magazine and refilled the clip to full capacity. He safed the weapon, wrapped it in a towel and secured it in a locker in the fore stateroom. Britt was sleeping fitfully as he stood over her. He quietly closed the teak door to the cabin.

The sun was sinking as he set up the satphone. He moved quickly, familiar now with the phone. He plugged the satphone line into the data port and initiated the Internet connection. His E-mail box was full of old messages from Susan, concerning the things they had discussed earlier that day. There was nothing from Cindy. No news was good news.

Coltrane retrieved the CD-R from its hiding place in the bilge. He removed it from the plastic jewel case, and slipped it into the CD-ROM drive of the computer. Then he went to his address book, and pulled down Susan's E-mail address. He composed a brief message.

E-mail
June 27
9:31:56 PM
From: WmColtrancMD
To: SKerr

Susan

The file that is attached to this message should be copied and given directly to Scott Lynwood immediately. IMMEDIATELY. Get a signed, dated receipt from him. The file may have information of interest to him. I will contact him in the AM with further details. Please E-mail confirmation of this ASAP. Do not tell anyone else about this message or file.

How are things?

Thanks Coltrane

Coltrane attached the file containing the data on the CD-R, and sent the message. He watched as the file was read and sent off into cyberspace. It took just five minutes for the entire file to be sent. When it had been sent, he shut down the computer and satellite phone, and went topside. He made a bed for himself with cushions on the cockpit bench, and settled in for the night watch.

Chapter 57

Tampa
June 28

Susan Kerr woke up at 5:30 AM, and was at her office by 7:15. The last week had been increasingly hectic and demanding for her, but she was finding that she was enjoying it more and more each day. Susan Kerr was born and raised in the heartland, the middle daughter in a large Catholic family. Money was scarce when it was her time for college, and she had tried to put herself through the nearby state junior college. But like many young girls away from home for the first time, her attentions soon drifted from her studies. Before she knew it, she was married to her high school boyfriend. Her marriage didn't stand the harsh realities of life and parenthood, and she found herself with two baby boys, and alone. Traveling to the Sunbelt in search of a better life away from the gray bitter winters of the Midwest, she settled her young family in Tampa.

Answering a newspaper ad for a secretary, she had joined the society staff five years ago. Staff attrition and her native intelligence and Midwest work ethic resulted in her rise in the organization. As the assistant to the president, she was subordinate only to the Medical Society Director and the physician President. Prior to Coltrane's election, her principal function at the medical society had been to oversee the secretarial pool, and perform mundane tasks for the director. In her thirties, without a college degree or marketable skills, she had settled into a stable, but dead end career.

The Director of the Medical Society, Floyd Gainer, normally ran all functions of the organization. For as long as she could remember, the society was not much more than a social organization. Gainer was a retired Navy man, an alcoholic, and his presence was scarcely felt. Everything ran smoothly, quietly, uneventfully. In every past instance, the physician president of the society had been only a figurehead. The president would open every meeting with a short speech, then drink, enjoy dinner and socialize. In fact, she rarely remembered anything of any consequence ever being done by the society other than the annual health fair. Now, in contradistinction to all presidents in the past, Coltrane was enacting policy, and making waves. Coltrane had changed everything.

The whirlwind of activity that had descended upon her and the society in the last month had energized her, spiritually and intellectually. She now had become the de facto director of the society. Coltrane had given her guidelines and direction, and Gainer was completely out of the loop. For the first time in her life, Susan Kerr was in control, running a dynamic and powerful entity. She was ecstatic.

Arriving early this morning, Susan found Coltrane's E-mail on her computer, along with the attached file. She pulled up the file, and opened it. All she saw was pages and pages of numbers, all in continuity without any punctuation or breaks. Not wanting to know anything more, she transferred the file onto a CD-R disc, and slipped it into a blank jewel case. She read through her messages from the day before, and contemplated how to deal with her most pressing problems.

For two days now, she had been getting calls from CNN and journalists with the major television networks. The reporters wanted to interview Dr. Coltrane about the medical society meeting and the accusations that the insurance plans had made. The story was on the verge of breaking into the national news. Susan had stonewalled them, promising an interview in the near future. Coltrane was aware of the pressure being brought to bear by the five major television networks, and had sent out a gag order over *Caduceus*. He didn't want every publicity-happy doctor telling his story on national television. He knew there were doctors who couldn't resist the urge to pontificate and blather on, blinded to their stupidity by their delusions of self-importance. Coltrane knew how a television camera could make someone instantly stupid.

Susan began taking calls after the rest of her staff arrived at 9AM. First she phoned Lynwood, and told him about the message and file from Coltrane. She respected and admired the man, having met him when he examined the society minutes. He promised he would pick up the file that morning.

Her phone was ringing non-stop. The news media was hounding her mercilessly. At one point, CNN asked if they could send over a team to interview her and the director. Kerr vetoed that suggestion, but promised to fax them relevant position papers immediately. When this failed to appease the news director, she told him that she would try to arrange a phone interview with Coltrane that afternoon. She quickly sent Coltrane an E-mail message informing him of the interview request and to call her ASAP.

Her anxiety continued to build as time passed without a response from Coltrane. By late morning, she was feeling the pressure physically affect her. Using relaxation techniques she had learned at a recent management seminar, she took a short walk in the park across from the society office. As she returned, she noticed the dark car with white government plates parked in the visitor's space. She found Lynwood in the waiting area, and led him back past the reception desk to her office. She pulled a brown sealed envelope from her locked top desk drawer, and gave it to the FBI attorney. He signed a two part receipt, and kept the carbon copy.

"Did Dr. Coltrane discuss the nature of this file with you? He hasn't contacted me yet." Lynwood was puzzled.

"No, sir. This is completely out of the blue. I have no idea what that file is about. I haven't discussed it with Dr. Coltrane yet today, but I will be communicating with him via the Internet shortly. Do you have his E-mail address?" Susan gave Lynwood the address, hoping that cooperation would turn the FBI agent into an ally. He thanked her and left the building.

Shortly after she returned to her desk, one of the secretaries came in, visibly upset. She had just gotten off the line with a state senator who had berated her for failing to connect him with Dr. Coltrane. Despite her explanations that Coltrane was out of town, the man had accused her of lying and threatened her with a congressional subpoena and warrant if she failed to get Coltrane immediately.

"Get me his number, I'll call him back." Susan calmed her down.

"The jerkoff is holding on Line 3," the distraught woman answered, and left the office.

Susan took three deep breaths, then let him wait for several minutes more before she picked up the receiver. "Susan Kerr here," she intoned.

"Susan Kerr? Why did she put me through to *you*? Where is Coltrane?" The senator was angry.

"I am sorry, but who is this please?" Susan asked sweetly.

"Susan, this is State Senator Thompson. I demand to speak with the president of your society. I believe that is Dr. William Coltrane. How can I contact him?" The senator calmed down somewhat.

"Senator, Dr. Coltrane is not available at this time. He is out of town at a medical meeting, and left instructions not to be interrupted during the conference. I can, however, take a message from you and relay it to Dr. Coltrane." Susan was firm.

"Miss Kerr, what is going on down there? I am hearing that the physicians are staging an illegal strike and that the area hospitals are unmanned and patients are not being treated. Apparently the county medical society is instrumental in organizing this strike. Can you confirm or deny these reports?" Thompson ranted.

"There certainly is no strike occurring here in Tampa, Senator. The society is having a strategic planning conference at this time, but patient care is not being impacted in a negative way. I would be glad to send you the position papers of the society if you desire." Susan hoped that Coltrane was staying within the letter of the law. She knew the power state senators could wield, but resented the man's pompous tone.

"Send me your position papers and…" Thompson ordered.

"Senator, your name is not familiar to me. Do you represent constituents in the Tampa or in the St. Pete area?" Susan interrupted him.

"I represent District 29 in Orlando." Thompson slowed down, regretting his belligerent tone.

"Your constituents are a hundred miles away. How can our problems possibly affect them?" Susan continued leading him into a debate he could not win.

"Anything that negatively impacts Florida healthcare is of interest to me. Please have him call me as soon as he returns." Thompson cut short the conversation, gave his office number, and hung up.

Susan wrote his number on a piece of scrap paper, then crumpled it into a ball and threw it into the trash. She opened the P4 laptop, and turned the computer on as she connected the data line. Within moments she was online with *Caduceus*. She sent off a short confirmation E-mail to Coltrane, acknowledging that Lynwood had received the data. Then she returned to the many tasks at hand.

Chapter 58

Nassau
June 28

His alarm woke him at 5:30AM. The Cuban savored his slumber, but today he had too much to do to waste time in bed. Picking up the Yellow Pages, he turned to Boat Hire and read the ads. He called the concierge, and got the names of two outfits that catered to the bonefishermen. He was told that no one opened until 7AM. He ordered breakfast, and drank his coffee as he considered his options. In reality, he thought, there was only one way that this could end. He finished his meal, and headed down to the casino. He forlornly wandered up to the cashier's window, and playing the losing gambler, took a $3000US advance on his MasterCard. The young lady sympathetically counted out the cash for him, and he shuffled off. He stopped at the concierge's desk, and arranged for a seaplane scenic overflight of the Exumas that afternoon. Satisfied, he strolled out the huge portico sure.

The Cuban walked out past the manicured tropical gardens in the circular driveway of the resort. He crossed the arched bridge to Nassau, and made his way to the commercial section of the wharf and docks. Stopping at a marine outfitter, he purchased a set of charts, a waterproof flashlight and a long bladed, serrated dive knife. He chatted with the salesman about prime flats for bonefish, bought a pair of polarized sunglasses and left.

The powerboat charters were located nearby in a shallow water section of the marina. The Cuban looked carefully for an outfit with clean new boats and their own repair facility. He selected the charter service with two 21 foot Boston Whalers in good condition. The hulls were clean and undamaged, and the MerCruiser outboards looked relatively new. The center console craft was well equipped with VHF radio, gimbal mounted compass and dual gas tanks. Seeing the twin circles of the MasterCard emblem on the window, he stepped inside.

The proprietor was a weather-beaten Irishman, his ruddy skin showing the effects of time and sun. He smiled as he looked the Cuban up and down, amused at his brand new boat shoes and embroidered polo shirt. Another filthy rich American to fuck up his precious boats, he thought. The beauty and clarity of the Bahamian waters deceived these fools. The reality was that the local waters were treacherous, and errors in judgment could be fatal. He raised his shoulders up off the glass counter to see what the man wanted.

In ten minutes of casual conversation and sea tales, the Cuban had dispelled any doubts the man had about his experience with the sea. Both Whalers were available today, and the Cuban chose the one with a clean, new 150 horsepower outboard. He rolled out the chart of the island, and asked about prime bonefishing spots. The flats on the far side of the island were the best this time of year, and the owner gave him tips on tide and bait selection. The Cuban rented a pair of binoculars and gave him a cash deposit, saying he would need the boat for three or four days. After checking that the fuel tanks were topped off, he cast off and motored toward the casino boat dock. He could leave the boat there while he took his plane ride.

The plane ride was noisy and rough. Updrafts and air currents caused by the tiny islands buffeted the single engine Aviat Husky seaplane as they flew outbound from Nassau. The pilot took him in a long sweeping arc toward Eleuthera and the Exumas. The Cuban had explained that he was looking for an area for a swimsuit photo shoot, and wanted to find a secluded cay in the outisland chain. He wanted a low level survey so he could assess each tiny coral island.

The Cuban knew the boat that he was searching for. It would be hard to miss the forty foot yacht, and he knew the Hunter logo on the sails and hull. He knew the name of the sloop as well. It only took them forty-five minutes before he spotted the sloop, lying at anchor in the lee of a saddleback island. The Cuban quietly marked the spot on his chart, and scanned the island with his binoculars. He mechanically went through the motions for the remainder of the flight. They were back in Nassau by sunset.

Chapter 59

Saddleback Cay
June 28
5:45AM

Coltrane was up before the sun. He stirred in the predawn darkness and lay on the bench, serenely gazing at the endless expanse of shimmering waters. As the sun rose behind the island, he slowly got up and surveyed the boat. The anchor had held well, and the boat floated lazily in the center of the little bay. The seas were flat, and the tide high. Coltrane went below and checked on Britt, who was sleeping soundly. He went back topside.

Putting on mask and snorkel, he slipped into the warm water off the transom, and swam along the side of the sloop. The boat was fine below the waterline, no trash or seaweed caught on the prop or rudder. He reached up and grabbed the nylon anchor line as it entered the water from the bow pulpit, and swam forward. The water was crystal clear, and he could easily see the anchor ten feet below. The blades of the Danforth had buried themselves deeply in the white, rippled bottom. Coltrane dove down and firmly set the anchor, then slowly swam back to the boat. The visibility was incredible and Coltrane watched as small schools of bait fish darted out of his way, and curious yellowjack swam beside him. He pulled himself out of the sea, and sat in the transom for several minutes, gazing out to sea.

Coltrane carefully rethought his original plan of action, and factored in the additional time that they had been granted. He knew that the Cuban may have trouble getting money or help in Nassau, but didn't want to assume too much. In the worst case scenario, the Cuban could get to their position by late today. Coltrane had to prepare for that eventuality.

Climbing up into the cockpit, Coltrane made a list of supplies he would need. As the sun rose, and the temperature climbed in the cabin, Britt stirred and woke. Coltrane greeted her and brewed a pot of coffee. He let her gather her wits, then discussed the list with her as they sipped their coffee. Today would be the most important day of their lives.

The Coltrane's knew Saddleback Cay very well. They had discovered it together seven years ago, when it was first designated as a Bahamian national wildlife preserve. The cay was privately owned, but uninhabited since the end of the eighteenth century. Stone ruins sat atop a hill as the mute testimony of the past. Legend had it that the ruins were the remains of a pirate lookout, the final outpost of the Barratarria pirate Jean Lafitte. Tales of ghosts and a woman singing beautifully at midnight only added to the idyllic allure of the tiny isle. The couple had found it on their first trip to the Exumas, and spent a week combing the five sparkling beaches and snorkeling in the pristine waters offshore. They had made love on the white sand beaches, and had never wanted to leave.

Saddleback Cay was strikingly different from all the other cays in the Exumas. Unlike the low scrub covered coral islands in the chain, Saddleback Cay's twin peaks rose over one hundred feet above sea level. The cay was shaped like a dumbbell, with the south peak towering over the smaller north peak. The narrow waist of the island was flanked on the east and west by twin bays, each with a sparkling sand beach. To the far north, a third wide beach curved along the edge of the island.

Like all the cays in the chain, Saddleback Cay was the remnant of an ancient limestone formation, created one million years ago by centuries of deposition and erosion. The cay consisted of limestone, coral and sand, nothing else. The coral was razor-sharp and jagged, cut by wind and water and time. It jutted out of the blue water on all sides of the island except the five small sand beaches, and the ancient limestone formed ragged black cliffs. Covering the rocky surface, impenetrable low scrub covered the island. The maze of brambles and thickets were passable only by narrow overgrown trails, left by the colonial settlers. In many places, nature had reclaimed even these pathways.

While Britt cooked a sumptuous breakfast, Coltrane set up the satphone and his notebook computer. He checked his E-mail first, and pulled up several messages from Susan Kerr. She was starting early today, he thought as he read through the series of notes she had sent that morning. Concerned about the urgency of her notes, he disconnected the data port, and lifted the telephone handset. He dialed her private line, and was surprised as she answered on the second ring.

"Susan Kerr." she said quickly.

"Susan, this is Coltrane. What is happening on the home front?" Coltrane started cheerfully.

"A bit too much action to please me, Dr. Coltrane. I am glad that you called. Let me bring you up to speed." Susan felt relieved to pass on the responsibility of the morning's events. "First, I was able to get the file to Agent Lynwood, and got a receipt per your instructions. But he has no idea what the data is about, and asked you to call with clarification if possible. Uh, I also gave him your E-mail address… before really thinking. Was that a mistake?" Susan just realized that Coltrane may not have wanted that information given to anyone. Especially the FBI.

"Hmmm...We have to assume from now on that our E-mail may be monitored. Nothing we can do about it now." Coltrane considered the ramifications of her error.

"Shit." Susan cursed. She hadn't considered that when she passed on the E-mail address. "I'm sorry, Dr. Coltrane. I didn't think of that."

"Don't worry about it, it may show good faith on our behalf. I welcome anything that helps to get Lynwood off my back. Please call him when we get off and tell him that I will be contacting him within the hour. It is very urgent." Coltrane said.

"Certainly. Another thing. I got a call from a Senator Thompson in Tallahassee. He's raising hell about what he thinks is a strike organized by the medical society. I am not sure how he became involved, but he is demanding that you call him immediately to discuss the situation." Susan explained.

"I've heard of the guy before. He's from central Florida somewhere; he has no business calling you in Tampa. But what worries me is that sooner or later, *our* elected representatives will be calling, and so will the Joint Committee on Healthcare. Then we'll have to answer their questions. Time may be running out. How is the membership holding up?" Coltrane wondered which way to take the conference.

"Very well. The practice management page in *Caduceus* is getting heavy usage, and the members are constantly updating it with their own experiences. The members are shocked to discover the actual reimbursement they are receiving for services. I think that the vast majority of our doctors have no idea of how little the HMOs are paying them. Their office managers collect and commingle the payments from all insurance and third party sources. Prior to *Caduceus*, few physicians were able to compare what they were being paid for, say, an office visit or an admission to the hospital. Now they can do that easily and they are very angry at what they are finding." Susan knew that Coltrane had anticipated that reaction.

"Good. The failure of our profession is our inability to come together and circle wagons. How is public opinion shaping up?" This was Coltrane's greatest fear. If the public felt that medical care was compromised, he would immediately and without hesitation end the conference. Patient confidence in physicians was the keystone of his profession, and he would not risk it in any way.

"So far, it has been favorable. I have taken it upon myself to ask Elizabeth Volk to interview David Strahan about his son's death. Strahan would not talk, on advice of his attorney. Elizabeth was able to interview the Diaz family, and got information from the Miami Police as well. The HMO refused to respond. The article was in yesterday's paper, and discussed on the evening news as well. I think it will help if you talk to Elizabeth again. She has too many questions that I can't answer, and the public needs clarification of our demands. We are holding our own so far, but I don't know how long it will last." Susan answered.

"Fine. Tell her that I will correspond with her via E-mail, maybe IM her today. In fact, call her and tell her I will be online and IM her within the hour."

"Thanks, boss. That will make my life so much easier."

"You're doing good work. You're taking to this like a duck to water. Can you hold out for a few days more?" Coltrane asked.

"I can hold out. I am finding that I enjoy the pressure and the responsibility, but I truly think that we are on the edge here. If a patient, even one patient suffers from our actions, I will never be able to forgive myself. How long do you think we can continue?" Susan knew the intricate back-up schedules that Coltrane had arranged to safeguard patient care. But she also knew that no manmade plan was infallible.

"I share your concerns, believe me. I, too, am unable to see down the paths that lay before us. Please trust me when I tell you that the Tampa area has complete coverage for both medical emergencies and for routine patient care. The physicians that draw call for the day will be working harder than usual, but everything will get done. Everyone will suffer inconvenience, but nothing more. Also realize that the alternative is to continue *as is*, with high school graduates making medical decisions for patients like John Strahan. Who knows how many lives like his will be damaged or lost. And remember, the vast majority of diseases take years, maybe decades to develop. Even cancers probably take ten or fifteen years to grow to a detectable size. Nothing is going to change in one or two days." Coltrane had always been perplexed by the layman's perception of health and illness.

"I'm sure you are right. I just hope some catastrophe doesn't mar the progress of the conference." Susan couldn't shake her foreboding.

"Maybe you're right. Give me the names of the HMO directors for PatientsChoice Florida and AthenaHMO. I am going to make an attempt to contact them today and discuss our agenda. Please call them and try to arrange a time for a teleconference ASAP. Maybe they are willing to make some changes. It must be clear to them by now that both patients and providers are unhappy with the current system." Coltrane hoped some resolution would occur soon.

Susan gave Coltrane the names and phone numbers of the two regional directors for the HMO plans. He discussed some minor details, told her to stall the CNN reporters, and thanked Susan for her confidence and hung up. Coltrane switched the satphone to standby, and sat back in the settee, and contemplated his next move. Britt fed them a huge breakfast of eggs, hash brown potatoes and onions finished with fresh squeezed orange juice. Coltrane resisted the urge to comment on the condemned man's last meal. They sipped coffee in silence, each deep in their own thoughts.

As Britt cleared the dishes, Coltrane picked up the satphone again. He dialed Lynwood's number from memory, and waited as the line rang. Lynwood picked up on the fifth ring.

"Agent Lynwood," He said tonelessly.

"Lynwood, this is Coltrane. I assume that you have received the file I sent you?" Coltrane started slowly, not precisely sure how he wanted to take the conversation.

"Yes, Doctor. I have examined the file, and it seems to be a long sequence of numbers. Is that what you sent me?" Lynwood asked.

"Yeah. My computer put it at 648 MB. The entire file is just one long number. Before I tell you anything more, I need to have your assurances on several points. Is that agreeable to you?" Coltrane wanted to get some of the weight off his chest.

"That will depend entirely upon what you are asking. What is the significance of this file, and where did you get it?" Lynwood pressed.

"Can you tape record this conversation? I would like a record of our discussion." Coltrane said.

"You are already being recorded, Dr. Coltrane. Continue." Lynwood was matter of fact.

"I believe that the file I sent you was the property of AthenaHMO and that it was stolen by Dr. Stephen Hendricks. More than likely, it contains damning evidence against Athena. I obtained the disc from a friend of Hendricks'. He claims that Hendricks stole the data on that disc. Hendricks then encrypted the data in the form of the continuous string of numbers." Coltrane paused.

"Dr. Hendricks died in a recent boating accident, didn't he? I remember reading about that a while ago." Lynwood recalled.

"Right," Coltrane answered, wondering how much to reveal to Lynwood about the circumstances surrounding Hendricks' death.

"Go on." Lynwood was clearly interested.

Coltrane related the chain of events that started with Strahan's death and the discussion of the case with Hendricks. He mentioned his theory that Hendricks had feared for his job as a result of his negligence in the transfer of Strahan. Further, Coltrane felt that Hendricks meant to hold the data on the file over his employer in an attempt to salvage his career. Coltrane waited for a response, sensing that his story sounded like a paranoid fantasy.

Lynwood said nothing.

"The man who gave me the disc told me he was sure that Hendricks had been murdered, and that his murderers were after the data. In fact, there were two CD-R's stolen by Hendricks. One disc was recovered and destroyed. Somehow, the killers have found out that I now have the remaining disc. I believe that they intend to kill me, and destroy the disc. I have sent you a copy for two reasons. First, once it is in the hands of the government, I hope that the chase will be over. The cat will be out of the bag, and therefore no reason to pursue or kill us. Two, you may be able to decode whatever the encrypted data means. Send it to the FBI lab in Washington, maybe they can decode it. I have looked at it for hours, and can find no clue to its meaning. But whatever the data is, it must be incriminating for them to go to such lengths to suppress it."

"You think that it is evidence of criminal activity by an insurance company?" Lynwood was incredulous.

"Possibly criminal activity. More likely deceptive business practices that would leave the plan liable for massive damages in a civil case. I am not sure which…" Coltrane was cut off by Lynwood's interruption.

"Listen, Coltrane. I don't know what kind of game you are playing here. First you set into motion a conference that may be a thinly disguised work stoppage, in violation of federal anti-trust law. Then you tell me that you are in New York, while you skip out of the country and play this charade from the Bahamas. You think you are so clever, fooling everyone with a satellite phone and E-mail. Now you lay this outrageous fable of hired killers and coded data on me, trying to stall me further. No more bullshit. Giving false information to a FBI agent is a federal offense. I want you back in the States in twenty-four hours or I will issue a warrant for your arrest. This is my last communication with you." Lynwood began to hang up.

"Wait. Wait. Wait. I know it sounds like fantasy. I didn't believe it myself. Except that a couple of days ago, I got a message that two men were asking questions about us in Marsh Harbor. They were asking about us at the charter base there. I have taken great effort to keep my itinerary secret. No one knows that we are in the Caribbean, not our friends, not even our families. How could anyone find us, and more importantly, who would be looking for us?" Coltrane demanded.

"I have known where you are for days." Lynwood said, matter of factly. "I checked your MasterCard statement and found the yacht charter payment. You must know that when Customs scans your passport, the barcode embedded below your photograph records your point of exit and your destination. And you were on the American Airline passenger manifest to Marsh Harbor on June 23rd. People are easy to find, Doctor."

Coltrane cursed. He had forgotten about the charter deposit, months ago when they had first planned this trip. Now he was forced to play one of his trump cards. But which one? The things Resendez had claimed? The details of Hendricks' death? Or the tape of Hendricks' conversation? All the lies were beginning to pile up in his mind, he didn't know what he had said, or hadn't said.

"The man who gave me data on that CD-R claimed that Hendricks was murdered. He also was the one who broke into my office last month. He knew exactly what was in my top desk drawer. He knew what photographs I have on my credenza. So I took him at his word. I went to the assistant county coroner, and told him that I had a bad feeling about Hendricks' death. He did a preliminary autopsy, and found duct tape adhesive on his wrists and ankles. Someone killed him, no question. You can check all this with Dr. Ken Jasper, at County Hospital. Ask him to describe our discussion, in detail. Tell him I sent you." Coltrane was frustrated, but relieved to get the burden off his chest.

"You are getting deeper and deeper into trouble, Coltrane. Now you are admitting that you've been withholding material information in a murder case. And protecting a witness or possible accomplice in the killing as well. What is your informant's name? Where can we find him?" Lynwood was angry.

"The man who gave me the disc is named Resendez. Juan Resendez. He was a friend of Hendricks, probably his drug dealer. He will verify everything I've told you. Just tell him that he will have to cooperate in order to get any whistle-blower reward. That should free his tongue." Coltrane was negotiating from a weak position.

"Whistle-blower?" Lynwood asked.

"If there are federal penalties involved with the HMO's criminal activity, whoever discovers the crime is entitled to a reward based on the amount of the fines. Is that not true?" Coltrane asked.

"True."

"I want to establish my claim in any action against AthenaHMO and related to this data I have provided to you."

"So noted. For the record, I am acknowledging your claim to those fees. Let's hope you will be out of jail in time to enjoy it." Lynwood now seemed to find the whole story amusing.

"Look, Lynwood. You may think that I am fabricating this entire story, but you are still a public servant and have a responsibility to check it out. Give me the benefit of the doubt. Call Dennis at the charter base in Marsh Harbor, call Resendez or the Tampa police, and even call the HMO to see if Hendricks stole anything from them, data, computer files, whatever. Call

Dr. Jasper and ask him if there was freshwater in Hendricks' lungs. You'll find everything is true. Which means that my wife and I are in grave danger." Coltrane ran out of ideas, breath and patience at the same time.

"I'll make some calls right now. But if you think you're in danger, I suggest that you notify the Bahamian authorities immediately. I am sure you realize that the FBI has no jurisdiction in a foreign country." Lynwood responded.

"We are in the Exumas. It is a two day sail just to Nassau. I don't think we have that much time. Call me right back. I don't know what to do." Coltrane lied.

"I am going to tell you exactly what to do. Radio the Bahamian Defense Force immediately and request assistance. They can send a cutter to pick you up in several hours. I can notify the American Embassy in Nassau as well. Give me your satphone number and keep it on twenty-four hours." Lynwood ordered.

Coltrane agreed, and gave Lynwood their approximate position. He deliberately miscalculated by fifty miles to give himself time. He didn't want rescue. He had to finish this in the islands. As he hung up with Lynwood, he wondered how it would all end.

Dead tired, with a pounding headache, Coltrane was physically and mentally exhausted. Only years of experience operating all night and day saved him from collapse. He shook his head to clear his mind, and opened the laptop to sign on to AOL. Within minutes he had established an IM connection to Elizabeth Volk.

WmColtrane: thanks for communicating with IM, the satphone bill is killing me

LizzyVolk7: no problem

WmColtrane: how are things in tampa-st pete?

LizzyVolk7: very hot for you, I'm afraid. public wants to know details of your plan, and when the docs are going back to full schedule

WmColtrane: as soon as we get some answers from the HMOs and the insurance industry

LizzyVolk7: the public wants to know your plans

WmColtrane: give them my position papers

LizzyVolk7: I have reproduced them, word for word, in the paper

WmColtrane: how did the public react?

LizzyVolk7: very well, especially to your comments that we need universal health care

WmColtrane: that is my personal view, not the official view of the society. I have a very radical approach to healthcare. But this is not the position of the society. Just my own demented scheme. Please note that distinction.

LizzyVolk7: I made that clear. But that stand makes you very popular with the community

WmColtrane: I won't be so popular when they hear the details

LizzyVolk7: please explain

WmColtrane: I think every American should be provided with basic healthcare. And I mean BASIC. No Viagra. No cholesterol lowering agents for people who continue to eat bacon and eggs every morning. No fertility procedures for people who can't have children. Judicious use of transplants. And everyone will also have to participate in the process. 61% of Americans are overweight and 30% are severely overweight, and clinically obese.

LizzyVolk7: whats the difference between overweight and obese?

WmColtrane: overweight is 10% above normal and obese is 30% above normal. obese people have 36% more health care costs, and 77% more prescription costs. Heart disease, diabetes, arthritis are the major costs in the system, and all are directly related to obesity. obesity has a greater cost to society than alcohol and cigarettes, which, by the way, are taxed via sin taxes

LizzyVolk7: are you advocating a tax on Doritos?

WmColtrane: maybe. or insurance criteria on all Americans to compensate for risk factors, just like any insurance is set up now

LizzyVolk7: what do you mean?

WmColtrane: when you apply for car insurance, the insurance company will factor your age, sex, driving experience, type of car, etc. and calculate your premium. It's not discrimination, simply actuarial science. a 19 year old boy pays more than a 35 year old woman. higher risk. why shouldn't that work in health insurance? a 5'2, 285 pound female is going to have health problems, more so than a 5'2, 125 pound female. regardless of race, creed or age. That is just fact. So why should the woman who walks every evening, watches her diet, doesn't abuse her body, why should she have to pay for the care of people who are couch potatoes? Not fair. And it's more than just medical costs. I had a woman in my office last week who was over 200 pounds and was on disability for 3 years because she claimed to have "nerve damage" in her ankle. Some idiot chiropractor had written her disability papers. Absolute fraud. I'm going to pull her disability and get her back to work. If she loses 30 pounds, her "ankle pain" will disappear.

LizzyVolk7: Man, you're harsh.

WmColtrane: People need to be responsible for their own health. We are going to really, truly empower Americans with their own healthcare. Make everyone carry their own weight. Pardon the pun.

LizzyVolk7: How do you intend to apply this in practice?

WmColtrane: Yearly physical exams. mandated. on your birthday, you get the day off by law. you have to go to the doctor, get an exam, height, weight, electrolytes, etc. etc. Basic, thorough physical exam. If you don't show, you automatically get fined $1000, added to your IRS bill, and get assigned the highest risk category. They do this kind of thing in other countries, for other programs. It will work.

LizzyVolk7: Annual weigh-in? Us women will love that.

WmColtrane: sorry, ladies. but it will be confidential. the good thing is that it will give everyone a real, financial motivation to stay healthy. nothing works better than hitting someone in the wallet. We tried the President's Council on Physical Fitness. President Kennedy started it and even Arnold Schwartzenegger tried to motivate us, but the country's health has been on a steady decline for fifty years. I never personally realized the extent of it until I went to Europe for the first time two years ago. Seems like everyone is trim over there, they walk everywhere, eat well, live healthier despite the fact that the US has a far better healthcare system.

LizzyVolk7: you are trying to legislate health. that is as impossible as legislating morality. good luck

WmColtrane: I'm not legislating health, I am just trying to provide uniform healthcare to everyone, and to distribute the cost equitably. I honestly believe that a byproduct of this system will be a general improvement in the nation's health. Does any of this help you?

LizzyVolk7: Yes, it all does. Thank you. Can I contact you at this E-mail address for further questions?

WmColtrane: Certainly. Thanks for your time. I hope you keep an open mind, and show the conference in a fair light. Later.

LizzyVolk7: Bye for now

Chapter 60

Saddleback Cay

It had taken them two hours to select their provisions and gear to go ashore. Coltrane had given Britt a long list of supplies and food which she collected and boxed up for transfer in the dinghy. Coltrane packed up the satphone and antenna as well as the weapons and assorted survival equipment. He put the medical kit and pistol with the ammo into their waterproof fishing tackle box along with a small hand-held VHF radio. Throwing everything into the dinghy, he made one last check of the sailboat. He secured the anchor line, and locked the companionway hatch. Throwing a towel and his swimsuit over the cockpit lifeline to give the appearance that the boat was occupied, he helped Britt into the inflatable Zodiac.

The outboard coughed to life, and Britt cast off. They drifted with the current until the tiny motor caught and pushed them toward the beach. Coltrane looked at the sloop as they pulled away. The sailboat was beautiful, tall and brilliant white in the sun. It appeared to be suspended in air as it floated in the transparent blue water. Behind the yacht, the horizon was empty. Before them, the beach and the dense tropical vegetation loomed in the bright sky. Coltrane was mesmerized by the beauty and solitude of the place. He daydreamed until the Zodiac landed on the beach.

They pulled the light boat up onto the sandy beach and tied it securely to a palm tree, safely out of reach of the rising tide. Coltrane shouldered the seabag and began the long trip to the ruins atop the high peak. Britt followed with the cooler of food and drinks. The path was narrow, and strewn with jagged chunks of sharp coral. The brush and brambles cut their flesh as they struggled to the top of the path. It took them two trips to move all the gear to their lookout point. They collapsed in the clearing amid the stone remains of a cottage.

The local lore had it that the island had been a privateer base after the American Revolution. Calvin had told them that the island was settled by the McGinnis sisters, two young girls who fished and dove for turtles there about the time of the Civil War. They claimed the seas around the island, and demanded tax from all those who landed or fished their waters. They reputedly spent their entire lives there, alone but for a dog and a gun, until the hurricane of 1889 destroyed their stone house and gardens. No one knows if they died on the island, or where they are buried. It is said that on stormy nights at a sliver moon, their plaintive voices can be heard, crying on the wind.

The colonial settlers had chosen the site of their cottage well. They had cleared the crest of the peak and erected a one room stone building overlooking the sheltered west bay of the island. Parts of the sturdy structure still stood, but the roof and most of the walls were gone. Still, the site was popular as a lovers' rendezvous, as evidenced by broken bottles and initials carved in hearts into the stone.

Coltrane rubbed the sweat from his eyes. He had chosen the highest point on the island because of the spectacular vantage point. Unfortunately, the small clearing had no protection from the blazing midday sun. He knelt behind a chest high rampart and scanned the horizon with his binoculars. Out to sea, the Atlantic rolled in six-foot swells, and was barren of vessels. Far offshore to the south in the shallow inland sea, Coltrane could see several sailboats. He could make out the luff of their sails, and knew that they were moving away from them. Relaxing somewhat, he scanned the shore of the cay from his lookout. He satisfied himself that he could see every approach to the island. From one spot or another, he could see down onto the two beaches in the waist of the island. The only area hidden from view was the far north beach.

"Hey. Robinson Crusoe. When are you going to tell me what you got planned?" Britt interrupted his watch sarcastically.

"Sorry, sweetheart." Coltrane laughed. "I didn't have time this morning to explain. The Cuban may get here today, and I think we are much safer up here than on the boat like a couple of sitting ducks."

"Shit. You want to stay here all day?" Britt asked.

"Yeah. And maybe all night too. I got all the gear we need to camp out for a while." He could see she was not happy with the idea. "Just bear with me for a while. I need to contact the States and Calvin."

Coltrane unpacked the satphone, and set the antenna on the walls of the ruins. He powered up the unit, leaving it on standby to conserve the battery's power. Taking the small handheld VHF radio out of the waterproof box, he switched the channel to 63. He hailed Calvin on channel 63 several times without response. He sat and listened for other traffic on the main band, channel 16. Transmissions were weak and intermittent. Coltrane realized that the compact unit did not have the range he needed to communicate with Calvin, twenty miles to the north. He cursed to himself.

Coltrane swatted at a mosquito as it buzzed near his ear. "Britt, help me rig up a shelter before we get fried out here."

Coltrane chose the corner where two stout walls remained and stacked their gear against the walls. He opened his seabag, and found their sleeping bag and the sheets that he had pulled off the bed in the yacht. He cleared an area in the corner, and lay out the sleeping bag on the rough dirt floor. They stretched the sheets from the walls to a nearby bush, forming a simple shelter from the overhead sun. Coltrane pulled the cooler under the shelter, and covered it with a beach towel. From their primitive lean-to, Coltrane could scan the Exuma Sound and the Banks. He picked up the binoculars, and settled in to maintain his vigil.

Time passed slowly in the sweltering heat. The wind was light, and the sky cloudless. Britt propped herself up in the corner against the cold plastic of the cooler, and tried to sleep. Coltrane watched the panorama intently, following each passing boat with interest. Small wooden fishing skiffs shot past the island all day long, ferrying lean black fishermen to their favorite spots. In the distance, two small barges passed on the way to Georgetown with their vital loads of supplies, fresh produce and meat from Nassau.

Realizing that there was no immediate threat, Coltrane began to rethink his plan.

From their position, they commanded the high ground and could easily watch the island's approaches. But Coltrane had not really given much thought to what he would do once the Cuban got ashore. Temporarily safe, he began to plan for that eventuality.

The island had several trails leading between the beaches and the ruins. Because landing from sea was impossible on the coral ledges that formed the rest of the shore, all the paths started at one of the beaches. The trails converged into a rocky stairway that wound up to the summit. This last pathway was overgrown with sharp bush and spike palms all along its length, as it bent and snaked up the coral hills. Anyone coming after them would have to ascend that trail.

Coltrane scanned the horizon intently. Satisfied that there was no immediate danger, he gathered up all the discarded beer and wine bottles from around the ruins. Evidently, this was a popular spot for the local kids to party, far from the prying eyes of their elders. Moving slowly so as not to disturb Britt, he pulled the half empty bottle of Myers's out of the cooler. He emptied it into the bushes before he could change his mind. Taking his dive knife and a backpack of other gear, he headed down the steep trail.

The path took two sharp bends as it descended to the west beach. Coltrane climbed all the way down to the water, and turned to look up the trail. He scaled the rocks, all the way to the top, pretending to be an attacker. Coltrane knew that the Cuban would expect them to be prepared. The Cuban must also assume that he now had Johnny's weapon. Coltrane tried to put himself inside the Cuban's head.

He chose the final bend in the trail to place the booby trap. Coltrane knew that as the Cuban approached the bend to the right, he would be wary of an ambush. He would be concentrating on the dense vegetation along the trail, searching for an unseen enemy. Coltrane chose a sand ledge between two large coral rocks, and began to dig. He excavated the sand from the trail, and embedded upright beer and wine bottles in the hollows he dug. Stepping forward, he repeated the process across the trail until a wide area had been mined. Standing up, he surveyed his work. Unless the Cuban walked on the coral outcroppings, he could not traverse an eight foot passage without stepping into the glass. And if anyone stood on the coral, Coltrane would have a clear shot at his silhouette from above.

Satisfied by the strategy, Coltrane took a large, flat rock and shattered the tops and necks of the glass bottles, leaving shards of jagged glass pointing upward from the sand. He hurriedly covered the exposed fragments with loose vegetation and palm fronds. He sprinkled sand over the entire area.

Coltrane retreated up the hill, and viewed the impasse from in front of the ruins. He searched among the ruins for loose stone blocks, and slowly built a small bulwark behind which to hide. From his foxhole, he would have a clear shot at anyone ascending the trail. He returned to the ruins where Britt scanned the seas with the binoculars.

"See anything?" Coltrane asked.

"No, but the little red light on the satphone is flashing." Britt had just noticed the blinking LED.

"Shit. I missed a call. It must be Lynwood." Coltrane flicked the power switch from STANDBY to ON. He dialed Lynwood's number.

"Agent Lynwood." His tone was urgent.

"Lynwood, this is Coltrane. Did you call me?" Coltrane asked.

"Yeah, about half an hour ago. Keep that phone on, will you?" Lynwood sounded irritated.

"Sure. It is hard to hear from above decks." Coltrane lied.

"Listen, I investigated your story. Have you contacted the Bahamian Police?" Lynwood inquired.

"Not yet. The nearest sub-station is in Georgetown, eighty nautical miles away." Coltrane stalled.

"You had better do it now. I contacted Dennis at the charter base in Marsh Harbor, and he confirmed that two men had approached the dockhands looking for you. He also told me that a young couple on another of his chartered yachts was found murdered yesterday. They were bound hand and foot, and shot in the back of the head." Lynwood said.

"My God." Coltrane was stunned.

"They were on the boat that you were scheduled to be sailing. Were you supposed to be on the yacht *Wanderlust*?" Lynwood asked.

"Yeah. Dennis switched us at the last minute." Coltrane was sick.

"That's exactly what he told me. It is possible that those two men found the *Wanderlust*, and believed that couple to be you and your wife. I also spoke with Dr. Jasper. Like you said, he did some preliminary tests on Hendricks, and found chlorine and freshwater in his lungs. He now thinks that Hendricks died elsewhere, maybe in a pool or hot tub, and then was dumped in the bay. You may not have much time, Coltrane." Lynwood was genuinely concerned.

"I don't know what we will do. I don't think the Bahamian Police can protect me way out here. You have no idea how remote an area the Exumas are. I may just head out to sea. There is no way he can follow me into the Atlantic." Coltrane continued to stall.

"He? I thought you said there were two men?" Lynwood was suddenly suspicious.

"*He. They.* Fuck, I don't know. What about Resendez and the HMO?" Coltrane tried to change the subject.

"I'm running a FBI database search for Resendez now, but so far nothing has come up. The name may be an alias. And the HMO has not returned any of my calls. My guess is that they will refer me to their legal department in Atlanta. Don't count on much return from that approach." Lynwood answered.

"What have the police turned up in the case?" Coltrane was grasping at straws.

"I haven't spoken with the Tampa Police. My guess is that since the death was originally ruled as accidental, very little has been done. I can call them tomorrow. In the meantime, get you and your wife in the protection of the Bahamian authorities. They can get you to the American Embassy in Nassau. I will notify the security section that you are enroute. Contact me anytime." Lynwood gave him his cell phone number, and after wishing them luck, hung up. Coltrane switched the satphone to standby, and leaned back against the stone wall.

He had been so intent in his discussion with Lynwood that neither he nor Britt had seen the seaplane fly by, almost a mile offshore.

Chapter 61

Saddleback Cay
June 28
8:34PM

The sky was aflame, the sun setting into a burning sea.

They sat watching the glorious sunset together. The crimsons and pinks and purples never seemed so spectacular. Coltrane suppressed the thought that it may be their last sunset. He pulled his wife closer, hard. The globe sank inexorably into the Caribbean Sea, pulling the light from the sky.

Night comes very fast in the islands. The sky turned purple, then black. Tonight was a quarter moon, and the crescent gave pale light to the island. Coltrane relaxed somewhat, knowing that the silence that descended upon them would protect them. They would be able to hear an engine for several miles. He knew no one had landed on the cay today.

As the sweltering day had passed, Coltrane had gone over every possible scenario in his mind, over and over. No matter how the Cuban approached the island, in the end he would have to climb the trail to reach them. The ruins were at least sixty feet above the distant opposite crest, and well out of range of the short barreled pistol. Even if a rifleman was positioned on the low hill, they were safe behind the scrub and stone of the ruins. Coltrane doubted that the Cuban would be able to obtain or transport a rifle easily.

They had spent the majority of the day resting, and taking turns on sentinel watch. Activity in the heat and humidity had been difficult and exhausting. They saved their energy, preferring to labor in the cool of nighttime. Britt scanned the horizon while Coltrane moved about the clearing, cutting brush for camouflage and prying stone blocks from the remnants of the ruin walls. He covered the shelter with branches and palm leaves, making it invisible in the moonlight.

The vegetation that covered the entire cay was typical Bahamian tropical scrub. Palm trees were rare, the coral rocks being matted with a dense impenetrable bramble of spike bushes, thorn trees and juniper. An occasional stand of causarinas offered some shade from the burning sun. Coltrane had tried to create a tunnel in the thicket as an ambush site, but found it impossible. The tough wiry stalks of the bushes were slow to yield to his serrated dive knife. Their sap was thick and tarry, and the razor sharp knife became uselessly gummed after the fifth stroke. Frustrated, Coltrane had abandoned his effort.

Satisfied that he held the high ground and could not be flanked, Coltrane concentrated on improving his advantage. The son of a high ranking US Army officer, Coltrane had studied military history since boyhood. He had read chronicles of Alexander the Great, the Art of War by Sun Tzu and many firsthand accounts of the senseless waste of life in the Civil War and WWI. His two tours of combat in Vietnam had only served to strengthen his philosophy of war and life. He knew that battles were won and lost on the most trivial of errors. Who would have thought that the accidental replacement of the Allison engine with a Rolls-Royce V12 Merlin would dramatically improve the high altitude performance of the P51 fighter, and alter the course of WWII? Or that the Soviets' crude T-34 tank would prove superior to German Tigers, driving the Wehrmacht from the steppes of Russia? He knew preparation and patience could overcome superiority in manpower and armament. He knew that he held the high ground, and that he was fighting for his bride and his life. In perhaps the final struggle of his life, Coltrane wanted all the advantages he could get.

The shelter was formed using a far corner of the stone ruins, facing toward the trail head. Coltrane's position lay at the opposite end of the same wall, but the center portion of the wall was completely destroyed by wind and time. Coltrane carefully stacked blocks and coral rocks to repair the wall to a height of two feet. He wanted Britt to be able to move freely from the shelter to the firing position under cover. If something happened to him, she would still have the speargun but might need to be able to retrieve the pistol.

Coltrane prepared his position at the top of the path, where the trail ended in the clearing. From behind his little stone rampart, he could see straight down the incline to the point where the trail turned. The vegetation angled away from the rocky trail, with the water of the bay in the distance. Anyone coming up that hill would be silhouetted on the bright surface, directly in his field of fire.

As Coltrane sat watching the water and the approach routes to the island, he realized that he had put too much faith in the pit trap on the trail. He had no warning system, or tripwire to tell him that someone was ascending the path. He promised himself to set one up in the morning. He scanned the horizon.

They took turns all night, one sleeping restlessly while the other stood guard. The night was hot and sticky. Mosquitoes from the brush swarmed by the hundreds to their bodies, attracted by the heat and the smell of blood. They particularly loved Britt, attacking her exposed face, ears, wrists and ankles. Almost immediately, the bites raised welts. The itching was maddening. She wrapped herself in the sleeping bag, preferring the suffocating heat to the incessant attack of the mosquitoes and sand flies. Coltrane tried to comfort her, wishing he had saved the Myers's. The night dragged on.

In the dark and still hours just before dawn, Coltrane strained all his senses. He willed his mind to become part of the night, to listen to the regular lap of the waves, and the soft stirring of the brush in the onshore breeze. Human strength, both physical and spiritual, is weakest just before the dawn. Warriors have instinctively known this since the dawn of time, and Coltrane knew the medical biorhythm studies that confirm it. Coltrane knew the Cuban would come at them now if he was on Saddleback Cay.

The mosquitoes buzzed in his ears and nose, biting him continually, mercilessly. The salt and sweat on his face ran constantly into his eyes, burning them. He held the pistol loosely in his right hand, safety on and round chambered. In his left hand, he gripped the boat's flashlight. Not wanting to put either down, he brushed the insects with his shoulder or wiped his face on his sleeve. From his position, he watched the sun rise in the eastern sea.

As light pierced the blackness, the sun cast a peach glow over the cays, and Coltrane relaxed. The sea was flat and still, barren of craft as far as the eye could see. To the east the Atlantic was calm, with three foot swells coming through the cut. Coltrane scanned both beaches as the early light bathed them. No boats or footprints. Coltrane glanced towards Britt, who had finally dropped off to sleep after a tortured night. He let her rest, and dug into the cooler for a cold breakfast.

As the tropical sun rose, the weather began. The intense heat of the day began to warm the water and the isolated cays, sending thermals up into the atmosphere, and creating movement of those air masses. Coltrane scanned the horizon for clouds, for the early signs of storms. Scattered high cumulus clouds dotted the brilliant blue sky. Coltrane hoped the weather would hold.

Coltrane shifted his position on the hard sand. His right leg had fallen asleep during his watch. He rolled away from his foxhole, and sat behind the ruins' walls where he could see the expanse of water before him. Propped against the cool stone wall with the warm sun on his face, he thanked his God that the night was over. Gazing at the peaceful scene before him, he fell into a deep sleep.

Chapter 62

Nassau
June 29
4:45AM

The Cuban awoke in the early morning darkness, and checked out before dawn. He carried his gear in the plastic laundry bags he found in the closet, and strode down to the marina dock at the casino. Within minutes, he had fired up the throaty outboard and was proceeding out the Nassau ship channel.

He followed the channel buoys out into the deep water, then turned southeast, bearing 149 degrees. He pushed the throttle down, and the boat surged forward. The MerCruiser easily brought the hull onto plane, and the boat flew over the dark water. The Cuban opened a Coke, and leaned back for the long ride. He cursed softly to himself, then laughed outloud. He had called his employer from a bar in Nassau last night, and was amused at their conversation. The man had told him that a copy of the second disc had been obtained by the Federal Bureau of Investigation. Therefore, circumstances dictated that the balance of his contract was canceled. They no longer wanted the disc, and felt that if Coltrane were to disappear in unusual circumstances, too much attention may be attracted to the matter. He was told to return to the States immediately. The Cuban was disgusted by the man's lack of professionalism. He told him that once set into motion, these matters were impossible to control. They develop a life unto themselves, he explained. He explained that he could not leave unfinished business here and just return to Miami. He told him not to speak any further on the telephone about sensitive matters. Angry and disgusted, he hung up as the other protested.

The Cuban reached into the little compartment in the boat's center console, and retrieved a small, heavy package. He hefted the gun, and smiled. If all went well, he would find and kill his quarry this afternoon.

Chapter 63

Saddleback Cay
June 29
11:32AM

The high pitched whine of the tiny outboard shook Coltrane from his sleep. Terrified that he had dropped his guard, he leapt to his feet and scanned the island. Three hundred yards offshore, a small aluminum fishing boat skimmed over the azure water. Two black men in the boat gazed intently forward, oblivious of Coltrane's presence.

Coltrane checked his watch. It was late morning, and Britt had had a good sleep. He roused her, and told her that he must go to the sloop for supplies. They arranged hand signals for danger, and Coltrane sprinted down the trail and took the Zodiac to the sailboat.

He grabbed a gallon of purified water, food, some essential cosmetics for Britt, and the flare gun from the life pack. Unarmed and unable to see the horizon, he felt exposed as he rummaged below the boat. Coltrane finished as quickly as he could, and dinghyed back to shore. He was glad to be back on land, struggling up the coral cliff trail.

Britt felt much better after cleaning her face and brushing her teeth. They applied insect repellent, preferring the thick oily layer to the constant sting of the ravenous insects. Coltrane didn't know how long he could wait on the coral plateau. He was beginning to doubt his plan.

Unable to sit uselessly any longer, Coltrane rose and surveyed the path, and the ruins, looking for a weakness in their defenses. He went into the cooler, and collected all the empty aluminum Coke cans. Then finding two more littered out in the brush, he walked down past the bend in the path. He selected pea sized, round gravel stones, and placed several in each can. Using a length of four pound test monofilament fishing line, he strung the cans up in the branches, rigging a trip line across the trail at different heights and spacing. Satisfied that a man could not move through the web without jostling the cans, he returned to the crest of the hill.

The battery on the satphone had ninety minutes of talk time left. Coltrane wanted to save an hour in the event of emergency in the event he or Britt needed medical assistance. That left thirty minutes. He debated how to best use the time.

Coltrane powered up the Iridium satphone, and after several tries he got through to the executive secretary of PatientsChoice Florida HMO's regional director. She informed him that the director was in meetings all day, and unavailable until later that week. He explained to her that he was returning his call, and would be on a sailboat for the next two weeks. Now was the time to talk if the insurance plan was interested. He gave the satphone number, and she promised to bring it to the director's attention.

Coltrane was surprised when the satphone rang an hour later. He answered, and a secretary put him on hold as she went to find the director. Coltrane suppressed his annoyance at the tactic, designed to position Coltrane as the supplicant. Eventually, the director picked up the phone.

"John McKinnon here," he announced.

"Dr. William Coltrane. I understand that you called Susan Kerr. What can I do for you, Mr. McKinnon?" Coltrane was pleasant.

"As you may know, we have filed charges that you are holding an illegal…" McKinnon started on a tirade.

"Look, Mr. McKinnon," Coltrane interrupted. "I'm not going to discuss the conference with you. Your claims are being investigated by the FBI, and I am confident that the allegations will be dismissed out of hand. I am on my vacation with my wife in the islands, and talking to you on a satphone. Don't waste my time. If you wish to discuss the concerns of the society with regards to improving the quality and efficiency of your HMO product, I will be glad to talk all day with you."

"There is very little to discuss, Dr. Coltrane. All our participating physicians have signed contracts that specify the fees and the procedures for patient care. Our plan delivers high quality care by reducing physician error and redundant expenses. Returning to the old system of unlimited, helter-skelter consultations and over-usage of specialists is never going to occur. You can't fight progress." McKinnon repeated the company line. He knew it by heart.

"Really? Tell me exactly how you reduce physician error." Coltrane demanded.

"By our oversight procedures. By proper use of specialists. Shall I go on?"

"Tell me about your oversight procedures. Who implements them?"

"My medical director, and a competent staff of nurses."

"One physician. You have one physician to supervise all fifteen hundred of us in the Bay area? What is his specialty?"

"Internal Medicine."

"Fine. Assuming that he has been keeping up with the evolving specialty, then I'll grant that he could be competent in Internal Medicine. But what about Surgery? Pediatrics? OB-GYN? Psychiatry? There is no way in hell that he can sit in judgment on my decisions as a surgeon. And I've never been able to get through to talk with him, anyway. It is always one of your RNs, and they are in even less of a position to be making those decisions for my patients. This is one of the main issues that I want to discuss with you."

"You doctors are always resistant to any form of supervision. You can't operate in a vacuum; there must be some governing agency. We are simply looking out for our enrollees."

"I agree completely with you on many points. I agree that an efficient governing body is lacking. I agree that specialists are sometimes overused. But to deprive a patient of the opportunity to be seen by an expert is criminal. I agree that many tests are unnecessary, but the only recourse to improve that problem is to have significant tort reform, or put medical malpractice in the hands of a compensation board run by educated professionals, not the jury system. Our membership would probably agree with many of your concerns, but not about how the insurance industry goes about achieving those goals. We are ready to initiate a discourse about our concerns at any time." Coltrane paused, hoping for some movement from McKinnon.

"We will not bow to extortion from the society. All you want is higher fee schedules. This whole charade is transparent." McKinnon was not going to budge.

"Yes, we do want higher fee schedules. You are absolutely correct. That seems to be a point that the news media is harping on mercilessly. This is where we have failed as a profession, in the business aspect of practice. We spend college in the sciences, and there is not a single course in business in the medical school or residency curriculum. We are like lambs to the slaughter, and have been for years. Stockbrokers send their kids to college on the mistakes of physicians and dentists. Our lives are consumed with our professions. And it is not ethical to allow business concerns to influence treatment options. If you were the patient, would you want the correct procedure? Or the one that gave me the best reimbursement? Business and medicine do not join easily."

"Of course I would want the appropriate procedure. And our procedures are reimbursed at a reasonable market rate."

"I disagree. Who determines your fee schedule?"

"I can't disclose that process, but it is done very carefully and equitably."

"Again, I beg to disagree. Take carpal tunnel release. Three years ago, Medicare was paying $575 for a unilateral exploration and release. That included the pre-op exam and physical, the surgery, the follow-up for three months, bandages, phone calls, the whole nine yards. The infamous 'universal fee' that you insurance plans love."

"And?"

"Does that sound fair and *equitable* to you?"

"I don't know the procedure. I cannot comment."

"Are you a lawyer, by any chance?"

"No, MBA. Harvard."

"*Jesus.* See, this is the problem. I am totally outclassed in trying to deal with you. Like the Japanese say: *Business is War.* You are trained in negotiation, I am trained in surgery. I will always lose."

"Hopefully," McKinnon laughed.

"Right. Well, let me describe the surgery. Forget the consultation, the history and physical, the consent process, the follow-up and all the paperwork and office visits. Let's just concentrate on the actual surgery. I travel to whatever OR the patient is at, I see her in the holding area, check the labs, talk to her, get a second informed consent signed, talk to the family, talk to the nurses, go over the patient with the anesthesiologist. Then I wait in the surgeons' lounge while the OR is prepped. Then, if I am lucky, the procedure will go on time. Usually, it is delayed by the operation before it, or an emergency, or whatever. Now, a taxi driver gets paid for that wait time, or a lawyer, but not a surgeon."

"Christ, Coltrane. You want to be paid for OR delays? You must be insane!"

"No, just making a point. Relax. Then I get in the room, and very carefully dissect, using special loupes and magnification, down to the nerve. I do the release, and put on a special cast and dressing. The whole procedure takes one, maybe two hours. Depending on the anatomy. Everyone has different anatomy, unfortunately."

"Your point?"

"My point is that your plan pays $177 for that procedure. Down from $350 last year. I know this because it is one of the most common procedures in my practice. That works out to about $25 an hour, before my overhead, which is about sixty per cent of my gross. So, let's see, what is that for me before taxes…about $10 an hour. After the government, federal state and local get their fair share, I am left with maybe $6. Now, my plumber gets $55 an hour, and he even gets to drink on the job."

"I don't know what the fee for that operation is, but it is in line with all our other fees, Dr. Coltrane." McKinnon answered listlessly.

"That is exactly my point. How do you explain the drop from $350 to $177? The procedure has not suddenly become twice as simple to do. My overhead is increasing, not dwindling. My malpractice is going up. My rent is going up. Inflation is going up. How is it that your fee schedules can defy all the other trends in costs in our society?"

"Like I said, our schedule is based on our research, our market analysis and the time involved in each particular procedure."

"Well, please tell me why, specifically, carpal tunnel release now is worth half what it was last year?"

"I'll look into that for you, Dr. Coltrane."

"Let me tell you what I think, Mr. McKinnon. I had a practice management consultant come to my office, and train the staff on coding and insurance policies. She had worked in one of the huge HMO headquarters in New York for years before going out on her own. She told us that what they did was determine the top two hundred most commonly utilized procedures, and simply decrease the payment on those procedures. So if hip replacements were being done frequently, then just cut the reimbursement by ten percent, and the savings were dramatic. Who cares about a procedure that is being done rarely. From an accounting standpoint, you can pay that at any fee you want, with no impact on the bottom line. That company just juggled the frequency and the payment until a good bottom line, *for their accountants*, was achieved. Right?"

"That's not how we do it, I can assure you of that."

"What is your objection to using the McGraw-Hill RBRVS?"

"It's outmoded. It was published in 1994."

"It has been revised, and can be revised yearly. I don't care what multiplier you use, I just want to know what I am going to be paid by your plan, so I can decide if I can afford to participate. Is that unfair or unreasonable?"

"We give our fee schedules, they are in the Provider's handbook, and in the contract you signed."

"No they are not. You give us a teaser, one page of selected fees, covering all specialties. And you give only the good fees, not the common procedures that I do, and not the ridiculously low fees like the carpal tunnel release. I know. I have asked for a full fee schedule from every HMO that I participate with, *and every single one has refused*."

"We will not release our entire fee schedule. Other plans can utilize it."

"Who cares? These schedules should all be out in the open. Medicare's is. Medicaid's is. We have a right to know what you will pay us. Where else in the world will a laborer accept a job, complete it, and then take whatever payment the client decides is just? Nowhere I know of."

"What, now you are a laborer? You think you can sell that to the public?"

"Look, let me make something real clear to you. There are two, totally separate, components of our movement. The primary issues are patient care and ways to improve the delivery of healthcare to the people of the Bay area, and the nation as a whole. If we're lucky. The secondary concern is correcting the criminal abuse that insurance plans, and various well meaning but ineffectual governmental and societal entities have perpetuated upon our profession, as a whole, for years. We have been weakened and divided by our independence, our obligations to our patients, and our ignorance. My intent is to educate and inform all the Bay area physicians on how best to deal with the myriad, non-medical aspects of their practices. And I don't give a damn what the public thinks about *these* issues. If they don't want to see me, I will not be offended if they go see a chiropractor. Or an acupuncturist. Or a holistic practitioner. Or an aromatherapist. Or a witch doctor. Whatever works for them. There are many other options out there, and they all accept cash payments. But I am a laborer, no question about that. I don't make a software program that I can duplicate and sell a hundred thousand times. If I do a procedure once or ten times, it still takes me the same amount of time, each time. You try to apply economies of scale to medical practice, like I'm manufacturing motorcycles or something. It doesn't apply. It works on paper for you to justify decreasing my fees, but it is false science. The logic doesn't apply to a labor intensive pursuit like medicine."

"I understand your frustration, Dr. Coltrane. But you're asking me to change the world, and I just don't have that power," McKinnon patiently refused to give ground.

"I am not asking for miracles. But you are a Florida HMO, and not responsible to some national headquarters in another state. You must have some leeway to change policy. Let me send you all our position papers. I am sure that Susan can get you our position papers. These address the issues that confront physicians and patients every day, day in and day out, week in and week out, year in and year out. The conference will continue until the membership has adopted a unified vision on how to best approach the problems as we see them. The goals of the conference are three pronged. One, to streamline the protocols for patient management. It is absurd that a physician must spend several hours daily, pleading to multiple layers of untrained and undereducated customer service representatives for permission to admit a patient to the hospital. That has to be improved. Two, improved access to medical and ancillary services. It is impossible to provide quality care to an ill or injured patient when there exists a maze of approved or participating providers, therapists, pharmacies, home health care, and on and on. I have had many patients simply give up rather than fight through the confusion of who and what is covered. Three, we want a published, complete fee schedule based on the McGraw-Hill scale. That's very simple to do. All you have to do is state a conversion factor. I am tired of the bait and switch game that has been played for years. Be happy that we have been so stupid for so long." Coltrane felt the blazing Caribbean heat affect his composure.

"I don't have the authority to make any of these changes, Coltrane. I would be willing to meet with your committee and discuss healthcare issues at your convenience, however," McKinnon responded.

"Really? I was told that you were able to make significant changes in local policy, Mr. McKinnon. I only wish to speak with someone who can effect change. Too much gets lost in the translation to do it any other way. If the society is unable to negotiate change with the insurance industry, we'll form an IPO or IPA and try it ourselves. We probably should have done that years ago, anyway."

"Dr. Coltrane, I will have to get back to you with details about a representative to your conference. You are asking for a radical overhaul of our entire insurance plan and delivery system. That cannot be done overnight, even if we wanted to make the changes you request." McKinnon left the door open for further talks.

"We need to meet soon and deal with the basic issues. Our demands are not unreasonable. The entire American healthcare system needs reform, and together we can make great changes. But we have to start somewhere, somehow. I will be waiting for your call. Thank you." Coltrane was hot, tired and unsure whether this executive was sincere or stalling. He exchanged pleasantries, and hung up.

"Dickhead," he muttered to himself.

"Was he shining you on?" Britt asked. She had heard his half of the conversation.

"I think so. I am getting jaded when it comes to these insurance executives. They are always talking out of both sides of their mouths. But I think he woke up when I mentioned the IPO." Coltrane leaned back on the stone wall.

"IPO. What's an IPO? This is the first time I heard of that." Britt was interested.

"I haven't mentioned it because the society has not really considered this option seriously. Jack Ferrara has looked into the possibility, but we are just in the planning stage now," Coltrane answered. Realizing that he had not answered her question, he continued. "IPO stands for Independent Physician Organization. Same as an IPA, Independent Physicians Association. That is basically a HMO, but owned and run by the physicians that are also the participating providers. My goal is to form our own IPO, and have every physician in the society enrolled. That will solve many administrative problems, simplify and improve patient care, and save money."

"The drawback is that IPOs are very difficult to set up. The federal and state governments have mindboggling bureaucratic bullshit that lawyers have to wade through. Critics will say that the physicians will minimize treatment in order to decrease expenses and improve the bottom line. Furthermore, the concept is relatively new and has no track record. Even though it looks good on paper, no one knows if it will work in actual practice. The insurance plans will do everything they can to weaken us, because an IPO would be very strong competition. A well established and organized IPO could effectively render insurance plans useless." Coltrane personally loved the idea, but doubted it would come to fruition.

"Why haven't IPOs been formed everywhere?" To Britt, they were the obvious solution to the multitude of problems.

"I really don't know, but I think it's because physicians are very difficult to organize. We are too independent, too stubborn and too..." Coltrane searched for the right word.

"Arrogant? Pompous? ... Shall I go on?" Britt asked, eyebrows raised, half mocking him, half serious.

"Sweetheart, you know that weakness and indecision are not attributes patients look for in a surgeon. But you're right. Every committee of physicians has too many chiefs, and no indians. That's why we get nowhere. Until now. Speaking of that, I'd better call Susan."

Coltrane checked the battery charge, and dialed the back line at the society office, his mind tired, his body cramped.

"Susan Kerr here," she answered immediately.

"Afternoon, Ms. Kerr. How are things on the home front?" Coltrane asked.

"God, am I glad to hear from you. It is getting very intense up here. I'm afraid everything is degenerating, disintegrating. When are you coming back?"

"Soon," Coltrane lied. "Bring me up to date, please."

"I've spoken with the physician relations spokespeople from the major hospitals in the Bay area, and they all publicly express concern about the potential bottleneck in the ERs. Privately, however, they agree with our positions with regard to insurance plan interference in the delivery of healthcare. The hospitals will not publicly come out in support of the society's action, but I think that they will support us in subtle ways. There is one glaring exception, however."

"What's that?" Coltrane asked.

"AthenaHMO."

"We expected that. What are they doing?"

"They've had their hospital administrators on the evening news for three straight nights, tearing us apart. Supposedly, all their facilities are swamped. They have two facilities in Pinellas County, and one in Hillsborough County. The main facility is Athena General, of course, and then they have a rehab hospital and a long term mental health facility. They claim they can't provide adequate medical care without the doctors."

"No shit. That is my point exactly. The sooner those idiots realize that, the better off we'll all be."

"Well, I don't think that the public is with us at this point. People needing to see a doctor are angry about being inconvenienced, and even those who are well are anxious about themselves and their loved ones if they become ill. There have even been disgruntled patients showing up at the conference trying to talk to their doctors. I'm concerned that it could get ugly."

"I'm equally concerned. But being sick is always inconvenient, and I can assure you that taking care of sick patients twenty-four hours a day, seven days a week, three hundred sixty-five days a year is even more inconvenient. In fact, my whole career is one long series of inconveniences. But that's the nature of the beast. This conference isn't making it any worse, but I agree that it may seem that way to some patients. Maybe it will make them more responsible in caring for their own health. Or maybe they will take stop taking us for granted, thinking that they can drink, and smoke and party their lives away, and then get a pill or a treatment or a magical cure on death's door."

"Don't hold your breath waiting for that," Susan laughed grimly.

"Right. Then maybe we should increase the number of physicians on each rotation. That should alleviate the strain on the ERs considerably, and reassure the community. Call that in to Elizabeth, and see that she puts it in the morning edition."

"Actually, we already did that. Due to public concern about prompt access to treatment, the committees decided to double the number of on-call physicians available, and to open additional offices for patient appointments."

"Perfect."

"But it is still a very unstable and volatile situation. I just wonder when we should call this thing off. It's getting too big for me, too much stress. There are people calling all the time, from all over the country. CNN, MSNBC, CBS, all the networks have commentators that want to talk with you. Some reporter from Germany even called yesterday. I don't know how long I can take it," Susan's voice wavered.

"Susan, be strong. This is like rolling the boulder up the mountain. If you quit, you have to start all over again, after the rock rolls right over you. Don't falter. No one is getting hurt but the HMOs. The longer we stay the course, the better chance we have at success. The only thing they know is profit and the bottom line. Please stay with us. I need you. I can't do this without you."

"I promised I'd finish this, and I will. It's wearing me down, though."

"Assign one of the girls to answer all incoming media calls, and just have her fax out our position papers all day long. Don't talk to those people, it is just a waste of your time. Ignore them. You'll do just fine." Coltrane's forceful tone raised her spirits.

"I don't know…"

"How are the docs holding up?" Coltrane changed the subject.

"The feedback from the doctors has been good. For the most part, their patients were tolerating the triage system for office appointments. The office staffs are straining to handle the huge volume of telephone calls efficiently, but they all understand the momentous nature of the effort. And office managers are amused to find that patient no-shows, usually at thirty percent or greater, had dropped to five percent. And collections for office visits is at eighty-five percent, almost unheard of before. I have never seen physicians put aside their differences and rivalries to come together in this way. Hopefully, some good may come of it."

"And the logistics? Is the conference running smoothly?"

"We have had to secure all entry points with off-duty Tampa police officers after several angry patients crashed the meeting in protest. The security has been further tightened because one of the protesters is a disabled mental patient with a long history of bizarre, violent behavior. I hope that things will quiet down."

"And is the hotel backing you in this?" Coltrane knew that the hotel was very sensitive to controversy, and would cancel the conference if they felt that the situation was dangerous or unsafe for their employees and other guests. He also knew that by hosting the conference, the hotel was getting tremendous local and national exposure. Corporate management of the hotel, both locally and at the national office, would be ambiguous as to whether hosting the conference was negatively impacting their public image. He knew they would cave under the slightest public pressure.

"So far, yes. But their PR woman is checking on us all the time, and she's as jumpy and irritable as a cat on a hot tin roof. Only time will tell." Susan finished.

"Ask our anti-trust attorneys to speak directly to the hotel manager, and the national headquarters as well. Have them assure the hotel that our conference is legal, and that it will be concluded soon. And have them reinforce the terms of our contract with the hotel, but in a subtle and friendly way. Okay?"

"Got it."

"*Carpe diem*."

"Easy for you to say, *El Presidente*," Susan laughed and hung up.

Coltrane secured the handset in the cradle, and felt it click into place. Looking up, he scanned the water slowly and intently, horizon to horizon, wondering if he had missed anyone during the long conversation with Susan.

"Do you think he will come today?" Britt quietly asked, following his gaze out to sea and spotting a small sloop on a beam reach, three miles out. She wished she was out there now, instead of on this sweltering coral rock.

"He has to come today. Even if it took two days to get a boat, he could make it here by this evening. He'll come today or tonight. Are you rested? Are you ready?" Coltrane had tried to give Britt as much sleep as possible. He was used to long nights without rest.

"As rested as I can be in these conditions."

Britt passed him the speargun and picked up the orange box containing the flaregun. Coltrane had reviewed the use of the flare gun with her earlier, and they had agreed to use it only as a last resort. It posed a serious fire hazard, and Coltrane himself wasn't sure if it was a parachute flare, or a starburst flare. Either way it would make a mess of someone at close range, if it didn't start a bush fire first. And if it did start a fire, they would be trapped in the inferno that resulted, unable to escape down the trail.

Coltrane looked lovingly at his wife of ten years. He had come to learn that she was very strong, both emotionally and physically. He had no doubt that she would endure this trial and weather it better than he would. Turning, he pulled the three bands back on the speargun, and engaged them into the notches in the steel spear. Checking that the safety was on, he set it on the stone wall. Britt opened the plastic case containing the flaregun, and set it by her side.

They both turned silently toward the shimmering waters, watched and waited under the pitiless sun.

Chapter 64

The Flats
June 29
9:14AM

The Cuban had been pushing the boat hard for two hours, and his knees were sore from the constant rhythmic pounding as the hull slapped against the swells at twenty-five knots. He had strapped two jerrycans of gas onto the teak transom of the boat, specifically to avoid having to refuel at Highburn Cay. He didn't want Calvin to be able to warn Coltrane of his presence.

He cut a path straight across The Flats, straight for the southern islands. He knew that Coltrane did not go back to Nassau, he would have seen him on his way out. He had carefully checked every yacht he encountered, and none was Coltrane's. The Cuban knew that the boat was not equipped or prepared for a long blue water passage, and he doubted that Coltrane had the charts to enable him to safely make his way to the Florida mainland. That left his quarry with two choices: either head further south in the Exuma chain and try to get lost in the hundreds of tiny cays, or make a run north, past him to Eleuthera or Nassau. Given the slow speed of the yacht, five to eight knots maximum, the Cuban knew that he would have crossed Coltrane's path had he run. He smiled grimly to himself. Knowledge is power.

As the low-lying chain of islands came into view, he swung to take a bearing on the northernmost key. The process would take time, but now he had all the time in the world.

Chapter 65

Exumas
June 29
2:36PM

He spent five hours weaving through the maze of tiny coves and bays that faced the Banks before he found the island he was looking for. Every three or four islands he had to venture out into the rough water of the Exuma Sound, just to be sure that the small sloop was not hiding in a little day anchorage on the Atlantic side of the chain. He knew Coltrane would have to anchor on the west side of the chain overnight; the weather was far too rough, and the east shore rocky and bleak. But he could be hiding out to sea by day, hoping to elude him. So the Cuban checked all possible anchorages, moving inexorably southward.

In the cove of a high crested saddleback island, the Cuban found the forty-two foot yacht, lying quietly at anchor, with a huge beach towel draped over the transom. The Cuban knew it was the Coltranes' yacht instantly, he remembered the number painted on the sides of the dinghy. He was amused that they had not moved since his flyover. Maybe this would be easier than he had anticipated. Smiling to himself, he continued his path south for two miles, then put out to sea and doubled back to the island. As he approached from the south, he scanned the charts for a topographical view of the small cay. It was a prominent feature of the Exuma chain, its two hills separated by a narrow waist formed by wide, curving sandy beaches on opposite sides of the island. At the northeast end of the island, another small beach sparkled in the afternoon sun.

His binoculars allowed him to view the scrub covered island with crystal clarity. He could see that the beaches were deserted, and the Coltranes were nowhere to be seen. A series of small trails ran up and over the crest of the saddle, but they were very narrow and overgrown. The Cuban saw no motion, no activity. Only at the top of the higher peak was there any evidence of a manmade structure; a cairn or stone ruins. He knew that the Coltranes would be there.

The tide was rising, and the flow was onto the flats. Even from six hundred yards out, he could see the turbulent flow through the twenty foot wide channel. He would have to wait for an hour or so to make it through the cut to the northeast tip of the cay. He cut the motor, and slumped lazily in the boat, pretending to fish with the drifting current. He cleaned and oiled his pistol, and calmed his nerves for the impending kill. No matter how many times he had killed, it never got easier, and never lost its thrill. He could taste it in his mouth, his blood up, a palpable intense fear entwined with exhilaration encompassing his entire body. He waited for the tide to change.

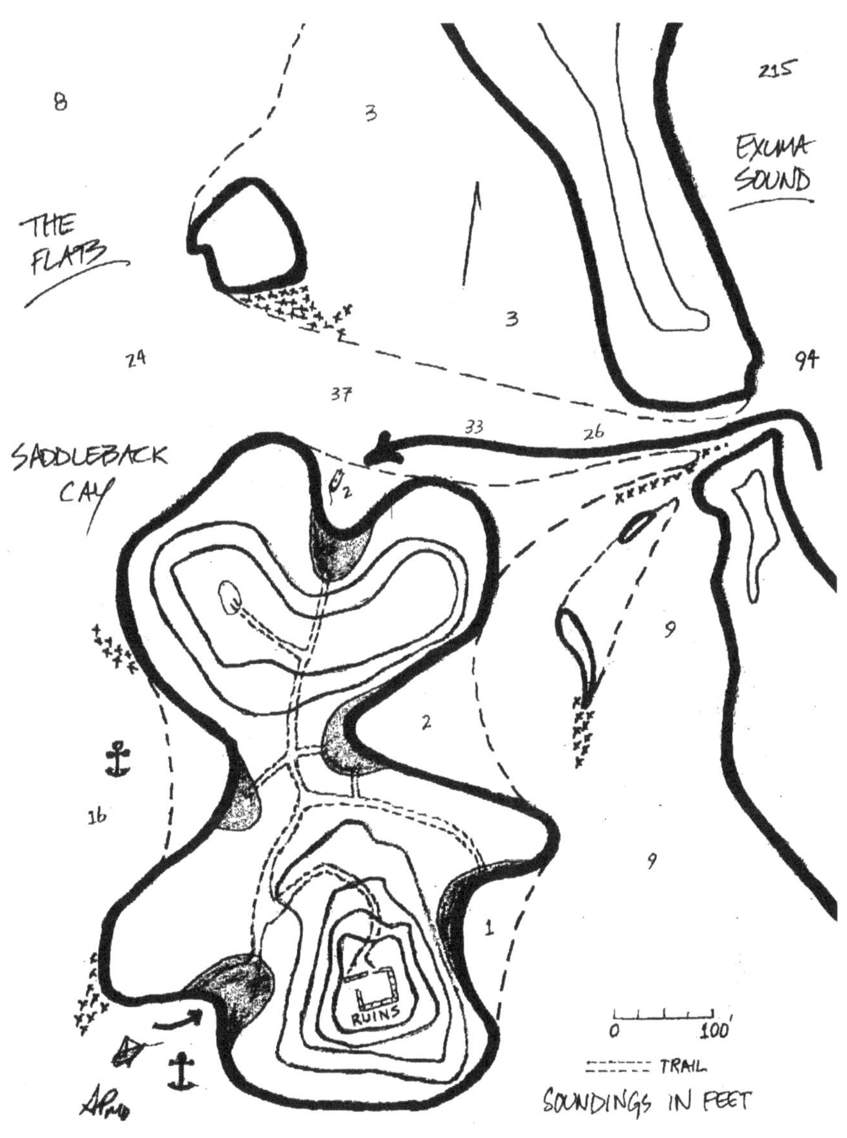

Map of Saddleback Cay

Chapter 66

Saddleback Cay
June 29
4:55PM

It was almost dusk, and Coltrane had seen nothing suspicious all day. A man in a center-cockpit powerboat cruised by earlier, but he had just been a sportfisherman. Coltrane had watched him offshore casting and trolling that afternoon. Coltrane wondered if the Cuban perhaps had decided after all to give it up and head for home. Certainly there were easier ways to make his dime.

Coltrane's wistful expectations were shattered as he saw the lone fisherman slowly and cautiously negotiate his way through the narrow channel northeast of the island. Coltrane lifted his Steiners and focused. The helmsman was nondescript, a floppy khaki hat covering his head. On the port side of the white fiberglass craft, he could barely make out faint blue lettering. He squinted through the powerful binoculars, sweat running in his eyes, burning them. The gunnel of the boat rolled and fell in the waves, obscured by seaspray. Suddenly he got a clear view of the words "*Royal Marina, Nassau*". He cursed softly.

He knew then that this was the Cuban, and that he would soon be on the blind side of the island, out of sight and range. His heart racing, he quickly checked his weapons as they lay on the stone parapet before him. Britt, sensing his agitation, crept to his side and followed his gaze out to sea. She watched as the small boat plied its way carefully through the channel.

"The Cuban?" she asked.

"Yeah. I think so. If he comes ashore, then we will know for sure." Coltrane raised the binoculars.

Coltrane watched as the boat cleared the narrow cut, and turned slightly northwest. Now the channel was fifty yards astern of the boat, and he still motored agonizingly slowly. If he was going back to Nassau, he'd have powered up and got up on plane by now, Coltrane thought. As if hearing his thoughts, the man in the boat looked up at the ruins on Saddleback Cay, and gently turned toward the northern beach. Coltrane followed the boat as it disappeared behind the opposite crest of Saddleback Cay. Coltrane could swear that the man was smiling.

Chapter 67

Saddleback Cay
June 29
6:05PM

They sat in the dusk, cross legged, facing each other. Coltrane had drawn a map of the island, and the path up to their redoubt. He marked the booby-traps on the winding trail, and the perimeter alarm he had stringed out around the ruins. They went over the tactics, again and again.

"There is only one way to reach us here, and that's straight up the trail. No one could penetrate this dense scrub without being cut to pieces, and if he tries we'll hear him long before he gets to us. He has to come right up here, right through our traps. He can't survive it. The only way he can kill us is if we do something stupid."

Coltrane traced the path of the attack. Coltrane had the high ground, and a clear field of fire at anyone ascending the trail. He hoped that would be enough.

Near the rear of the ruins, at the base of the mass of coral and stone, Coltrane found a small depression in the earthen floor. There he helped Britt build a small wall of large stones to shield her as she lay in the shallow pit. He set the open flaregun case against the rock wall by her side. He kissed her gently on the lips, tasting the cool sweetness of her mouth, loving her for her strength and faith. No words were spoken.

Coltrane went forward to his nest. He lay down in a rifleman's prone position, rolled slightly on his left side with his right leg up and out, knee flexed. He dug in, moving sand and brush to form a perfect contour in the ground for his body, padding his hip with a folded old shirt. He knew he would be waiting for hours in that spot, motionless as a coiled serpent.

They lay, silently, watching as the sun set gloriously in the west. The rose and peach hues spread from horizon to horizon, bathing the tiny cove in a luminescent glow. Coltrane remembered Venice, the special rare light that had inspired the brilliant work of the Renaissance painters. He was transfixed by the sunset, the brilliant azure waters, the white sand. If he had to die there could be no better place than here, he thought.

Time passed slowly.

Chapter 68

Saddleback Cay
June 29
7:12PM

The Cuban cut the throttle as he drifted into the shadow of the island's lower crest. He was hidden out of view from the ruins, and he had all night. The boat glided into the shallow bay, and he anchored in three feet of crystal clear water. He saw starfish laying on the sand bottom, and hundreds of bright silver and blue fish darting through the calm water. As the boat settled on its anchor, he rested and stretched, massaging his sore back and knees.

In the twilight, he scanned the nearby beach. He listened to the quiet lapping of the waves against the beach, strained for the sound of someone moving through the scrub that bordered the half-moon beach. Nothing. There was only one path away from the beach into the interior of the cay. The narrow, overgrown opening was nestled among jagged coral and rock. One way in, one way out.

The Cuban regretted that he had gotten to this point. He should have retrieved the disc long ago. Now it was more than just a job, more than just the disc and his fee. Now the stinking Yankee had his face, knew what he looked like and maybe even his name. That moron Johnny could have told him everything. Now, he would have to kill the doctor. And his wife. Maybe have some fun with the woman, first. Then there would be plenty of time to search for the disc. He looked up. The sun was almost gone.

Now the Cuban's thoughts were racing. Would Coltrane be stupid enough to venture out against him? Would the doctor try to strike first? Could he be racing to the beach even now? The Cuban doubted that. Yet, as a lifetime of experience had taught him, anything is possible. The Cuban ceased his reflections, and reaching for his pistol, sprang over the gunnel and waded through the warm water to the edge of the bramble scrub. Lifting a thorny branch out of his way, he moved cautiously onto the trail.

The trail was steep and littered with sharp coral shards. The sun had set, but the hard ground stored the intense heat, radiating it back as the air cooled. Flies and mosquitoes covered him, hungry for the first blood meal of the day. They feasted on him, attacking every exposed inch of his sun burnt skin voraciously. He ignored them, pushing quickly to the crest of the lesser peak. He lay on the reverse slope of the path, and looked up out over the saddle towards the ruins.

The narrow trail meandered down into the saddle, then branched as it traveled to the four curving beaches on the south half of the island. It ran straight across the narrow waist of the island, then curved up to the west as it reached the ruins. The Cuban saw no movement in the fading light. He defocused his eyes and listened to the wind, the birds and the insects; a tribal ritual he had learned in Angola as a young soldier decades ago.

Nothing. He crawled backward down the trail a few feet, cradled his head on his arms and waited for darkness to descend.

Chapter 69

Saddleback Cay
June 29
8:48PM

The last rays of sunlight had long since departed, and night enveloped the island. Coltrane could see down the trail thirty feet to the bend, but as the light faded he had to strain to make out the outlines of the rock and scrub. High overhead, fast moving evening winds pushed the clouds in front of a bright moon. Coltrane hoped that the sky would clear for him, letting the moon light the path.

They had lain quietly for two hours now, the initial surge of adrenaline wearing off and the metallic taste in their mouths remaining. Neither one spoke, each watching the small patch of earth before them, each deep in their own thoughts.

Coltrane had spent countless hours like this; as a boy hunting on his uncle's ranch in the Texas Hill Country and on the Mogollon Rim in Arizona, and more recently on the guided hunts he took two or three times a year. Once in Arizona he had waited along a narrow stream, nestled among huge granite boulders for eight full hours, never moving, never stirring. A herd of grazing cattle had drifted in to within feet of him, unaware of his presence. He had slipped into a state of peaceful meditation in the solitude, aware yet unaware of his surroundings. Hours later, movement attracted his eye and brought him out of his reverie. A flock of wild turkeys were thirty yards away, cautiously drinking from the stream, aside and among the cattle. He had carefully selected and killed two from the flock. The noise of his shotgun had stampeded the cattle all around him, and only the boulders saved him from being trampled to death. It was a day and an experience he would never forget.

But over time, Coltrane hunted less and less. Disgusted by weekend hunting trips with his buddies that amounted to nothing but binge drinking and shooting deer with a high powered rifle from a pickup truck, finally he just quit altogether. Then, five years ago, a surgeon buddy introduced him to bowhunting. He quickly realized that bow hunting was a completely different sport. To get a clean kill with a bow required the stalker to close to within ten paces of the prey. No blasting away from a pickup truck stopped on the road. Bowhunters had to camouflage their entire body, face, hands, bow and gear. They had to cover their human scent with foul, animal musk, and be able to approach prey cautiously and agonizingly slowly, from downwind. They had to be quiet, to remain motionless when the deer looked straight at them, unable to discern what the bizarre creature was that appeared before them. They had to be able to draw an eighty pound bow, slowly, smoothly, and noiselessly. All with adrenaline pumping through their blood, high on buck fever. Then find a flight path for the arrow through the thicket, as the slightest brush with a leaf or branch would deflect the shaft's true path. For Coltrane, this was hunting. The playing field was leveled. He loved the stalk far more than the kill, and rarely took the shot. He was a natural, and enjoyed the solitude of the hunt. His prowess sharpened with every hunting season. It was a thrill that was difficult to experience in any other way.

Vietnam had been a different story. Why had he joined when he had a college deferment? Patriotism? A thirst for adventure? Bloodlust? His uncle had said that a man only gets one good war in his lifetime, and Coltrane had figured that Vietnam would be his. When he landed at Camh Ranh Bay in January of 1971, he was euphoric. He was a green second lieutenant, lean and hard from boot camp, full of unearned confidence and impatient to cover himself with glory and the blood of his enemy.

In the beginning, he had scorned his small brown foe as ignorant, uncivilized. He laughed at stories of eviscerated VC crawling into the jungle to die slowly or be eaten alive by feral pigs rather than surrender or seek aid. Once, on a night ambush his platoon had slaughtered a column of VC while they were singing to ward off the spirit demons of the night. They mocked their victims for weeks after that ambush, singing their version of the happy tune whenever superior officers were in the vicinity. Through the hardship, the backbreaking toil of humping eighty pounds of gear through unbearable heat and humidity, razor sharp elephant grass cutting his skin, sweat encrusted fatigues rotting off his body, the weeks without a decent bath or fresh food, the warm beer, the dysentery; he reveled in it all.

But as the months wore on, the closest of friends died, the original members of his platoon were killed and maimed and torn by metal and shell; the casualties of war. The luster of glory faded. He had thought he was fearless, the Marines had taught him that. But fear had found him, and though he had dealt with fear and death well, he always doubted if there was not a better path, a better way he could have gone. Maybe some of his dead comrades would have lived. In the last two months of his thirteen, he refused leave for R&R. He knew if he left his unit, something bad would happen. Some fuck-up officer in Saigon, living on cold Pabst and fifty cent blow-jobs, would send his platoon out on a clusterfuck and get his men killed. For nothing. So he stayed until the end, finally turning over the platoon to a new brown bar, bittersweet in the parting with comrades with whom the bond was stronger than brothers, deeper than the shallow loves of his life.

Coltrane stirred from his reverie, and glanced over at Britt. She could barely be seen over her little rock pile, and didn't notice his glance. His heart flooded with love for her, and the desperate need to protect her from harm. Strengthened, he turned back to the trail. He would kill the fuck if it meant driving a sharpened stick through his eye with his last dying breath.

Chapter 70

Saddleback Cay
June 29
9:32PM

The Cuban was a battle-hardened veteran of four guerrilla conflicts spanning three decades. From Angola to Central America, he had served Communist Cuba in the struggle to free the oppressed peoples of the world. He was a seasoned jungle fighter, a professional in the savage, deadly and personal business of war, and he moved as one now. With every cloud that obscured the face of the moon, he advanced forward quickly and silently. Within an hour he had moved down the face of the lower hill into the saddle, and began his ascent up the trail to the ruins. He stayed in the shadows of the scrub border of the trail, switching from side to side as the trail snaked up the hill, always out of view of his quarry at the crest. The going now was very slow. The Cuban knew he would have to watch for booby-traps. The doctor had been waiting for them on the yacht, hadn't he? He moved with slow and deliberate caution, inching forward with his fingers lightly sweeping the air and ground before him.

Three hours passed as he slowly crept up to the ruins. He saw nothing unusual on the trail. A scorpion bit him, and he promptly crushed it in his fingers. Small rodents and lizards skittered in the bush. Then, just before him, the trail took a sharp turn to the right, and vanished out of sight into a large coral outcropping. The Cuban felt an old, familiar, uneasy feeling in his gut. He paused and scanned the trail with his peripheral vision, allowing his retina to register faint images with better acuity. Several passes over the area gave him the feeling of a presence above him. He gently stretched his bare arm up, and felt a taut wire against the hairs on his forearm. He froze.

The Cuban didn't take the time to disarm the booby-trap. He simply rolled onto his back, and carefully shimmied under the wire until his feet cleared it. Then he continued forward. Several yards further up the path, he hesitated again. Heaps of vegetation littered the trail, covering the full width of the path. There had been very little litter on any other section of the trail. The Cuban saw palm fronds mixed among the debris. He looked up and around for a palm tree, but saw none. He stopped.

The Cuban reached down to his right calf and drew the dive knife from its leg sheath. With gentle, methodical sweeping motions he probed the area directly in front of his face. Moving inch by inch, he shoved the debris and palms out of his path. The coral and sand gave way, and he discovered a pit dug deep into the floor of the path. His hand grazed across a shard of glass, slicing open the skin and muscle on the edge of the palm. He exhaled sharply through clenched teeth.

As he applied pressure to the cut on his hand, the Cuban looked at the bend in the trail. He estimated that he was very close to the ruins, maybe twenty feet. He could see the sky as the scrub thinned out and opened up at the top of the trail. He knew the doctor had dug a pit across the trail, and filled it with broken glass. His soft leather boat shoes would be no protection against the glass. He might as well be barefoot. To the right and to the left, the scrub was impenetrable. Before him, the pit straddled the path, probably stretching from side to side. Further up the trail were three large coral outcroppings, one on the left edge of the trail and two along the inside curve as the trail turned to the west.

In the end, the Cuban knew what he had to do. He lay still for several minutes, allowing the blood to clot on his right hand, his gun hand. He said a quick Hail Mary, then pulled the pistol and flashlight from his waistband. He released the pistol's safety, and slowly came to a crouching stance, just under the cover of the scrub along the right side of the trail. Creeping to the edge of the pit, he waited and listened.

Chapter 71

Saddleback Cay
June 30
1:25AM

It was well past midnight, but Coltrane was wide awake. He knew that the Cuban had landed on the far beach, and was working his way toward them right now. He strained his ears to catch the faintest crunch of coral beneath a footstep, the lightest brush of bush against fabric. He heard nothing.

His field of view covered the steep path of the trail down to the coral rock formation, but little more. Coltrane focused on a spot off to the right of the trail, using his knowledge of retinal anatomy to maximize his night vision. Coltrane knew that his central vision was primarily for color perception, and that peripheral receptors were far superior for motion and light sensitivity. As he studied the trail, he memorized every leaf, every twig, every rock in sight.

Coltrane also knew that when the shooting started, the muzzle flash from his weapon would temporarily blind him if he wasn't prepared. Left unprotected by a widely dilated pupil in the darkness, the brilliant intensity of the yellow-red fireball would overload and bleach the retina, and the recycle time for the delicate receptors was several seconds. Long enough for a man to reach him while he was blinded, and kill him in his defenseless state. Fearing this, Coltrane kept his non-dominant eye squinted shut as he stared down the trail.

It had been peaceful for a long time, the wind gently rustling the low scrub and the waves lapping on the beaches below. Now the wind was picking up, with weather rolling in from the southeast. Coltrane instinctively sensed the shift and he scanned the sky. A huge cumulus cloud formation was moving rapidly to blanket the moon. Suddenly Coltrane felt uneasy. The fine hairs on the back of his neck tingled, and a chill ran down his spine. He quickly looked back to the trail, and sighted the gun down the center of the path just as the clouds quenched the moonlight.

Chapter 72

Saddleback Cay
June 30
2:51AM

With a savage lunge, the Cuban pushed off with his right leg and leapt up the path. He used the coral rock on the left edge of the trail as a stepping stone to bound over the glass-filled pit. As he jumped, he pointed the flashlight straight up the hill and began firing into the ruins.

The coral buckled under his heel, and he slipped wildly to the left against the bramblebush that bordered the trail. The dense shrub held his weight, and lacerated but still upright, he continued uphill. His short, muscular legs churned wildly beneath him, but he lost his footing on the decomposed coral. Again he slipped and fell, cutting his hands and elbows as he landed in the second bed of upright broken bottles. Still he came on, screaming and firing his weapon into the gray mass of stones at the crest of the hill. He didn't feel the torn flesh on his arms and face, nor did he sense the small bullets as they tore into his stocky frame. The adrenaline was fueling his body up the hill at his unseen foe. The end was near.

Chapter 73

Saddleback Cay
June 30
2:51AM

Coltrane heard the crunch of coral gravel as the cloud bank plunged the islands into darkness. He saw the beam of the flashlight swing up the trail, then arc wildly out into the night sky. Squinting his right eye shut, he aimed the small pistol down the trail at the pale mass that appeared from behind the coral outcropping. He gently squeezed off a round, watched the bright yellow fireball mushroom out of the barrel and then disappear. Now he was blind. The Cuban had appeared exactly where Coltrane knew he would. Coltrane heard the bellow and the noise of the bushes, and fired at the sound.

Suddenly the path was illuminated with light, shining through the bushes from Coltrane's right. He saw the Cuban hurtling up the trail toward them, firing wildly, his face contorted, his arms covered with blood. Coltrane locked on the center of the Cuban's chest and fired. As he aimed again, one of the Cuban's shots hit the stone palisade by Coltrane's head. The ricochet sent metal and stone shrapnel into the side of Coltrane's face and right eye. A wave of blinding, excruciating pain hit him, momentarily paralyzing him. Coltrane howled in pain and anger, and turned his good eye to his attacker. He fired round after round into the onrushing figure. The gun jammed after the fifth shot, a spent casing stovepiped in the slide.

Coltrane dropped the gun, and reached back for the speargun. His hands were trembling as he fumbled with the clumsy weapon, and brought it to bear down the trail. His chest was heaving so wildly that he couldn't keep the speargun steady.

But his field of fire, where he expected to see the Cuban just feet away, was empty. The light that Britt had providentially supplied wavered as it shone with an eerie glow through the brush, the shadows dancing on the coral. The Cuban sat slumped, his legs twisted awkwardly beneath him, and his torso embedded in the brush. He had collapsed back toward where he started his rush. His head dangled forward on his chest, rising and falling with his labored breathing. He still held his pistol loosely in his right hand.

Coltrane raised the speargun to his shoulder, and twisted his face to sight with his remaining good eye. Keeping the ugly weapon centered on the Cuban's belly, he called to Britt to crawl to him. She set the flashlight on the rock ledge so its beam illuminated the Cuban, and scrambled into his foxhole. With his free hand, he passed her the pistol, and told her how to clear the jammed casing. She performed the maneuver quickly, reloaded the clip and chambered a round.

"If he makes the slightest move, shoot him. In the belly. Right in the navel." Coltrane rose up, keeping the speargun centered on the Cuban's abdomen.

"*Where are you going? What are you doing?*" Britt screamed frantically at him, still pointing the pistol at the moaning Cuban.

"He's alive, but he won't be for long. Only he knows what this is all about. Only he can give us any answers. He is the key to it all. I have to talk to him. Just shoot him if he moves." Coltrane stood up, and felt the pain in his face and shoulder for the first time. He had paused to step over the stone wall just as Britt began firing. She fired deliberate, measured shots into the Cuban's shuddering body until the gun was empty. Five rounds.

"Now go talk to him." Britt smiled grimly at Coltrane.

"Shit, woman. What the fuck is wrong with you. Now we'll never know what the disc is about." Coltrane cursed.

"First of all, that asshole knows less about that disc than we do. Secondly, he was in no shape or mood to tell you anything. Thirdly, he still had a gun in his hand and could have shot you in the process. That was a dumb-ass idea. Now please take me back to the boat so we can... *Shit!... Fuck!* You're bleeding. Are you hurt?" Britt jumped up and grabbed the flashlight.

Suddenly the strength drained from him, and he sat down hard on the stone wall, feeling weak and nauseated. Britt shone the light on his face, and gently brushed the dirt and sand from his wounds. Coltrane winced. His right eye was filled with blood, and Britt couldn't see the iris or the pupil. The light she shone into his face was blinding, and painful. He pulled away, pain shooting through his blood soaked shoulder.

"Get me to the boat. We can take care of this shit later," Coltrane indicated the gear strewn about them by waving his left arm. "Get the medical kit and the cooler lid and let's get to the boat." Coltrane put the speargun on safe, then laid it carefully on the ground. He painfully bent down and gathered the pistol and the box of ammo, putting them in his sea bag. Britt picked up the flashlight, and with some puzzlement, removed the molded plastic lid from the cooler. She followed him carefully down the dark trail.

Coltrane stopped at the corpse of the Cuban, and stooped to retrieve the weapon from the fallen man's hand. He safed it and shoved it into his waistband. When they reached the booby-trap, he turned to Britt. Taking the hard plastic cooler lid, he laid it across the bottom of the pit, crushing it onto the broken glass. Using the lid as a stepping stone, he crossed the bend in the trail. Then he helped Britt across. Together, they slowly made their way down to the beach. Britt sat in the sand while Coltrane waded out to bring in the dinghy. They started the tiny outboard, and puttered out to the yacht without speaking.

Chapter 74

Saddleback Cay
June 30
3:27AM

After getting aboard and quenching their terrible thirst, Coltrane stripped and surveyed himself for wounds. He tried to wash off with the transom shower, but his shoulder pain was excruciating. The injury to his right eye sent searing pain straight through his skull. Exhausted, he pulled three Vicodin tabs from the medical bag and washed them down with white wine. Britt fired up the diesel, and within ten minutes, they had hot water for the shower.

Britt quickly undressed, and bathed in the transom shower. Her shower over, she went below and returned topside with the medical kit and a huge battery operated lantern. She set them on the cockpit table, and turned her attention to Coltrane.

For three hours, she attended to his wounds. First she gently bathed him, soaking off the encrusted blood and stanching the bleeding. Coltrane had three long gashes on his face where rock shrapnel had struck him. They were bloody, but superficial. She cleansed them with bottled water, and applied Steri-Strips to close the skin.

In his right shoulder, Coltrane had a much more serious wound. Either a stone or bullet fragment had penetrated his chest just below the collarbone. The entrance wound was bruised and swollen, and there was no exit wound. Coltrane couldn't raise his elbow, and his shoulder was too tender to move. He told Britt to wash and bandage the wound, and made himself a sling from a pillowcase.

The right eye was exquisitely painful. Coltrane directed Britt to use a drop of local anesthetic to numb the cornea, then had her flush his eye thoroughly with water. She held his lids open with a bent paper-clip she found in the chart desk. Coltrane had to be held down for the unpleasant procedure. The anesthetic, meant for local anesthesia for minor procedures, burned the eye, and the pupil dilated, making it sensitive to the bright light of the lantern. The irrigation of his eye loosened and flushed out blood clots and stone fragments. There were tiny shards of stone embedded in the eyelids, and several small lacerations of the upper eyelid. Mercifully, Coltrane's cornea and vision were intact. She tenderly patched his eye with ointment and squares of cotton gauze.

Coltrane was getting weaker by the minute. He wondered if the shell fragment had lacerated his axillary artery or punctured the apex of his lung. Quickly, he checked for his radial pulse. But he was too weak and shaky to discern it. Fading fast, he described to Britt the clinical signs he would exhibit if the bullet had pierced his lung, and told her to check the pulse in his right hand every hour or so. Then he slipped into unconsciousness.

Chapter 75

Saddleback Cay
June 30
6:04AM

Coltrane awoke as the sun rose behind Saddleback Cay. Night on board had been agony. His shoulder hurt, his eye hurt, and he had an intense pounding headache from the Vicodin and wine and dehydration. He lifted his head from the cockpit cushion, and saw Britt sleepily watching him from the opposite bench. He remembered passing out, hours ago. She must have stayed up all night with me, he thought. Shit.

Coltrane bolted upright, shocked by the realization that they still had to dispose of the Cuban, and clean up the mess on Saddleback Cay. He scanned the horizon. No boats. But this time of year, the Exumas were extremely popular with charter sailors, and cruising yachtsmen. Someone could be along at any time.

He went below, popped two Vicodin and drank a liter of Gatorade. Still parched, he opened another liter bottle of Gatorade, and drained it in three long swallows. He stuffed some gear into his nylon sea bag, and climbed on deck.

"You scared the shit out of me last night. I wanted to call for help all night." Britt was weary and angry, but grateful to see him moving about easily.

"You didn't call, did you?"

"No, you seemed to be breathing fine, and your hand was warm. I always got good pulses. But we have to get you to a hospital today, baby. You have a bullet in your shoulder, for Christ's sake!"

"No. I'm fine. If things get worse, maybe. But I'll decide that. I'm a surgeon, I know how to deal with this. And if we notify any authorities, we are in deep shit. The Bahamians have no tolerance for criminals. We could spend the rest of our lives in a Bahamian jail." Coltrane was adamant.

"That's better than dying from that wound."

"From what I have heard about Bahamian prisons, maybe not. Now I have to go ditch the Cuban before some picnickers find his rotting corpse. Stay below, but keep an eye out for anything unusual. I will be back in about two hours." Coltrane climbed down into the dinghy.

"What are you going to do with the body? Let me help." Britt was worried about his strength.

"Nothing fancy. I'm going to sink him offshore. You need to stay here and watch the boat. Say, do you remember what kind of shirt he was wearing?" Coltrane couldn't picture the man's body for some reason.

"I think a red polo shirt. Why?"

"Get me a red shirt, any red shirt. And one of the sheets, please." Coltrane started the outboard, and checked his gas tank.

Britt came back to the transom, and handed him a white bedsheet and one of his red T-shirts. Her face was lined with concern.

"Don't worry, I am going to take his Whaler. They are indestructible. You can cut them in half and they don't sink. Don't worry. I'll be right back. I love you." With that, Coltrane cast off and whipped the dinghy around, heading for the beach. He waved as he passed by the yacht, and Britt went below.

Chapter 76

Saddleback Cay
June 30
10:04AM

Coltrane climbed up the trail, and stood over the Cuban. Already, the intense heat of the Caribbean was putrefying the corpse. The skin was a mottled purple where the blood had settled and coagulated. Despite the 100 degree heat, the body was cool to the touch. Coltrane shuddered. He found the keys to the Whaler in the man's shorts, and dragged the corpse down to the beach. After covering the body with the sheet, Coltrane ran along the trails to the north beach. There he donned surgical gloves and the red T-shirt, and waded out to the boat.

The 150 horsepower motor fired up instantly, and within minutes, he brought the powerboat around to their little cove. He beached the boat next to the dinghy, and with some effort and struggle, manhandled the corpse into the Whaler. Coltrane scanned the horizon, and saw nothing. Thinking he was safe for awhile, Coltrane climbed quickly to the stone ruins. He collected their critical gear: the speargun, flaregun and satphone. He searched the ground, and recovered nine of the spent brass shell casings. The rest he would have to find later. One last look over their campsite revealed nothing obviously incriminating.

Coltrane stood atop the highest coral rock, and scanned the horizon in all directions. Far to the north, two yachts were on a beam reach, and headed this way. They were sailing very close, probably friends traveling together. If they were coming here, they would take an hour to arrive. Out to sea, Coltrane saw one small inter-island freighter steaming for Eleuthera. Nothing else was visible, horizon to horizon. Satisfied that he had time to leisurely dispose of the body, Coltrane climbed down the trail.

Coltrane took the Whaler around the south tip of Saddleback Cay, waving toward *Blue Pearl* as he sped out of sight. He powered through the cut, and headed for the open ocean. He motored at top speed until he was almost five miles offshore, and land had vanished from sight. The swells were three feet, the seas calm. The Exuma Sound was six thousand feet deep here, and dark blue. He was completely alone, a solitary craft, for as far as the eye could see. He put the boat in neutral, and let the motor idle. For five minutes he sat slumped in the captain's chair, bone-weary and exhausted.

Finally, he rose to complete the grisly task. He tore the bloody bedsheet into strips, and used them to bind the wrists and ankles together. Then he pulled his filet knife from his sea bag, and sliced the Cuban's belly open to release the intestines. The stench made him gag and turn his face away. He performed a similar procedure on each side of the rib cage. He wanted the fish to have easy access to the tissue, and avoid the bloated corpse surfacing at some inopportune time in the future. He wasn't going to take any chances. Finishing the gruesome task, he wrapped the Whaler's anchor rope around the corpse's ankles and neck, and pushed the carcass overboard. He watched as the shrouded corpse slipped into the dark water, and drifted deeper. Within seconds, it was gone.

Coltrane washed down the decks of the Whaler repeatedly, until all traces of blood and gore were gone. He disassembled and broke down both of the pistols, and threw the parts overboard along with the ammo and filet knife. Satisfied that he had sanitized the boat and destroyed any links to the death of the Cuban, he washed his gloved hands and arms in the cool saltwater. All the evidence was gone. He cranked up the boat, and headed for the cut.

Chapter 77

Saddleback Cay
June 30
3:44PM

Coltrane left the boat on the northeast beach where he had found it, beaching it where it would not float off on the next high tide. He disabled the motor to discourage anyone from stealing the valuable skiff. He removed the red T-shirt and pocketed his surgical gloves, and waded onshore. When he emerged from the trail onto their little beach, he was startled to find the dinghy missing. Panicking, he searched up and down the shore of the small bay, finding nothing. He had tied it well, the tide could not have floated it off. He cupped his hands, and yelled for Britt.

Presently, she appeared in the cockpit. Then he noticed that the dinghy was tethered to *Blue Pearl*, just hidden from his view. He motioned for her to come and get him. While she dinghyed in, Coltrane climbed to the ruins again. He was amazed to find the area pristine; the blood stained coral was gone, the trash and supplies were packed out, the stones replaced and the booby-trap filled in and resurfaced with large coral rocks. He retraced his steps to the trailhead just as Britt pulled the dinghy ashore.

"I got tired of hiding belowdecks. It just got too hot. I cleaned up." Britt was dead-tired, but felt cleansed.

"Nice job, sweetheart. Any trouble?" Coltrane asked.

"Nope. No one came all day. Two sloops sailed by earlier, but they didn't stop. What did you do with the body?"

"He sleeps with the fishes. Let's get out of here."

Within minutes, they had weighed anchor, and were sailing on a gentle breeze, southward.

Chapter 78

Hawksbill Cay
June 30
6:25PM

It was almost sunset when they dropped anchor at Hawksbill Cay. Winds were from the east, and they were protected by high rocky bluffs that surrounded the inlet. A fine, shallow sandy beach lay at the base of the bluffs. Coltrane anchored in twelve feet of crystal clear water, and let the boat drift backward to snug up the line.

The sleek boat weathervaned with the light easterly breeze, turning so that the cockpit and transom faced directly into the sunset. It was a spectacular blaze of crimson, peach and red. The water shimmered and sparkled, its turquoise depths showing the shallow sand bottom of the Great Bahama Bank. They both sat basking, reverent, in the glow of the magnificent scene. For the Coltranes, this beauty was the reason they continually returned to this place. For the solitude, for the untouched pristine beauty of nature and God. Coltrane had circled the world twice, and seen many things, but never had he seen nature quite as magnificent.

Coltrane went below, and brought up the brown Myers's bottle, and set it on the cockpit table. He sliced a lime wedge, crushed it between his thumb and forefinger, and dropped it into Britt's tumbler. His shoulder hurt, but the warm buzz of the rum gradually numbed his pain. Peacefully, they sat in the stern of the boat as the sun set. When Coltrane drifted into sleep, Britt gently covered him with a blanket, and stretched out on the opposite bench, watching over him as long as she could remain awake. Soon, she too was in a deep, peaceful sleep.

Chapter 79

Hawksbill Cay
July 1
5:54AM

The rising sun woke them as it crested the bluffs of Hawksbill Cay. Britt went below to prepare breakfast before the heat made the cabin unbearable. As she made coffee, Coltrane went to the transom shower and rinsed his shoulder wound. During the night, the wound had bled, leaving his chest covered with caked blood. Carefully, slowly, he cleansed the blood from his body. He inspected the entrance wound, and gingerly pressed the swollen tissue. He winced. Clear fluid mixed with blood clots drained from the ragged hole in his tanned skin. He was grateful that there were no signs of infection. He knew that if the drainage became purulent, he would have to surgically explore the wound. He smiled grimly at the irony; a surgeon's last procedure being performed in primitive conditions and upon the surgeon himself.

They ate a breakfast of eggs with red potatoes and onions sautéed in butter from Wisconsin. Meals were always more intensely flavorful on the yacht, the scenery gorgeous as the morning developed. Britt went below and cleaned the dishes as Coltrane enjoyed his coffee.

"Now what? Back to Tampa?" She asked.

"Probably. How many days do we have left on the charter?" Coltrane answered.

"I think four or five. I don't even really know what day it is." Britt realized.

Coltrane came above decks with the computer and satphone, and set up the antenna. He dialed Lynwood's number.

"Agent Lynwood."

"Lynwood, this is Coltrane. What have you been able to find out?" Coltrane started.

"You know, Dr. Coltrane, the more I investigate your claims, the more questions are raised. Your story is becoming increasingly bizarre. Have you notified the Bahamian authorities of your position? Are they on the way to escort you to the American Embassy?" Lynwood was perturbed.

"Listen, we're doing fine. I haven't seen a soul in two days, and we have had some boat trouble that kept us from getting to Georgetown. These islands are beautiful, and I'm enjoying the company of my bride. Maybe this was all just a false alarm. I probably watch too much TV." Coltrane lied, hoping to placate Lynwood.

"Coltrane, where are you? Exactly!" Lynwood demanded.

Coltrane glanced at Britt, who was piecing together the conversation. She looked concerned.

"In the Exumas," he answered.

"Don't bullshit me, Coltrane. I have access to US Customs Intelligence satellite overflight photographs. I can find you and read the label on your beer can. Now I want you to make your way to Nassau immediately, or I'll have the Bahamian authorities arrest you and seize your craft within an hour." Lynwood threatened.

"On what grounds? Who put a bug up your ass?" Coltrane was taken aback by the vehemence of his attack.

"On the grounds that you are a material witness in the Hendricks' murder case. You were right. Forensic examination of the body here in Tampa has shown that he was drowned in fluorinated city tap water, probably in a bathtub. That evidence alone is not proof of murder. He could have accidentally drowned, and the body dumped to avoid embarrassment. But he also had several subtle but definitive indications that the drowning was intentional, possible during prolonged torture by immersion. As you said, we found evidence of duct tape adhesive on his mouth, wrists and ankles." Lynwood softened his tone. "I want you back in Tampa where the Bureau can protect you. I genuinely believe that you are in grave danger, Dr. Coltrane."

"Yeah, yeah, maybe you are right…" Coltrane's voice trailed off.

"Do you want me to send a boat for you?" Lynwood asked.

"No. I'm responsible for this yacht and have to return it to the marina in Abaco. It's worth half a million dollars, I can't just leave it where I want. I'll be in Tampa in two days. Have you had any luck with the file? Can your cryptologists in Washington decode it?"

"No, we have had no luck with it at all. The HMO is very angry about the data, and is demanding the original file back immediately. Do you still have the original CD-R?" Lynwood asked coolly.

"What? You told them about the file? Why the hell did you do that?" Coltrane was furious.

"First of all, by your own admission, the data was stolen from the HMO's administrative offices. I am required by law to return stolen property to the rightful owner. As far as I know, the data has no significance with regards to any criminal activity. But this is one reason that I want you back in Tampa. There are many unanswered questions surrounding this matter."

"Alright, we are on our way." Coltrane thanked him, and pressed the red END button on the phone handset.

"Something is wrong. His whole attitude has changed. I don't get it." Coltrane looked at the phone, and then raised his eyes to meet Britt's.

"He's going to give them back the data? That doesn't matter, we can keep a copy of the disc. Why would the HMO admit that the data is theirs? Why not just deny any connection?" Britt wondered.

"Good question. Who knows? Maybe they are unsure of exactly what files Hendricks stole. Maybe they want to try to cover their tracks before someone decodes the files. They may not even know that the files are encrypted. Shit, I don't know. None of this makes any sense." Coltrane leaned back against the bench cushion and slowly exhaled.

"Lynwood wants us to go to Nassau?" Britt asked tentatively.

"To the American Embassy there." Coltrane replied.

"You refused?"

"We're not in danger any more, and we still need to work out what that data means, and settle some loose ends with the insurance plans. I need to find out what's happening with the society. Christ, this is giving me a headache. Would you check my E-mail while I get some aspirin?" Coltrane went below for aspirin and a glass of cold water.

When he returned to the cockpit, Britt was intently scrolling through a long series of messages from Susan Kerr. She looked up as Coltrane sank wearily onto the bench.

"You should have a look at these. And then you better call Susan." Britt said quietly.

Coltrane moved around the wheel, and sat next to Britt as she opened the E-mail messages. He read them outloud.

E-mail
June 28
7:24:41 AM
From: SKerr
To: WmColtraneMD
Rec'd data attachment. Will contact Agent
Lynwood at AM.
sk

E-mail
June 28
3:26:53 PM
From: SKerr
To: WmColtraneMD

Data given to Agent Lynwood, and receipt obtained per instructions.
sk

E-mail
June 29
11:33:32 AM
From: SKerr
To: WmColtraneMD

Conference going extremely well. HMOs are weakening, I think. Public is still behind us for the most part. Hospitals fine. Docs enjoying the respite, much deep-sea fishing going on.
Want you back here, please.
sk

E-mail
June 30
10:24:41 AM
From: SKerr
To: WmColtraneMD

Dr. Coltrane
Lynwood has been here three times this morning, asking questions about you and a man named Ochoa. He interviewed all of the staff, and showed them photographs of Ochoa, specifically asking if Ochoa was ever in the office, or if anyone had ever seen you and him together. Very serious, very stern. He interrogated me for half an hour about you, and Ochoa and Hendricks. He thinks that you and Hendricks were involved in something, I believe. Please call. I have many questions and things I need to discuss with you.
sk

E-mail
June 30
7:24:41 PM
From: SKerr
To: WmColtraneMD

URGENT
Dr. Coltrane

Ochoa, the man that Lynwood was asking us about, was murdered last night in East Tampa. I just saw it all over the evening news. Lynwood must have known about the murder when he was in the society office this morning. He thinks you knew the dead man. According to the TV news, Ochoa was a small time drug dealer and two time loser. Why does Lynwood think you would know him? Very strange behavior. The meeting is going well, should we extend the schedule? Want you back, please. By the way, where the hell are you?
Lynwood says you're in the Bahamas???????
sk

Coltrane read through several other E-mail messages from members of the society. The tone of the messages was somber, but the general feeling seemed to be positive. Only one diatribe was entirely negative, and Coltrane laughed outloud as he read it.

"What is so funny?" Britt asked.

"Joseph Carlsten ranted on for two pages about how we are abrogating our responsibility to the public by placing financial pressures on the insurance plans. If I didn't know that he is a moron, the letter would upset me. How does that asshole survive in the real world?" Coltrane mused.

"I don't think that he has much of a practice." Britt answered quietly.

Britt's comment jolted Coltrane back to reality, back to thoughts of his very busy practice. Immediately, he recalled his pending surgical schedule. He remembered Mrs. Davis, who needed her joint reconstruction when he returned. His island frame of mind dissolved. He picked up the phone and dialed Susan Kerr.

"Medical Society." Susan answered, her voice tired.

"Susan, how are things going? I got your E-mails, and I am sorry about the delay in responding to them. Things have been hectic here, and I have had problems with the computer and the phones." Coltrane lied.

"Thank God you finally called. I really need to talk with you. All hell has broken loose here, Doctor. What bad news do you want to hear first, the society's pending injunction or your pending arrest?" Susan was extremely agitated.

"Susan, Susan, calm down. Everything will eventually work out. Now listen carefully. I am talking to you on a non-secure satellite phone, and there is a high probability that this phone and our society phone lines are being tapped, as well as your home phones. Do you understand?" Coltrane spoke slowly and deliberately, then paused for her answer.

"Yes." Susan responded, surprised.

"Good. First of all, the society is simply holding a perfectly legitimate medical conference, one of literally tens of thousands held every year. There is absolutely nothing illegal or unethical about the conference. The society in general, and you in particular, are perfectly innocent. You must be confident of this, and you must remain confident of this."

"Yes, I am. And I will." Susan replied quickly.

"Good." Coltrane exhaled, and leaned back on the settee. "Now please bring me up to date with regard to the conference."

"The HMOs have been very vocal in the media about the diminished availability of healthcare as a result of the conference, but I believe that the public has not felt any significant impact. I know that several major trauma cases from the surrounding counties have been routed to Orlando or Miami, and that is costing the HMO very dearly. But locally, everything is going well. All the physicians assigned to cover the call rotations have pledged not to balance bill any patients they see on HMO plans with which they don't participate. So, really, the public is benefiting by having a wider choice of doctors at no extra cost. They seem to like the expanded choices. But I think that the physicians are almost finished with the business of the conference, and anxious to get back to normal."

"No doubt. How have the negotiations with the hospitals been going?" Coltrane asked.

"The hospitals claim that they are very limited in their options by federal regulations, and HCFA guidelines. There's not much they can do. St. Mary's has promised to establish a multi-specialty clinic to provide free care to uninsured patients in the county. The medical staff has volunteered to staff the clinic on a rotating basis. This should relieve some of the load on the ER, and the administration has created a fund to reimburse on-call physicians for all uninsured and no-pay ER patients. We are pressuring the five other large hospitals to co-operate or provide similar programs." Susan was upbeat.

"Outstanding. That's a step in the right direction. What the administrators say is true; their hands are tied by strict federal regulations. Any significant change in our hospital system would probably require Congressional action. What about the insurance plans? Have you made any progress with regard to the fee schedules?" Coltrane carefully worded the question.

"As you expected, we have received nothing in writing from the national HMOs," Susan explained. "But there is good news. The two local HMOs *have* submitted proposals to modify their existing fee schedules so that they conform with the 2002 McGraw-Hill RBRVS schedule. The final details are not worked out, but the proposals look good on paper."

"When do the schedules go into effect?" Coltrane was skeptical of any promises.

"They didn't specify. The plan administrator told us that any changes must go before the board of directors." Susan began to think she had been too trusting, too gullible.

"Athena has been promising me a revised, uniform fee schedule for three years. I can tell you that lying and stalling is more than a tactic with them; it is an ingrained way of life." Coltrane could feel his anger rising. "Now I want you to give Athena and all the other plans the following message. Tell them that we will wait for their directors meeting, and when their proposal is formalized, I will present it to the conference committee for evaluation. But the conference will continue until the issues that necessitated convening it have been addressed."

"But I think their meeting isn't for another month," Susan pleaded.

"That is *bullshit.* I guarantee you they are having meetings daily. The decision rests with one man, anyway. You have to convince them that we can wait longer than they can."

"Yes, Doctor." Susan sounded embarrassed at her naiveté.

"Don't feel too bad. They strung me along for a while, too. That's what they are trained and paid to do, make money for the corporate accountants. I'm afraid to ask about Lynwood. What has he been asking you about?"

"Apparently he thinks that you are involved with this Ochoa man who was recently murdered. He seems to feel that Ochoa and Hendricks were connected in some way. He told me that the FBI is investigating both murders, and that he is requesting two more special agents from Washington to assist him. He warned me that Medicare fraud may be the motive for both killings, and that your absence from the country makes the investigation very difficult." Susan paused, and her voiced trembled. "He thinks that you are involved in this, or a suspect or something."

"In the organization of the conference? You mean in some anti-trust violation?" Coltrane had heard that before.

"No. In the events surrounding the murders of Hendricks and Ochoa."

"*WHAT?* He thinks I killed Hendricks... *and* this guy Ochoa? I've never heard of Ochoa. I have never even met anyone named Ochoa. He told you I am a suspect? What a fucking idiot." Coltrane swore bitterly.

"He wants you back in Tampa immediately. He told me to tell you that." Susan was shocked by his disdain.

"I'll call him right away. He must be trying this as a ploy to intimidate me, and you as well. I don't want you suffering under stress or pressure from anyone. Is the conference able to run without you tomorrow?" Coltrane asked, concerned and feeling guilty for leaving Susan in the crucible.

"I suppose...what do you want me to do?" Susan thought he had a different project in mind for her.

"Take a day off. Relax, get your mind off the job. And stay away from the office and Lynwood. If I need you, I'll call or E-mail." Coltrane needed time to think.

"Dr. Coltrane, I want to help." Susan offered.

"I know, and I am very grateful for everything you have done. But I just need time to sort all this out. I will be in touch." Coltrane thanked her, and hung up the satphone.

Coltrane's mind was racing, flooded with disjointed thoughts and doubts. How could Lynwood suspect him of murdering Hendricks or this Ochoa? He sat back and looked across the cockpit at Britt, who had been listening with intense interest.

"What the hell is going on?" She had deduced the essence of the conversation.

"Fuck, I don't know. I think Lynwood is just screwing with Susan's head. I'll find out right now." Coltrane picked up the satphone, and dialed Lynwood's number.

"Agent Lynwood." he answered, his tone flat.

"Lynwood, this is Coltrane. I just spoke with my assistant, Susan Kerr. Why are you harassing her and the society staff?" Coltrane demanded.

"Dr. Coltrane, you may not be aware that Carlos Ochoa was found murdered here in Tampa yesterday. How well did you know him?" Lynwood asked bluntly.

"I don't know any Ochoa. Maybe he is a patient of mine, but the name is unfamiliar." Coltrane lied. The name was vaguely familiar. Hadn't Johnny said something about an Ochoa?

"Coltrane, I will remind you only once that I am conducting a murder investigation. You would be very ill-advised to lie to me now." Lynwood said coldly. "What we know is that Ochoa was a small time drug dealer who was found burned to death in a remote area east of town. When we questioned his common-law wife, she said that Ochoa knew you. He had mentioned your name to her on several occasions. She thought he arranged several meetings with you. Any idea why he would do that? He must have known you."

"Maybe he was talking about an office appointment. I have a huge case load of trauma patients."

"No, he wasn't a patient of yours. We cross-referenced him against your office patient list, the Medicaid patients and the hospital records for the past two years. You never saw him as a patient."

"I keep telling you, I don't know any Ochoa."

"I think that you do," Lynwood paused, wishing he had Coltrane one on one, to judge his physical reactions. Telephone interrogations were almost useless. "How do you explain the fact that your fingerprints were found on an envelope that we found at his home. One of those bank envelopes specifically for cash deposits. From your bank. You must have paid him off for something. I just don't know…"

"*What? Bullshit!* You're jacking with me. I don't have time for this shit," Coltrane was exasperated, getting nowhere with Lynwood, and began to disconnect the satphone.

"We found your name and office phone number on notes at his home as well." Lynwood persisted.

"*Wait one…Resendez.* Juan Resendez. You are talking about Juan Resendez. *Christ.* They killed him. I told him to get out of town." Coltrane interrupted before he could think about what he was saying.

"Say again?" Lynwood was suddenly interested in what Coltrane had to say.

"Resendez *is* Ochoa. Same guy. He probably has a few more aliases, as well. I already told you about him. The encrypted data that I sent you was given to me by Ochoa. He came to me with the files, on a computer disc stolen by Hendricks from the executive offices of the insurance plan. He wanted money for it; for some reason he thought it would be worth something to me. He believed that it incriminated *me* in some way. I don't think that he knew what the data meant, but he was sure that someone wanted it badly enough to kill Hendricks for it."

"How did you find him?"

"I didn't. He found me. He paged me through my answering service. You can verify that with them easily enough. I think that it was one or two days after Hendricks was killed."

"And you believed him?"

"Not at first. But he convinced me. My office had been broken into recently, and he convinced me he had done it. He was telling the truth."

"Did you meet with him?" Lynwood wanted to know.

"Yeah, at Doctor's Hospital."

"Doctor, I will need some corroboration of your story. Was anyone else present? Any witnesses to your meetings?"

"No. The meeting was at night. Neither of us wanted to be seen."

"How much money did you give him?"

"A couple hundred dollars. Just to get out of town. I thought he might be in danger."

"You bought the disc for two hundred dollars? Is that all Ochoa blackmailed you for?" Lynwood asked immediately, his voice thick with sarcasm.

"Listen, I keep having to repeat this to you. Ochoa had no idea what was on that disc. He thought it incriminated *me*. I wanted it because I thought it contained evidence of wrongdoing by Hendricks' employer. I wanted it to use in the Strahan case. I never paid him for anything. I told him that if there was any government whistleblower award, I would split it with him. At the time, I really didn't hold any hope of anything coming of the matter. Obviously, I was wrong."

"So your statement is as follows: You were contacted by a known felon, someone who told you that he had previously burglarized your *own* office. This felon then attempted to blackmail you with data you knew to be stolen from AthenaHMO, and arranged clandestine meetings with you. And you attended those meetings, alone. You subsequently bought the data, and then paid the stranger to get out of town? You entered into an agreement with this felon to split potentially millions of dollars of federal whistleblower payments relating to the CD-R evidence. And now, both this man and Hendricks are dead, murdered execution style. And you are in the Bahamas, telling me that you are in New York. You don't look good in this, Doctor."

"You actually think I was involved in Ochoa's murder?" Coltrane asked.

"As of this moment, yes."

"For God's sake, Lynwood, how the fuck could I have killed anyone in Tampa? We have been out of town for almost a week." Coltrane bellowed.

"Ochoa's body had been sitting in the swamp for some time, and with the burns, the coroner can't place the time of death accurately. That's something that a physician, and in particular a burn surgeon, may be familiar with. Right, Doctor? And his girlfriend is an addict. She doesn't know what day *today* is, much less when she last saw Ochoa. He could have been killed quite a while ago."

"Maybe I should talk with my attorney." Coltrane felt a chill run down his spine.

"If you have something to hide, you had better have a damn good one. But if you're innocent, you will make life much easier on yourself, your practice and your family if you cooperate."

"Are you threatening me?" Coltrane bristled.

"Not at all. But if you cannot explain your connection to the murdered man, I will have no choice but to obtain a search warrant for your home and office. And the society offices as well. Don't make life hard for yourself, Doctor." Lynwood's manner projected confidence.

Coltrane felt his heart thump rapidly three times, slamming hard against his sternum and sending an odd sensation through his chest. His world was collapsing around him. Coltrane tried to envision the correct path to take. Some truths he would never be able to reveal. But his dealings with Ochoa were clean. Hopefully, he could lift the cloud of suspicion by revealing part of the truth.

"Everything I have told you is true. If I were guilty, do you really think I would be talking to you right now? You'd be talking to my attorney. Or, more accurately, you would *not* be talking to my attorney. I know what my rights are. And I don't expect you to trust or believe in me. But I do expect you to make a reasonable attempt to verify my story. Check it out. Call my answering service. They keep accurate, computerized records of all my calls. Check with the Tampa Police. They will have a record of the office break-in. I know that they dusted for prints, I told them where to dust, for Christ's sake. And if Resendez…or Ochoa spent time with Hendricks, certainly his neighbors could identify him. Take a little time to look into my story and you will see it's all true." Coltrane realized that the tale sounded wild.

"The Tampa Police are running a fingerprint analysis at the crime scenes and your office right now, checking your prints and Ochoa's and Hendricks' as well. They should be done within twenty-four hours. I'll check everything you mentioned, Doctor Coltrane. Now, when can I expect you back in Florida?" Lynwood persisted.

"Two, maybe three days. We're in a sailboat, with hundreds of miles of open ocean between us and the nearest island airport. This yacht is not equipped for night passages, and I am not going to endanger our lives by recklessly rushing back to port. I promise you that I will return to Tampa.

And I did not kill Ochoa or Hendricks. I would have no reason to kill either of them. What possible motive could I have?" Coltrane was drained, and wanted the conversation to end.

"Ochoa's death makes you the sole recipient of the whistleblower reward, doesn't it? That may be a very substantial motive. Partners and business associates have been murdered for much less, Doctor Coltrane. And you had a very intense and bitter relationship with Dr. Hendricks, by all accounts. There are too many unanswered questions. And your explanations are so bizarre that I have to look very, very closely at you." Lynwood's tone dripped sarcasm.

"Listen, I haven't told you everything." Coltrane paused, uncertain whether he should continue. "I have incriminating evidence against Hendricks. I taped a conversation with him about the Strahan incident, where he admits his negligent refusal to provide appropriate care for the boy. I had no reason to kill him. He had reason to try to kill me! You've got everything backwards." Coltrane tried to reason with Lynwood.

"Where is this tape?" Lynwood asked.

"My attorney, Davis Clark, has it. You can discuss all the details with him. You can listen to the entire recording. I'll tell him you will be calling." Coltrane replied.

"Good. I'll look into the tape tomorrow. But in the meanwhile, I want you to call me tomorrow with your position. Is that clear?" Lynwood demanded.

"Yeah, fine. Look, the key to all of this is the files... the data from Hendricks' CD-R. Someone at the FBI should be able to decipher the code. It can't be that complex, Hendricks must have encrypted the data within hours of stealing the discs and I doubt he was an expert in computer programming or encryption. Once you decipher the data, you will see that I wasn't being blackmailed. I know the insurance company is behind all this somehow. But I promise that I'll call you tomorrow," Coltrane finished wearily, and pushed the END button on the satphone.

He slumped back against the cockpit cushions, drained and frustrated. Before he forgot, he called Davis Clark, and left a message on his voicemail to cooperate with Lynwood's inquiry to the fullest, and allow him access to the recording. Then he disconnected the Iridium, and cursed softly.

Coltrane lay the satphone down on the console and looked over at Britt. She had been listening, and the concern was etched on her face. Coltrane reclined on the cockpit bench, and tried to compose his racing thoughts.

Britt was the first to speak. "They can't really believe that you killed anyone, can they? That's absurd. Lynwood is just trying to pressure you to return to Tampa and end the conference."

"I think you're right. But some of the things I did look real bad. All the phone calls, the money I gave him, my fingerprints on the bank envelope; all this evidence points to some kind of association between me and Ochoa. Resendez. Whatever his real name is. Or was. Now I remember Johnny mentioned the name Ochoa. I didn't pay any attention. Shit." Coltrane paused and racked his brain for any further links to the dead man.

"Even so, you were down here when he was killed. You have an air-tight alibi."

"Not really. Apparently he was killed and then his body burned. That, and the fact that he sat in a bayou for days, make it difficult to place the time of death accurately. Lynwood assumes I killed him before we left."

"Why would you give him all this information about Ochoa and Hendricks if you were the killer. What a load of shit. He's just trying to intimidate you."

"Well, it's working. He intends to search my office and our home if we don't return. I don't know how I can prove my innocence. In Ochoa's and Hendricks' murders, I mean. I killed the real murderers who are the only witnesses to any of this." Coltrane exhaled, long and slow.

"Actually, sweetheart, *I* killed them. We *both* killed them. And I assume that there is no evidence left on earth that they existed?" Britt was not sure how the bodies were disposed of, and didn't really want to know.

"Completely eradicated. Bodies cut into pieces, and passports, guns, clothes, everything, all on the bottom of the Exuma Sound. It is 900 fathoms deep out there. No one will ever recover them. There will be nothing left but bones after the fish are done anyway. *Shit!* I've burned all my bridges."

"Look, maybe you ought to call off the conference. That's all Lynwood wants. If he leaks this to the papers or gets a search warrant for the office, the adverse PR will permanently damage your reputation, and that of the society."

"No. Not yet, or it all will be for nothing. We can't quit now, we are so close to accomplishing something. If I end the conference, we're back to square one… no, worse…because the HMOs will know we don't have the balls to finish anything. No, I want some changes made. We only quit if patients suffer. Besides, if I terminate the conference for personal reasons, I would betray my colleagues." Coltrane paused. "God, I'm tired. I haven't slept in days. I can't think straight anymore."

"Why don't you sleep now. We can stay here for awhile." Britt scanned the horizon. There were no craft visible, and the little bay was serene in the twilight's glow.

"I don't want to stay here. We are too close to the BDF post in Georgetown, and I can't stand being here any longer. There's only one option." Coltrane turned to his wife, and gauged her resolve. He reached into the watertight case in the cockpit table, and pulled out the navigation charts. "Can you handle a night crossing? In the Atlantic?"

"You're insane. You know we are not supposed to be sailing at night; this boat isn't equipped for it. The charter company intentionally omits night sailing gear, just for that reason. And anyway, navigating through the coral heads would be impossible without sunlight. Those coral bommies would rip a hole in the hull before we got half a mile." Britt was getting exasperated.

"I know. That would be suicide. What I want to do is cut across Exuma Sound, swing east of Eleuthera into the Atlantic and then north to the Abacos. It is all deep water, no rocks except as we come around the southern tip of Eleuthera. Then a free shot all the way to Great Abaco. It's a little longer route, but much less difficult. Open ocean all the way." Coltrane studied the charts, and turned them so Britt could see the course traced by his suntanned hand.

"I don't know, Bill. The weather can get rough, we won't see rocks or coral heads, and if one of us goes overboard…" Britt was frightened.

"Did you hear the weather report today?" Coltrane asked.

"Winds 15 knots from the southwest. Seas 1.2 meters. I think that there is a cold front moving our way, but we should be good for another day or so," Britt's training as a pilot had left her with a sound understanding of weather and meteorology, phenomena that Coltrane had never been able to comprehend.

"Perfect, we can run a beam reach all the way to Abaco. What do you say? Up for a little adventure? But you've got to decide quickly; we are almost on high tide and better get out the cut in the next half hour." Coltrane smiled, gleefully.

"Fine. But only if you feel that this is our best move." Britt was unconvinced.

"Good. Start the motor and I'll pull the anchor." Coltrane pulled on his salt encrusted sailing gloves, and climbed to the pulpit to bring in the anchor. As Britt fired up the Yanmar diesel, the yacht swung gently about, and headed toward the narrow cut connecting the shallow sea with the Exuma Sound and beyond, the dark blue Atlantic.

Chapter 80

Exuma Sound
July 1
8:33PM

With Coltrane in the pulpit, they negotiated their way through the narrow cut between Hawksbill Cay and Little Hawksbill Cay, then broke for open water. Coltrane resisted the urge to drop a trolling line off the back of the boat. As the shelf fell off and the water deepened to a dark blue, Coltrane came back to the cockpit and reviewed the nautical charts. He calculated a bearing from the map, and verified it using his handheld GPS.

"Come to 045 and see how the winds are, sweetheart." Coltrane stood and checked his bearing with the LCD readout on the AutoHelm. Everything looked right.

Britt nosed the boat slightly to port, and watched the telltales on the mast shrouds. The wind was steady, and from the southeast. She knew she could sail easily under these conditions, and nodded to Coltrane.

He climbed carefully up to the housing of the main mast, and released the mainsail. Moving cautiously to avoid the swing of the boom, he cleared obstructions to unfurling the mainsail. Then he ducked down into the safety of the cockpit, and readied the jib as well.

When Britt saw that he was ready, she nosed the yacht into the breeze, and Coltrane winched out the mainsail, the wind catching it and flapping it hard against the mast and boom. He cranked furiously on the chrome handle until the sail was taut to the tip of the boom, then secured the main. The boat heeled to port as Britt brought it back to course. After relaxing briefly from the exertion, Coltrane pulled out the jib, and watched it billow in the breeze, then crack taut as it filled with wind. The gunnel dipped into the dark water, and the yacht immediately picked up speed, knifing through the waves. Within seconds, they were sailing at six knots, and Britt cut the diesel.

Coltrane scanned the horizon, seeing nothing but the slowly receding silhouette of the tiny coral islands in their wake. The only sound was the rhythmic pounding of the bow through the four foot waves. In the distance, he could see the swells became larger, but smoother. No whitecaps.

"How you doing?" he asked, settling on the settee cushions.

"Fine. You know I don't like this deep water sailing. Put on orangie before you fall overboard." Britt referred to the bulky orange life preservers stowed under the cockpit seats.

"Can you handle the boat if I take a short nap? I am dead tired." Coltrane slipped on a life vest, and went below to retrieve the helmsman's safety rig for Britt. He strapped her safety line to the heavy steel cleat in the cockpit, fondling her gently as he adjusted the harness.

"I can see just how tired you are, Billyboy." Britt smiled, watching the horizon. "I'll wake you if the wind shifts, or I need help. How far to Eleuthera?"

"About thirty miles, so about five hours. Nothing in the way but the US Navy buoy, maybe half way. We should pass way south of it."

"US Navy? Here?"

"I think they do high speed submarine runs out in the Sound. Practice sonar, stealth technology and anti-submarine warfare. The water is deep and protected, and no underwater obstructions. At least until I sank those two boats out here." Coltrane laughed.

"Shit. You mean that there are submarines out here? Can they hear us coming without the motor on?" Britt was not happy with the news.

Coltrane stared at her, and laughed so hard that he cried. Then he imagined a sinister, gray form rising out of the black water, and smashing into the small sailboat. He remembered the incident off Hawaii and the Japanese fishing boat disaster.

"You know, that isn't such a dumb question. I wonder how they surface at night. Turn your navigation lights on. Just for the hell of it, I'll turn on the stereo. Loud. Put Don Henley in the CD. I don't want to play JFK tonight."

"JFK?" Britt was puzzled.

"PT-109. Kennedy was rammed and sunk by a Japanese warship at night in the Pacific. WWII. Didn't they teach you *any* history in Catholic School?"

Britt shot him an ugly look.

"Never mind, I'm sorry I brought it up. We won't run into anything out here." Coltrane gave her a smile, and settled down on the cockpit cushions.

The bright, clear ring of an electric guitar filled the night, strong against the rich vibrance of the acoustic guitar. He could distinguish the tactile sound of a guitar pick, resonating on taut steel strings.

Coltrane leaned back, intoxicated by the deluge of exquisite sound, as Henley sang, *"Learn to be Still",*

It's just another day in paradise
As you stumble to your bed
You'd give anything to silence
Those voices ringing in your head

You thought you could find happiness
Just over that green hill
You thought you would be satisfied
But you never will...

Learn to be still...

Coltrane looked up at the stars, listened as the sound washed over him, the lilting guitar riffs flowing outward from the boat, over the jet black waters of the Sound. He reveled in the lyrical poetry and perfect strains as they reached into the depths of his anguished soul.

We don't know how to be alone
So we wander 'round this desert
And wind up following the wrong gods home

Coltrane drifted, faded, lulled by the song, bathing in the perfection of it all. Within minutes, he was dead asleep.

Henley sang on,

And one more starry eyed Messiah
Meets a violent farewell...

Chapter 81

Exuma Sound
July 1
11:47PM

Coltrane awoke three hours later. The sea was covered in darkness, the white sea spray flying past the gunnel of the cruising yacht. Britt stood steady behind the wheel, bracing her body against the heel of the deck. She smiled at Coltrane as he looked up.

"It's a beautiful night, babe. Look at the stars."

Coltrane looked up past the glow of the mast light, and saw a luminous sky, stars sparkling and clearer than he had ever seen before. Constellations shone brightly in the heavens, and as if on queue, a falling star streaked across the southern quadrant. He lay quietly, the only sound the rhythmic waves breaking against the hull, and took in the magnificent scene.

"How are you doing?" Coltrane roused his sore body, and stood beside his wife.

"Tired. We are about twelve miles from the southern tip of Eleuthera, according to the GPS. I never saw the Navy beacon. It has been a beautiful night, though."

Coltrane took the helm, and Britt removed the harness, and handed it to him. She stretched to relieve her aching muscles, moving like a cat. He watched her, admired the way she moved, her grace and strength, her lithe body fluid in the moonlight. His loins ached as he drank her in.

"Come sit on the captain's lap, little girl." He laughed.

"You sick pig. Just drive the boat. I'll get you some coffee, then I want to sleep too." Britt went below to brew some coffee.

The coffee was bitter, but awakened him. He scanned the horizon, his night vision adapting slowly. Night sailing is treacherous, much more dangerous than sailing in daylight. Distances are deceiving, and depth perception is lost. The water turns black and deep, and a sailor's imagination creates frightening visions. Even for an educated, twenty-first century sailor. Coltrane couldn't imagine the terror of the ancient mariner. The irrational fears are many, but the danger is very real. A sailor overboard is a routine exercise in daylight, but a sailor overboard at night has virtually no chance of rescue. A rogue wave, easily seen and crossed in daylight, can be disaster at night. Coltrane rarely sailed at night, and was not cavalier about the attendant risks. But he knew there was no other option. They needed to be in open, international water, and they needed time.

Britt had nestled herself on the cushions, and was sleeping peacefully. Coltrane watched her lovingly, grateful that he had found her years ago, and amazed that she loved him so completely and unselfishly. She had become his guiding light, his reason to live. As he watched her, his resolve hardened to end this quagmire in an honorable manner. The cost to them was becoming unbearable.

At 11PM, he rounded the southern tip of Eleuthera, standing three miles offshore and guided by the bright beacon on the rocks. Immediately, he felt the change as they entered the Atlantic. The swells increased in depth, and in interval. Huge rollers swept in, lifting the thirteen ton boat and tossing it about gently like a toy. As each subsequent wave passed, the yacht would surf down the crest, Coltrane seeing only water until reaching the trough. Then only dark night as the next wave lifted the boat skyward. He kept his fear barely under control, fighting to maintain the sails full and the boat under way.

The exaggerated heeling of the boat and the waves crashing over the sides woke Britt. She looked around, uneasy at the size of the seas. Coltrane motioned to her to take the helm, and secured her in the harness. Slipping on the wet deck, he crashed into the companionway, tearing a gash in his shin. He cursed and bellowed into the wind, and struggling with the jib sheet, released tension on the jib. The sail fluttered, and the boat slowed and came upright. He disengaged the mainsheet, and allowed the boom to loosen and move out. Ducking his head to avoid being hit by the boom, he squinted to see the faint outline of the eastern shore of Eleuthera. Barely visible in the distance, he saw land. He pointed a heading for Britt, and when the yacht came to that bearing, he tightened the sails somewhat. They would have to compromise by taking a slow but less punishing course.

As they gradually made their way along the coast and got further offshore, the swells diminished and the wind dropped off. Britt, now fully awake and unable to lie down on the pitching yacht, went below to try to read for a while. Finding that impossible in the low light, she brought the P4 notebook up on deck, and plugged it into the cockpit powerpoint. The green luminescence of the computer display bathed her in its glow, and she scrolled through the old E-mail messages. Finding nothing of interest, she opened the data file stolen by Hendricks, and scrolled slowly through the pages of numbers.

Britt Coltrane was fluent in the arcane language of medical CPT and ICD-9 coding, and in the methods of electronic medical billing. Over the course of their ten year marriage, Britt had gradually become immersed in the day to day affairs of Coltrane's practice. Initially, she had resisted being involved at all in the workings of the practice; it was completely foreign to her. But when a key, trusted employee was caught in a complex scheme of fraudulent billing and embezzlement, Coltrane had dragged her into the office to temporarily fill the vacancy. Subsequently, she became interested and challenged by the business aspect of the practice, and oversaw all the financial and administrative workings on a daily basis. The vast majority of her time was spent in discussion and electronic communication with insurance plans, and she was as familiar as anyone with insurance and medical billing documentation.

As she scrolled through the pages and pages of numbers, she could find no break, no punctuation, no change in sequence or repetition of sequence. For hours, she scrolled up and down the document without a clue revealing itself. The files were saved in an unusual format, but it seemed to be a slightly different version than the most current version on her laptop. She could edit and insert or modify the document using the pulldown menus. But nothing she did provided any answers.

"Do you know what format this document was created in?" Britt asked Coltrane, her eyes hurting from hours of staring at the tiny characters on the green screen.

"Good question. Probably a proprietary medical records system, or records management system. I bet that the HMO has their own, special software applications. I don't know. Why?" Coltrane knew very little about the mechanics of computers.

"I can navigate within the document, but it would be so much easier if I knew more about the program."

"You're asking the wrong guy. I don't know shit about programs." Coltrane looked down at her, shielding his eyes from the bright computer screen to protect his night vision. "Anything look odd to you?"

"Something is weird, but I can't place it... Wait a minute...You know, these numbers have to be social security numbers. First of all, that's the best way to identify patients, and secondly, it is the only method Medicare uses. These have to be SSNs, maybe mixed with procedure codes or internal insurance company codes. But how can we break them down?"

"If they are just SSNs, I mean SSNs only, then since there are nine digits in the SSN plus the A or B identifier, there are ten digits to the SSN and therefore ten possible different lists of numbers you could separate. We could send those ten lists to Washington, and they could find out if the SSNs match patients in Hendricks' HMO. But I think there must be more than that. That would be just too easy." Coltrane scanned the water and tried to put himself in Hendricks' place in those final hours.

Britt went back to the data. There was something there. Her subconscious mind had seen it, identified it. It nagged at her, but she could not bring the revelation to the surface. Tired from hours of staring at the screen, and the sea spray burning her eyes, she shut down the notebook, and stowed it belowdecks in the chart table. Exhausted, she kissed Coltrane goodnight and crept to the fore stateroom, curled up and within minutes, fell into a deep sleep.

Chapter 82

Atlantic Ocean
July 2
2:23AM

As the night passed, the seas becalmed. With the heat of the tropical sun gone, the ocean quieted, and the winds fell off. The giant rollers still came off the Atlantic, traveling all the way from Africa. But now they were smooth, and gentle, without the whitecaps of the earlier waves. Coltrane altered his course to angle slightly into the oncoming crests, and trimmed his mainsail. He played with the sail trim and the heading until he found the combination that harmonized wind and waves. After checking 360 degrees for other vessels or lights, and his distance offshore, he sat back in the helmsman's station and looked out into the night.

All around him, for as far as the eye could see, the ocean was black, and empty. In the impossible distance, the sea blended with the sky. Above him, the brilliant whiteness of the mainsail stood out, held tight in the breeze, radiant against the starry sky. Coltrane watched as the mainsail moved, pitching and rolling with the movement of the yacht, amplified by the height of the sixty foot aluminum mast. Above the masthead light, the stars flickered brightly.

Coltrane leaned back against the steel safety line, looking straight up into the night sky. He scanned the stars until he found Orion, and smiled. Always above, always watching over us, he thought. In this lonely, desolate seascape, the company of the celestial guardians brought comfort to him, as they had to the ancient mariners.

This moment was the essence of sailing for Coltrane. The thrill of mastering the elements, however briefly. The danger of an open ocean, blue water sail. The risk of night sailing. Coltrane gazed lovingly at the sleek lines of the yacht, the brilliant translucent white fiberglass hull, adorned with stainless steel and chrome winches and nautical gear. White bubbling water sloshed continuously over the port gunnel as it dipped into the waves, and ran back off the deck through the metal rails. Behind him, the waves created by each gunnel curved into each other to leave a perfect, soundless trail in the black water. The luminous wake glowed as millions of tiny, phosphorescent algae, disturbed by the turbulence of the huge craft, emitted blue-green light. As Coltrane look around at the majesty of sea and sky, he thanked God that He had created such beauty and perfection, and that His hand had placed Coltrane in the midst of such magnificence. An effusion of warmth and peace engulfed him, soothing his mind and body.

The hours passed quickly. Soon the sloop reached the northern tip of Eleuthera, and with some fear in his throat, they passed away from the protection of the land mass, and out into open ocean. As the reassuring bulk of the island gradually slipped behind them, the wind picked up, and the swells deepened.

The change in the boat's rhythmic motion wakened Britt, as the pre-dawn light began to show in the east. She made coffee and a simple breakfast, and they took turns eating and manning the helm. The winds were favorable, and light enough to make the passage comfortable. When the sun rose, they found themselves alone on a blue sea.

Coltrane rechecked his bearing and verified their progress with the GPS. He calculated from the bearing and the actual progress that the ocean currents were pushing them to the west at four or five knots per hour. He input the data into the AutoHelm, heading the yacht for the Abacos. Coltrane never sailed solely by his instruments. He always checked against charts, or compass. He had tried to learn celestial navigation, but found it almost impossible to understand. How the ancients and the explorers had navigated always filled him with awe. But then again, the ocean floor was littered with those who had failed.

At midday, they struck the sails, and drifted for an hour to relax and have lunch. In the distance, a huge freighter passed, from east to west, probably from South America, headed to Miami. Even miles away, the size of the vessel was huge, surreal. It seemed to take forever to pass from view. Coltrane set the sails, and Britt took the helm.

As they sailed, Coltrane went below and pulled his fishing gear from the sea bag. He took a steel leader, and selected a bass jig from his lures. Setting the spinning rod in a tube holder in the stern of the yacht, he let out a hundred feet of line. Every time that he had made this passage in the past, Coltrane had caught fish. Sometimes he caught barracuda, sometimes yellowtail snapper, sometimes mahi-mahi. Once, he even caught a five-foot shark. It had taken him forty-five minutes to pull the shark in, using his light tackle and twenty pound line. When the shark finally was pulled to the back of the boat, Coltrane realized that he would have to free the hook somehow. But the shark merely rolled on its side, looked up through the crystal clear water, and bit clean through the steel braided wire leader. In a flash, it had disappeared. As Coltrane let out his line, he remembered the battle, and hoped for a hit.

The day passed quietly. Coltrane had no luck fishing. He tried five or six different lures, with no luck. He even tried a local favorite, a blue and red spoon that certainly only the stupidest fish would hit. The speed of the sloop was not right, too fast or too slow, Coltrane thought. He decided to take a short nap and let the fish get hungry.

Coltrane was awakened by Britt's wild shouting. He bolted upright from the cushions, and saw her pointing excitedly to the sides and front of the yacht, and yelling at something in the water.

"Get the camera, get the camera!" Britt yelled.

Coltrane looked over the side, and saw an incredible scene. A pod of Atlantic bottlenose dolphin swam alongside the yacht, jumping and leaping into the air as they surfed the bow wave of the fast moving sloop. A huge male led the group, jumping and dancing out in front of the bow. His speed was breathtaking, and he flew from one side of the boat to the other, crisscrossing the bow, just feet ahead of the boat. The dolphins swam at blinding speed, hurtling under the boat, and running just inches below the surface, looking up at the startled humans yelling excitedly at them. Water glistened on their taut skin, the broad muscular sinews clearly defined as they flexed their powerful tails. They leapt out of the blue water, their entire bodies flying gracefully in long arcs, then slipping into the water again. Mothers with their young at their side swam further out, playing, but cautious with their babies. Britt watched one young dolphin, identified by a scar on his dorsal fin, do a tail walk behind the boat. Coltrane tried to capture their grace and speed on film. Then, as suddenly as they appeared, they were gone. Minutes later, Britt spotted them jumping, miles to the west. She was a little sad that they had left.

By three o'clock, it was clear that they would not make Little Harbor by sunset. The cut between the Sea of Abaco and the Atlantic was narrow, and very treacherous. Coltrane knew that to try to pass through at night or in failing light would be suicide. That left only one safe anchorage within reach. Hole in the Wall. They could make anchor in an hour. He corrected his heading, and made for Hole in the Wall, a small sheltered bay with a mangrove swamp and shallow inland sea on the leeward side of Great Abaco.

Two miles out, they turned into the breeze, and took in the sails. Coltrane cranked in the roller reefed jib, and secured the jib sheets. Climbing onto the deck, he released the heavy mainsail, and returned to the cockpit to wind in the roller-reefed main. Britt fired up the diesel, and they made directly for the southern tip of Great Abaco.

Refusing to accept failure fishing, Coltrane dropped their speed to five knots, and let out a long leader with three lures in series. The shoals and the shelf dropoff were prime spots to get a strike, and huge fish lay in the shadows waiting for prey. Within five minutes, the reel screamed as line flew out behind the sloop. Excited, Coltrane left the helm, and jumped to take the rod. Britt grabbed the wheel as he maintained pressure on the line and reeled in the hit. In the distance, just below the surface, a brilliant green and blue flash raced obliquely through the water, then dove deep. Coltrane knew immediately that he had a mahi-mahi, a good-sized fish and fantastic eating. He easily brought in the fourteen-inch mahi-mahi, and threw it in the deck cooler, covering it with ice. Dinner tonight would be outstanding, he thought.

They rounded the southern tip of Great Abaco at dusk, and found the bay completely deserted. Coltrane anchored in a protected cove, below thirty-foot sand dunes that ran into the sea. The water was shallow, and warm. Coltrane stripped off his shorts, and dove off the transom into twelve feet of sparkling clear water. He let the warm water caress his aching body, and support his sore limbs as he swam toward shore. The white sand bottom was perfectly barren, covered only with a thousand tiny ripples. He crawled on shore, and half-buried his naked body into the fine, powder like sand. Intending to rest for a moment, he let the dying sun bask upon his face. He fell into a trance-like sleep.

Her touch woke him gently. He opened his eyes, and saw her kneeling naked over him, the sun behind her head, sparkling through her wet strawberry blonde ringlets. Her breasts were dusted with the fine white sand, the pink of her nipples showing through. She bent down, pressing her nude, wet body onto his. He tasted the salt on her full soft lips, felt the cool wet texture of her mouth. They rolled in the surf, and gently made love with the bubbling, warm water lapping against their skin. Lying on the beach in the afterglow, they watched the sun set in a crimson sky.

They swam back to the boat as the sun sank into a flat sea, the peach and coral brilliance of the sunset almost obscuring the shape of the yacht. Coltrane showered her off on the transom, and washed the salt and sand from her smooth skin with the handspray. Unashamed, she turned her back to him, and held the spray over her head, closing her eyes and washing the salt from her hair. Coltrane stepped back, and watched the water cascade off her shoulders, down her back arched like a cat, sheening off her round, hard buttocks. The glow of final light bathed the scene in a luminous pink hue, her body perfect and exquisite. He stiffened so hard it was painful. She smiled peacefully at him, and before he could embrace her, she turned and went below.

Britt mixed a pitcher of Myers's and pineapple orange juice, adding coconut milk and the juice of two limes to the blender. While he sipped on the cocktail, Coltrane assembled the stainless steel brazier on the stern of the boat. The barbecue was held out over the water by a long metal arm, so that the typical drunken yachtsman would be less likely to torch the boat. He started a small pile of briquettes, and prepared to grill the mahi-mahi he caught earlier that afternoon. He filleted the bright green and blue fish, and soaked the white pieces in lime and melted butter as the fire settled. Britt prepared a salad and rice and fresh island vegetables. They ate dinner in silence, enjoying the fading sunset and the delicious flavor and texture of the fresh mahi-mahi. There was nothing quite like freshly caught and prepared gamefish, and Mahi-mahi was one of the finest.

Britt went below to clean the kitchen, and Coltrane cleared the cockpit. He moved back down the broad steps of the transom, and rinsed off the dishes in the cool seawater. Hundreds of tiny, translucent bluefish darted in to devour the morsels of food, moving together in schools as one living thing. He dumped the ashes from the grill, and dipped it in the seawater, steam hissing as the metal cooled. Stowing the day's gear in the lockers, he set up the laptop, and connected it to the Iridium phone. He logged on to *Caduceus*, and downloaded messages and E-mail. As the datalink continued, Coltrane poured himself another rum drink, and sat in the cockpit, gazing out over the calm water. Perfect time for a cigar, if he had one, he thought. Maybe he could pick up a Cuban Cohiba before he left the Bahamas.

The pale flickering of the computer screen stopped, and the download was finished. Coltrane scrolled through the several messages from physicians, and from Cindy about next week's surgical schedule. A message from Susan Kerr caught his eye.

E-mail
July 1
3:24:41 AM
From: SKerr
To: WmColtraneMD

> Agent Lynwood is looking for you.
> Sorry, I couldn't stay away from the office. He found me. He wants you to contact him ASAP. He wants to discuss the tape with you? He has been leaking to the press that he wants to interview you re: murder investigations. Very bad for your reputation.
>
> The conference is breaking up, all the sub-committees are finished with their reviews, and feel that they are just wasting time sitting around without any direction. If you are not back by Monday, they will all go back to work. Public opinion, as usual, is divided. No

advances on the HMO front re: definitive fee schedules or list of procedures and coverage.

Please advise.
sk

Coltrane's low curse brought Britt topside. His expression told it all, but she looked over his shoulder, and read the E-mail. They exchanged glances, and Coltrane exited *Caduceus* and disconnected the phone from the laptop. He dialed Lynwood's number from memory.

"Lynwood," he answered.

"This is Coltrane. Did you get the tape from Clark?"

"Yes, but Clark denies being your attorney. In fact, he says that he was only holding the tape for you in the hospital safe."

"What! Impossible! Don't pull this kind of sophomoric shit with me, Lynwood. I know what's on that tape, I recorded it myself." Coltrane was furious at the tactic.

"Clark gave me a copy of the tape, and I've listened to it many times. It clearly implicates you, Coltrane. Care to relive the relevant passages?" Lynwood replied, smugly.

"Yeah, I do."

Lynwood could be heard fumbling with the recorder over the speakerphone. After a few moments, the taped conversation could be heard.

"The policy is clearly outlined in the manual. The attending physician must contact the primary care doctor assigned to the patient and obtain authorization. Did you try to contact him?" Hendricks' whine was recognizable, even over the satellite transmission.

Coltrane recognized his own voice responding. "*Yeah, but that process takes time. It took me fifteen minutes to get through. And then the representative I spoke with didn't have the medical background to understand what I wanted or why it was important.*"

"*What was the patient's name, and what exactly happened*?" Hendricks asked.

"*John Strahan. He was shot in the face, and I wanted him transferred from Bayside to...*"

"*You were the primary physician in that case. I just saw something about him on my desk...Here it is. My staff has been talking with the family about his transfer. I spoke briefly with the father, I think. How did you get involved?*" Hendricks interrupted.

"*I was asked by his father to take on his care. I spoke with the physicians there at Bayside and tried to assist.*" Coltrane recognized his voice, but knew the tape had been altered. His inflection, his speech patterns didn't sound right. And he certainly didn't accept the care of John Strahan that night.

"*Why would you want to move him*?" Hendricks asked wearily.

"*I wanted him returned to Tampa*." Coltrane heard himself say.

"*Bayside is a fully accredited hospital, and a participating facility in our network. The hospital is brand new. I concurred with the written policy…*" Hendricks voice became distant and garbled. The tape ended.

Lynwood shut the machine off. He returned to the phone.

"Interesting, isn't it?" Lynwood commented dryly.

"That conversation never happened," Coltrane replied forcefully.

"John Alistair believes that it did happen."

"Alistair!! Why are you talking with that asshole?" Coltrane was livid.

"He contacted me when he heard about the second death. From the information in the newspaper and on the news, he came to believe that your tape was evidence in a capital murder case. In such a circumstance, he is obliged to offer it to law enforcement. He believes that the tape shows that you were at least partly responsible for the death of John Strahan by delaying appropriate treatment with your ridiculous demands to transfer the boy. You kept him in the ER too long, and he died when he could have been saved if promptly admitted and treated in their ICU." Lynwood finished, and the silence was unbearable.

"This whole thing stinks. Why would I make a tape of a conversation that incriminates me in Strahan's death, then keep it and distribute it to every attorney in town? How the hell did Alistair get a copy? Where did he tell you he got it?" Coltrane was outraged.

"He claimed that a copy was mailed to his office. His copy is exactly the same as the original I got from Clark." Lynwood answered, impassively.

"He has a multi-million dollar stake in this; he is suing me, Bayside Hospital and the HMO for malpractice and wrongful death in the Strahan case. He'd sell out his own mother for this case."

"I doubt that. Everybody's conspiring against you, right? Alistair, Clark, Hendricks, those guys in the Bahamas that are chasing you, who else? Everybody is crazy but Coltrane, is that it?" Lynwood sneered.

"Look, that tape has been altered. I didn't say any of that, or at least not in that context. Did you listen to the tone and inflection of some of those sentences? Clearly, the tape was dubbed. Your lab should be able to tell that, shouldn't they? You can check with Strahan, even he knows that I did not accept care of his son. The patient was in Miami, for Christ's sake."

"Quit trying to tell me how to run my investigation. You've got me sending discs to the lab in Washington, and now you want me to analyze this audiotape? You think the FBI lab is at your disposal? Does your balloon ever land, Doc? *YOU* are the prime suspect in this case now. You had better be back in Tampa by Monday AM, or I'm getting a warrant for your arrest and extradition, and a search warrant for your office and home. End of conversation." Lynwood curtly terminated the discussion, and hung up.

"Fuck!!!!" Coltrane howled into the still night air, shattering the silence. Britt had come topside when the conversation had become audibly tense. She had listened to the majority of the argument. He face showed visible concern, and the sudden violence of his curse shook her.

Coltrane turned to her and frowned. "Clark sold me out. He must have given the tape to the HMO or Alistair, or maybe to both, I don't know."

"Why?" Britt asked.

"Why do people sell out their friends? Usually cash. My guess is that he sold it to the HMO. The tape was altered, and you'd need very sophisticated equipment to do that well. And Alistair would have been delighted to have the original tape incriminating Hendricks and the HMO; he wouldn't have altered it. The HMO has far deeper pockets than I do. Yeah, that's it. Clark sold the tape to the HMO, and they sent the altered copy to Alistair."

"But why send it to Alistair? They're still responsible for Strahan's death. It occurred in their hospital, under the care of their doctors." Britt wondered aloud.

"Technically, yes. But the altered recording shows that I accepted care of the patient, and demanded immediate transfer. They will say that *my* demands were the cause of the delay in treatment. They will say that they were just following the directives of the physician in charge, like all good insurance people should. They can hardly be expected to make medical judgments, can they? That's the responsibility of the physicians." Coltrane began to see the Machiavellian brilliance of the strategy.

"They're turning our own arguments against us," she realized, stunned.

"Yeah. And in Florida, it's illegal to sue HMOs."

"What? It's illegal? Then why is Alistair suing them?" Britt was confused.

"Well, not illegal. There are only a few selected grounds under which suits may be filed against HMO plans. Alistair was alleging breach of contract and gross negligence, which is actionable. Any other action is forbidden by state law, and by the contract that the insured signs when he or she accepts the terms of the policy. You know, all that fine print on the application form. They will try to get off the hook on the grounds that they were just following HMO policy, and the main cause of John's death was my *interfering* with their normal ER protocols. It's a very good defense. It will spare them destructive and costly negative PR, and release them from charges of breach of contract and negligence. It may get them out of the lawsuit altogether. And that will make me the responsible party. Me alone."

"How do we fight this?" Britt challenged.

"I don't know, baby. We can't fight it. Only Hendricks and Ochoa could exonerate me, and they are both dead. And the only witnesses to Hendricks' and Ochoa's murder are also dead, and their remains are unidentifiable by now. My tape implicating Hendricks has been altered to provide evidence against me. My fingerprints are all over everything, including money Ochoa had and the audiotape. We fled the country, have been lying continuously to Federal agents for a week about our whereabouts, and killed two men. Shit." Coltrane laughed blackly, cynically. "At this point, only our mothers would believe us."

"Don't give up, goddamn it. There is one way out." Britt was undaunted.

"What?" Coltrane laughed, and filled his glass with Myers's and ice. He had always admired her indomitable spirit, but knew that this time there was no way out.

"The disc," she answered.

"Shit, we will never crack that. It is nothing but numbers. You need a program to count and calculate frequency of repetition of numbers, then frequency of repetition of sequences of numbers, and on and on. You need a mainframe computer, and a host of computer geeks to program it. All we've got is a laptop, and I can't even use Microsoft Works, for God's sake. Shit." Coltrane went amidships of the yacht, and sat below the mast, looking out across the Northeast Providence Channel. Over the horizon, miles to the south, was Nassau. Coltrane contemplated fleeing there, his mind too agitated to concentrate.

While Coltrane brooded quietly, sipping his rum, Britt curled up on the cockpit cushions, and plugged the notebook computer's transformer into the powerpoint. The bright glow of the screen illuminated her beautiful young face as she scrolled slowly through the endless chain of digits, searching for the elusive key to the riddle, lying just below the surface. Hours passed.

Chapter 83

July 2
Hole in the Wall
11:22PM

Nothing made sense. She scrolled down through page after page of endless numbers. She could find no pattern, no break, no punctuation at all. How had Hendricks encrypted the data? This mass of numbers had to be a series of Social Security Numbers and ICD-9 codes; she was positive of that. Insurance plans and Medicare used SSNs to identify patients, and Medicare further tagged the SSN with a letter, A or B, to signify inpatient or outpatient service. ICD-9 codes were a universal method of designating a clinical diagnosis, and were an essential part of any medical billing document.

Every time a patient visited her family doctor, or went to the ER, or to a clinic, or was admitted to the hospital, or had surgery, every time anyone had contact with the healthcare system, an ICD-9 code was generated. An ICD-9 code is a highly specific method to precisely identify a specific disease or symptom for which treatment has been sought. The disease is then cross-checked against the treatment, and verified.

A patient presenting with lung disease and subsequently treated with prostatectomy would red-flag the computerized billing system, and the bill would be rejected immediately. SSNs, ICD-9 codes, and treatment codes must all correlate, or payment will not be processed. In years past, in fact until just recently, all verification was done by hand at Medicare, Medicaid and major health insurance carriers. With the advent of mainframe computers and high-speed data networks, it is now all done digitally. Britt understood this system, and knew that if Hendricks wanted to download data that could incriminate the HMO, he would have to have SSNs to identify patients, and ICD-9 codes to identify specific billing events. Neither would be of any value without the other.

But no matter how she viewed the data, she just couldn't analyze it. She tried searching for a regular frequency of the number 1 or 2, thinking that would be the obvious code for A or B in the Medicare identification scheme. Additional digits were added to the nine digit SSN in some coding schemes. But there was no recurring sequence that suggested that had been used. Failing that, Britt looked for repeating pairs or sequences of numbers that might be used to separate individual patients' data. Nothing appeared to fulfill that criteria either. The flickering of the display and the endless array of digits was beginning to give her a headache.

Lowering the lid of the laptop, she leaned back on the cushions and gazed up through the stainless steel mast stays at the brilliance of the night sky. Directly overhead, the Milky Way stretched from horizon to horizon in a huge, sparkling arc. Above, Orion watched, his three starred sword perfectly aligned in his belt. The ocean sky had such depth, such clarity. She lay on her back for a full hour, mesmerized by the infinite, pristine beauty of the spectacle. Never on land had she seen such a sky, even in the desolate Sonoran desert of Arizona. A shooting star brought her back from her reverie.

Britt reluctantly opened the laptop, and stared hard at the display. If she couldn't break the code by finding the key, then she would approach from another angle. Maybe she could reverse engineer a code that Hendricks might have tried. From what she knew about him, she doubted that he had the time or the background to devise a sophisticated encryption program. Whatever he had done to the raw data, it was probably quite simple. She knew that the data would have to consist of SSNs and ICD-9 codes, linked in some way. But since she didn't know the format of the data before Hendricks modified it, she was at a significant disadvantage.

Suddenly, she recognized the peculiarity in the sequence that she had sensed more than noticed. There seemed to be a high frequency of 0 in the number chain. Perhaps the memory of lost wagers at the roulette wheel sparked her recognition of the pattern. Quickly, she ran through line after line of digits, and found that 0 was very regular in repetition. Statistically, the odds of 0 appearing was one in a ten, but the actual frequency was much greater than that. With a loud yell, she jumped up and focused intently on the computer display. She had found the key to the code.

Britt's uncharacteristic outburst brought Coltrane down from the deck, rum in hand. He sat next to her in the cockpit, and looked at the brightly lit display with interest.

"I think that I've found a pattern here, maybe the way that Hendricks separated patients. I don't know yet. But the zeros repeat pretty regularly, with a frequency of fifteen digits. Odd. Let me see here… if I move the cursor to here…" Britt used the directional arrows to move the blinking cursor to the space after the first 00 she found, then hit the *Enter* bar. The huge mass of digits was moved down, leaving a line of numbers at the top.

7051537468300
860347015896350130857698078924870215 30764
858721037910443827951033920785721586 03468

07391423080579741238236930135846708269840
24508913748249538092409274287058769235485

She repeated the procedure again and again, until she had created a list of fifty or more individual clusters of fourteen numbers. She turned to Coltrane, who was watching closely.

7051537468300
860347015896350
254869529358793
265408957436290
239695485723180
935458793652837
515369582547130
857698078924870
215307648587210
379104438279510
339207857215860
346807391423080
579741238236930
135846708269840
245089137482495
380924092742870

"A ten digit SSN plus a five digit ICD-9 code equals a total of fifteen digits, but I don't know whether the SSN or the ICD-9 comes first. My guess would be the SSN, because ICD-9s are usually three digits with a decimal point, then one digit, like 301.9. He had to compensate for the possibility of the fifth digit that occasionally occurs, like 488.27. That's why the 0 and 00. See?" Britt excitedly explained the decoding to her husband.

"What about the first sequence? It's only eleven digits." Coltrane had had a few too many rums to follow her quickly.

"We don't know if this is the first or the second disc. I think it's the second, and those numbers are the tail end of the first disc. I'm just going to ignore them for the time being. I also don't think there is encoded Medicare A or B. That threw me for a long time. And I could still be wrong. But I think that we should E-mail the others to Lynwood and have him check and see if there are real patients to match those SSNs, and if they are enrolled in Hendricks' HMO. And if there are HMO patients with these SSNs, then were they treated for the corresponding medical diagnosis recently? That's what Hendricks was trying to hold over them; he had evidence of illegal billing or fraudulent billing practices." Britt organized the data of the first fourteen patients into easily readable form, and then hooked up the Iridium to the laptop and accessed *Caduceus*. She wrote a short note to Susan Kerr.

E-mail
July 3
1:44 AM
From: WmColtraneMD
To: SKerr

Susan,

Please contact Lynwood ASAP and deliver this list of patients to him. We feel reasonably certain that all are patients in Hendricks HMO, and had treatment for the indicated diagnosis within the past year. If true, the disc that you gave to Lynwood contains thousands of instances of illegal or fraudulent billing by the HMO.

Respond as soon as you have an answer.

8603-47-0158 ICD-9 Diagnosis code 963.50
2548-69-5293 ICD-9 Diagnosis code 587.93
2654-08-9574 ICD-9 Diagnosis code 362.90
2396-95-4857 ICD-9 Diagnosis code 231.80
8576-98-0789 ICD-9 Diagnosis code 248.70
2153-07-6485 ICD-9 Diagnosis code 872.10
3791-04-4382 ICD-9 Diagnosis code 795.10
3392-07-8572 ICD-9 Diagnosis code 158.60
3468-07-3914 ICD-9 Diagnosis code 230.80
5797-41-2382 ICD-9 Diagnosis code 369.30
1358-46-7082 ICD-9 Diagnosis code 698.40
2450-89-1374 ICD-9 Diagnosis code 824.95
3809-24-0927 ICD-9 Diagnosis code 428.70

Thanks,
Britt

Britt hit *Send*, and the message shot out into cyberspace. She saved all her work in a file folder, and shut down the laptop. Exhausted, she slumped against Coltrane, and they nestled on cushions in the corner of the cockpit. Within minutes, they were sound asleep.

Chapter 84

Hole in the Wall
July 3
6:02AM

The sun woke Coltrane. He looked over at Britt, sleeping peacefully in the queen-size bed of the main cabin. He had carried her below during the night, after awakening with his leg asleep in the cockpit. The fore stateroom was nicely sized, large for a sailboat. With the hatch open and fitted with a wind scoop, it made very comfortable sleeping quarters. He gently disentangled himself from her arms, and climbed above decks.

The tide was slack, and the small bay was like glass. Aside from the quiet lapping of waves against the hull, silence reigned. Not even a breeze fluttered the sails, or whistled through the stays. Coltrane smiled as he surveyed the horizon. Not a ship, not a single soul in sight for as far as the eye could see. No evidence of the hand of man. The soft pink glow of the dawn bathed the scene. Perfect. This was the experience he sailed for. Seclusion and peace in the most beautiful paradise of God's creation.

He slipped his fishing rod from the metal sleeve in the stern, and pulled the inflatable dinghy up to the transom. Grabbing his tackle box, he quietly stepped into the little boat. After making sure that he had an anchor and chain, he rowed steadily away from the yacht toward the huge, rusting old freighter beached at the entrance to the bay. The old relic had been there since 1954, when it ran aground during a hurricane gale. The ferocity of the storm had driven the eighty-foot steel vessel ashore, and embedded it into the sand dunes with such force it remained there to this day. He knew that he would find fish around the rocks and steel compartments of the wreck. When he was far enough from the yacht not to wake Britt, he fired up the outboard, and made for the broached hulk.

The sun was just barely above the horizon. Coltrane poked through his little traveling tackle box, and selected a blue broken back. The two inch lure had a big plastic lip that resembled an open mouth of the fish, and caused the lure to weave back and forth as he cast and retrieved it in the clear water. In addition, it had a hinge in the middle of its back that made the tail flip back and forth realistically. Coltrane was always impressed with the lifelike action of the lure, and always surprised that the fish weren't equally impressed. He flipped the lure out, using a radial pattern to test all the waters. When nothing hit, he switched to a red feathered bass plug, a lure that had been successful in Bahamian waters in the past. Why a fish would hit an ugly white and red ball with a plastic feather, yet pass on the artistic and lifelike broken back, never ceased to amaze him.

It seemed that he fished for hours. He tested all of the lures he brought, and even rigged a line that simulated a broken back chasing a small bass plug. Nothing hit. He saw a small yellowtail run right up to the broken back, then turn away at the last second. The fishing was peaceful, the water so clear that he could see the bottom in perfect detail; he could distinguish individual grains of sand. The act of casting and retrieving gradually hypnotized him.

His trance was broken by a loud splash, immediately to his right, three feet from the dinghy. His head snapped around, and he froze. Hanging in midair, at the zenith of its arc, was a huge Spanish mackerel. The kingfish was exactly parallel to Coltrane, and he looked directly into its round, black eye. Every scale shone brilliantly, radiant in the sun behind them. The muscular shape and broad, flat tail screamed speed and power. The cruel, downturned mouth was partly open, the many razor sharp teeth shredding the air. It seemed to be mocking him. In a flash, it was gone.

Coltrane scrambled to get the biggest lure he had, and fixed it to a steel leader. He knew that he had less than no chance to catch that predator, but what a battle it would be if he did! The fifteen pound line and light weight spinning reel made the contest fair, and if he got him in, it would take hours. He flipped the lure out in the direction of the mackerel, and tried bringing the bait across the fish's path. He watched the water for activity as the big fish ran down prey. But everything was dead calm. After an hour, he pulled anchor and dinghyed back to the yacht.

Britt sat on the back of the transom, a cup of coffee in her hands, her pretty little feet dangling in the cool water. She had a cup ready for Coltrane after he secured the dinghy and stowed his gear.

"Any luck?" she asked, knowing the answer.

"No, but I saw a gorgeous king jump. I think he was checking me out, because he only jumped once, right next to my boat. I could have grabbed him, he was so close. Just incredible. I think that predators want to know who is in their territory. You remember that shark we saw in the Turks last year?" Coltrane recalled the morning that he had maneuvered their sailboat toward a slick of feeding fish, thinking that he might catch some mahi-mahi for lunch. They had just pulled up anchor, and were in very shallow water, maybe eight or ten feet at the most. As Britt motored toward the frantic activity on the surface, Coltrane had grabbed his tackle and ran to the pulpit to cast out into the mass of jumping fish. Suddenly, a huge bull shark appeared in the water, directly in the path of the yacht. It was dark gray, and thick in girth, at least ten or eleven feet in length. The fish was swimming with that sinuous, lazy glide characteristic of the big sharks. It rolled slightly, and looked directly up through the clear water at Coltrane, then passed five feet from the hull of the forty foot yacht. Not the human on deck, not the massive hull of the boat, not the huge winged keel underwater, not even the hammering drone of the diesel motor bothered it. The fish knew no fear, dominating its world without question or challenge. Coltrane had been swept with a wave of awe and cold fear, even as he stood in relative safety on deck.

"Males marking their territory. Very typical behavior." Britt laughed, remembering the shark. She had radioed in to the marina because the huge predator was heading straight for the shallow hotel beach. No one had seemed concerned enough to alert the swimmers. Shark warnings were bad for business. They had spent the rest of the cruise venturing into the water only very timidly.

"If I could get that king on this light tackle, it would be like landing a marlin. I would be fighting him all day." Coltrane grinned with anticipation.

"You've got other things to do, Bill. We didn't check in with Lynwood as you promised. You had better contact him." Britt handed him a hot cup of coffee.

"Alright, fine." Coltrane put his tackle away, and sat down with the satphone.

The phone rang five times before Lynwood's secretary answered. Lynwood was on another call. Coltrane left his number, and was told the call would be returned within the hour.

It was twenty minutes before Lynwood called back. "Where are you now, Dr. Coltrane?" he asked.

"The Abacos. I can be on a plane to Tampa tomorrow, if necessary. Did Susan Kerr give you the Social Security Numbers?"

"I got them this morning," Lynwood answered flatly.

"Are any of those patients insured by the HMO?"

"We have no intention of calling American citizens and questioning them about their health insurance. I think that many of them would consider that an invasion of privacy, and I would have to agree. Despite what you may think, the government does not keep the SSN, address and telephone number of every citizen in a database."

"Sure you do. HCFA does. The Health Care Financing Administration has the numbers of all Medicare participants, and has all enrollment of secondary insurance plans as well. They have to, to keep track of the deductibles and co-payments." Coltrane was becoming angry. "Come on, Lynwood. Make an effort. I'm innocent until proven guilty, remember?"

"Don't tell me how to run this investigation, Coltrane. I'm not going to tell you that again."

"I know things you don't know," Coltrane stated quietly.

"What do you know? Are you withholding evidence?"

"I know that the tape was faked. That Hendricks was murdered. That Ochoa stole the computer disc from him after his death. I told you all these things, and still you don't trust me? Did you have that tape analyzed?"

"I sent the cassette to Washington by courier. It'll be a few days before they can tell me anything. But the tape had your voice on it, no question about that."

"I'm not denying that I recorded the conversation, or that that was my microcassette tape. What I'm saying is that the content of the conversation has been altered." Coltrane was becoming exasperated with the man's obtuse nature.

"I understand." Lynwood paused. "How did you say that I could cross-check these patients?"

"Contact the HCFA office in Washington, or Blue Cross and Blue Shield of Florida in Tallahassee. They're the Medicare administrators for the state. Either one should be able to cross-reference the patients against the HMO. I guarantee those patients are now, or were at one time, enrolled in Hendricks' HMO," Coltrane finished, and waited for a response.

"I'll call you this afternoon with my findings. But this is the last wild goose chase I run for you, Coltrane." Lynwood resented being taught how to pursue the case.

"Thank you for your help. I will be in touch, or call me on this phone anytime." Coltrane was conciliatory, left his number again, and hung up.

He looked across the cockpit at Britt, who had been listening to the entire conversation. He shrugged. They sat silently for several minutes, contemplating.

"There is one thing I don't understand." Britt broke the silence. "How does the HMO scheme work? How do they steal payments, and from whom?"

"They file inflated claims. Or they do what's called 'upcoding', which means increasing the severity of the DRG disease code on the hospital or office record. For example, say I examined a patient with a cold, but diagnosed him as having angina, and put him in the ICU overnight. I can code for angina, which pays much more than a common cold. Plus, I can bill for ICU visits. All in all, the fees would be ten, twenty times what they would be if I billed for a cold," Coltrane explained.

"Okay, but how would the HMO make any money that way? They don't bill for us. Could they bill for a doctor?"

"Maybe they bill for the doctors they employ as gatekeepers. I don't know…" Coltrane realized that he had never completely thought the scheme through. Something was missing. He had missed a connection somewhere.

"You think that the plan physicians are in on it?"

"No, that's impossible. Maybe one or two guys might be stupid enough to take such a risk, but that plan has thirty or forty doctors on staff. They would all have to be involved. It could never happen. And it doesn't make sense. Why involve your employee in a billing scheme when you are already paying him? No, I think that this is being done at a corporate level, with only the highest executives involved. The only ones profiting are the board of directors. Remember Enron? Remember Columbia/HCA?"

"You don't think that Hendricks was in on it?" Britt persisted.

"Maybe he did the actual upcoding. They'd need a medical professional to determine the higher level codes to use. A layman would not be able to manipulate the billing codes and DRGs correctly. Maybe Hendricks just stumbled onto the scheme during one of his lucent moments. Who knows?"

"That still doesn't answer my question, Bill. Exactly how does the HMO benefit from these patients?" Britt pursued her point with gentle tenacity.

Coltrane looked at her, puzzled. He frowned as he realized that she was right. There was no valid connection between the patients, the HMO and the fraudulent billing scheme. Only healthcare providers could generate Medicare bills, and insurance plans were essentially payers, not providers. That line had become blurred somewhat with the advent of HMO salaried gatekeepers, but insurance plans generally did not provide healthcare.

Then it struck him like a diamond spike, right between the eyes. He leapt up and grabbed the Iridium handset. He dialed a number by heart.

"What?" Britt asked, surprised.

"I'll tell you in a minute," Coltrane said as the phone rang on the other end.

"Athena ER," a woman's voice answered.

"Medical Records, please." Coltrane responded.

After a minute, a female voice came on the line. "Medical Records Department."

"Becky, this is Dr. Coltrane. How are you?" Coltrane, like all hospital based physicians, spent several hours each week in the medical records department, completing his charts. History and physical exam dictations and operative reports had to be complete and accurate before the hospital could process the patient's bill. Incomplete records meant no revenue for the hospital, and were cause for suspension from medical staff. It was tedious and annoying paperwork, universally detested by every physician in every hospital. Becky made it bearable with her cheerful personality, and a huge bowl of Halloween sized candy and chocolate bars she kept in the records room. Coltrane loved the Snickers and Butterfingers.

"Fine, Dr. Coltrane. I have about ten charts here for you, in your pile. You haven't been in for some time. Do you want me to set them out?"

"Man, you're tough. I'm on vacation. I promise I'll do them next week. But I need to ask you for a favor. I have two face sheets that I can't read the patient names. I left them in my pocket, and they got thrown in the wash. All I can make out is the SSN. Can you pull up a name for me?" Coltrane knew she had a computer terminal at her desk, and could access the hospital data bank.

"Sure. Patient information is input by name, hospital number and SSN. Give me the numbers." Becky knew Coltrane's voice, and it was very common for doctors to lose or forget patient numbers. She turned to her terminal, and typed in the SSNs that Coltrane gave her.

"Maryanne Stihl is the first patient and Joseph Ahrens is the second. These are old records, neither patient has been hospitalized this year. Are you sure that they were seen here?" Becky could tell from the records that neither patient had been hospitalized at Athena in the past twelve months.

"Maybe not, but I thought so." Coltrane lied. "I'm sure it was Athena, because they are both HMO patients. Double check for me, please."

"You're right, both are Medicare with an Athena Gold HMO secondary. They would have to come here for inpatient treatment. I can pull their files, if you like."

"No thanks, Becky. I will have my office track them down. I appreciate your help," Coltrane thanked her, and hung up.

Coltrane put the phone down, and stood up in the cockpit, letting out a yell that startled the shoreline seabirds to flight. Britt looked at him with wonder. He bent down, and kissed her hard on the lips.

"You were absolutely right. I guarantee you that all those SSNs belong to Medicare patients who are enrolled in the Athena Gold HMO. The hospital has been upcoding the DRGs or the ICD-9 codes on inpatients, and collecting a huge bonus of increased fees," Coltrane explained.

"Medicare pays the hospital fees directly to the HMO?" Britt asked.

"The insurance company owns both the hospital, and the HMO. They receive money from HCFA and Medicare through several different channels. The main source is direct billing for patient services like inpatient room charges, OR charges, ER charges, lab fees, the usual obvious medical bills. But hospitals also get grants based on the severity of diseases they treat, and the level of medical education the hospital provides to medical schools or residency programs. The greater the level, the more money given. And there are other factors that I don't even know about. I was talking with Jack Ferrara about the oncology unit at Athena last year. He said they got a ninety-seven million dollar Federal grant because of the cancer load there."

"You think that Athena falsified the cancer census to get the grant?"

"Probably. It would be easy enough to do, especially in an older Medicare population. Nearly everyone over sixty-five has a suspicious mole or skin lesion somewhere. Let me think…how would you set it up…" Coltrane sat down, and considered the possibilities.

"Doctors decide the DRGs and ICD-9 codes, don't they?" Britt knew that she always had Coltrane fill out those sections of the HCFA 1500 forms. Even if she knew what the diagnosis was, it was critical to get the code exactly correct because it went on the patient's permanent medical record. An error or inaccurate code could affect the patient's ability to get life or health insurance in the future.

"That's right, and the physician always has to sign the code section of the face sheet to verify that the codes are correct. But sometimes, if a patient has multiple medical problems or has been in the hospital for awhile, that list of codes is long. I've seen fifteen or twenty codes on face sheets, and they are often in pencil. The medical records people scribble in the codes, based on what they find when they review the chart." Coltrane realized that he had never given this odd arrangement much thought.

"So someone has been slipping in codes for non-existent medical conditions, and pocketing the upcharges. That would make sense. It creates the connection between the patient upcode and the HMO." Britt had completed the circle.

"Right. And the beauty of the scheme is that I think that the people doing the upcoding don't know they are committing a federal crime. In fact, I think that they believe they are doing the patient a great service." Coltrane allowed his mind to follow the trail to the obvious conclusion.

"Now you've lost me."

"Every hospital has to have a Tumor Board. You remember seeing those weekly meeting announcements? The Tumor Board is responsible for screening and cross-checking all medical records for any diagnosis of cancer, and following up on those patients. The medical records technicians go over every discharge summary and chart of every hospital patient, and pull any chart that has a diagnosis of cancer. A Tumor Board nurse reviews the charts, and presents them to the chairman. Together, they monitor the treatment and progress of the patient and the cancer."

"That's a good idea. It provides a fail-safe mechanism to make sure nothing slips through the cracks." Britt said.

"I think that it's a federal regulation, and it works very well. If you have four or five consultants treating a patient, sometimes communication gets difficult. Tumor Board ensures that a potentially life-threatening condition is not lost to follow-up. But my guess is that someone high in the HMO or hospital administration sent out a directive to intensify the search for malignancies. Made it a high priority. On the surface, it seems highly admirable to try to identify cancer. The technicians and the nurse reviewers probably attack their job with tremendous zeal, and think that the hospital executives are saintly in their concern for the patients. Meanwhile, they're coding every mole and cold sore as: Suspicious Lesion, Skin, ICD-9 Code 238.2, and inadvertently defrauding HCFA of millions. Shit, the scheme is fucking brilliant. The patient is never aware of his new, fraudulent diagnosis because it is in his hospital chart, and he is not allowed to view it. Even if he got his hands on the chart, he couldn't figure out what an ICD-9 Code meant. Who knows what a 238.2 signifies? And since he's a Medicare patient, and doesn't pay for his treatment, he doesn't care anyway. The doctors just look for the diagnosis that they admitted the patient for, so if they see anything else on the face sheet, they assume another attending physician made the entry, and will care for the problem. So they ignore it as well. Very elegant. You have to admire the mind that conceived such an exquisite and complex conspiracy."

"Don't admire the asshole too much. He tried to have us killed."

"I know. But the plan is perfect. Even if we know what was done, it's impossible to prove intent. The administrator simply says that he was doing his job, and following the federal mandate. How could monitoring cancer in hospital patients be a bad thing? Even with Hendricks' list of patients, I don't know how we can proceed from here." Coltrane's initial exhilaration at the discovery now faded as he realized the tortuous nature of the scheme.

"We have to get back to Tampa. Now." Coltrane began to pace and calculate the sailing time to Little Harbor.

"It's almost noon, and it's a good four hours to Little Harbor, and another two to Marsh Harbor. There is no way we can make that trip today. Why can't we just stay here and enjoy the afternoon? All I want to do is take a long walk on the beach with you. Make love in the sand. Watch the sunset together. Please? We haven't had a minute's rest since we set sail." Britt was exhausted, and angry.

"Yeah, you're right. Even our vacations are stressful. I'm sorry I got you involved in this, sweetheart." Coltrane put his arms around his wife, and rocked her side to side. Neither had slept well for days, and the tension was beginning to take a toll on their sanity.

Coltrane picked up the Iridium handset, and turned the unit off. He went below, and gathered up a cooler of fruit and juices and the half empty bottle of Myers's. Taking Britt by the hand, he helped her into the dinghy and headed for the most beautiful, pristine stretch of white sand beach he had ever seen.

Chapter 85

Hole in the Wall
July 4
5:52AM

Coltrane was up with the sun, and had pulled both anchors by the time Britt was stirring. He was under way within twenty minutes, and by ten o'clock they had navigated the narrow cut at Little Harbor, and were in the calm, sheltered waters of the Sea of Abaco. By 1PM, the boat was safely docked at the marina, and Coltrane saw Dennis jogging down the dock to greet them. The look on his face worried Coltrane.

"Doc, I hope nothing is wrong. The Bahamian Police want to speak with you, and I have been ordered to report to them as soon as you arrive." Dennis stepped onto the boat after requesting permission to board. Coltrane waved him aboard.

"What do they want with me?" Coltrane wondered, unprepared for more bad news.

"I don't know, but they wanted to be here when you docked. I didn't think you would like that, so I told them I never know when my charters get in," Dennis leaned close to Coltrane and whispered. "They will definitely search your boat and gear, so if you have anything illegal, you had better dump it off the side or give it to me right now."

"Thanks, Dennis, but we're clean. In fact, I would like you to be present while they search as a witness, please," Coltrane gratefully shook Dennis' hand, and began to lay out all their gear on the wooden pier. Now he was relieved that he had dumped the speargun and the shotstick.

"No problem, Doc. I gotta call the authorities and tell them you are here," Dennis replied with a wink.

Coltrane turned to see a worried look on Britt's face, and motioned her below. They discussed their strategy for the ensuing interrogation by the Bahamian Police. Within ten minutes, a small blue English Ford with a blue light pulled up to the street side of the marina and two Bahamian policemen slowly got out. Coltrane had had experience with Bahamian authorities before, and braced for what he knew would be a difficult and frustrating ordeal.

The Bahamian government, like many former colonial territories, is heavily steeped in the British tradition of government. The bureaucratic hierarchy is pervasive, inflexible and all-powerful. Bahamian citizens are prohibited from owning firearms, and the Bahamian police do not carry weapons. Crime is very rare, and as it is almost impossible to quickly escape the islands, the law enforcement agencies rely on patience and time to catch criminals. That was what worried Coltrane.

Dennis led the two men toward the end of the dock where Coltrane's yacht was docked. They were both impeccably dressed, and carried themselves in a ramrod straight stance. Even in the oppressive heat and humidity of the afternoon, their starched white shirts and epaulets were crisp, the creases in their trousers razor sharp. They were proud men, unquestionably professional, resplendent from the braided royal blue officers' caps to their patent leather shoes, shined in a mirror finish. Every brass buckle and button dazzling in the midday sun. Coltrane's eyes were drawn irresistibly to the brilliant Bahamian seal of woven gold on the men's caps.

"You are Doctor William Coltrane?" The tall, slender one asked sternly.

"Yes, sir," Coltrane stepped off the yacht, and faced the two officers.

"I am Officer Whalen and this is Officer Warderick," he nodded to his shorter, stout subordinate. "May I see your passports, please."

"Certainly," Coltrane answered, and went below to retrieve their passports. "What is this about?" He asked as he handed them to the man.

"We have some questions for you regarding a double murder that occurred here recently. Do you mind if we search your luggage?"

"In the States, that would require a search warrant. Do you have one?" Coltrane asked politely.

"Well, you are not in the States, now are you? You are in the Bahamas, and subject to Bahamian law. Here, we do things differently. I have the right to search and seize your property, and will do so immediately if you do not cooperate. Or would you prefer to continue this discussion at the jailhouse?" The policeman's tone was threatening.

"I see. Be my guest. I have no wish to spend Independence Day in jail." The irony was lost on the dour Bahamian policemen. Coltrane forced a smile, and stood aside to allow the men to inspect his gear and luggage.

They went through his fishing gear and scuba gear with great interest, and examined his knives closely. They demanded to see his fishing license, and scrutinized it thoroughly. The stout policeman asked if Coltrane had caught anything. They were particularly interested in where and with which knife the fish had been cleaned. Coltrane showed them the scaling knife, and the fillet knife that was in the yacht's kitchen. The tall man put both knives into plastic evidence bags.

"This looks like a dangerous knife, Doctor. What do you use this for?" The tall man held up Coltrane's double edged dive knife, frowning as he examined it.

"It's a scuba knife, officer. Nothing more." Coltrane answered.

"A vicious looking weapon," he muttered aloud, placing it into another evidence bag.

"Will I be getting that back before we leave?" Coltrane asked quietly.

"That depends upon when you leave, Doctor," the tall man said slowly, and turned toward Coltrane.

Coltrane felt a sinking in his stomach. He now fully comprehended that these men had no concern about detaining them on the island indefinitely, and would not hesitate to do so. With or without cause. He had to convince them that they were innocent. He glanced up at Dennis, who shrugged his shoulders, sympathetic but unable to help.

"Do you think that we had something to do with the murders?" Coltrane asked.

"Apparently, on the day of the murder, two men came to this marina and inquired about you and your wife. They said they were friends of yours, and planned to meet you here in the Abacos. Who were they?" The tall policeman demanded.

"They were lying, they were no friends of ours. Dennis told me about it. But no one knew we were here, not even our families. I have no idea who they could be," Coltrane explained, then suddenly stood up and reached for his wallet. "Look, this will clear us completely. I have a MasterCard receipt for diesel fuel from that day. I remember talking to Dennis about those guys, and I was in the Exumas, at Calvin's. There is no way that we could have killed those people. We were a hundred miles away." Coltrane pulled out the diesel receipt from Calvin's dock, and presented it to the tall man. He found several more receipts from Eleuthera, and showed the policeman them as well.

"We will verify these credit card bills, and test your knives this afternoon or in the morning. But you understand, there is a connection between you and the murdered couple. You see, they were sailing on *Wanderlust*, the boat that Dennis' dock man told the men you were on. These men may have been trying to kill you, and found the other people by mistake. You are our only remaining lead on this case, and I regret that I must detain you here until our investigation is complete." The policeman gathered up their evidence and the Coltranes' passports, and stepped up and off the yacht.

"How long do you think that will take? I have responsibilities at home that need to be considered." Coltrane began to feel both anger and frustration, but knew that he was walking a thin line. Antagonizing the Bahamian authorities would be a serious mistake. They could keep him here forever, or worse. He had no desire to be in a Bahamian jail, and the thought of Britt in jail made him physically sick. He bit back his anger.

"May I have your cards, please," Coltrane asked.

"My card and my badge number," the tall policeman gave Coltrane his card. "Where will you be staying in Marsh Harbor?" He asked politely.

"Great Abaco Beach Resort."

"We will contact you there if we have any questions. Good day."

The two officers strode back down the dock, chatted briefly with Dennis before returning to their car, and left. After he was sure that they had departed, Dennis came down the dock with two ice-cold bottles of Amstel, and his sincere apologies. He withdrew, leaving the Coltranes alone.

Coltrane sat in the cockpit, his belongings strewn around the yacht and on the pier. Britt sat down next to him, and put her arm around his shoulders. They sat quietly for several long minutes. Then they both got up, and without saying a word, gathered and repacked all their gear, carried it down the pier and loaded it all into one of the ubiquitous cabs roaming the marina, and headed for the resort.

Chapter 86

Great Abaco Beach Resort
July 4
6:55PM

After returning from a long cruise, the first night on land was usually a delicious luxury. Coltrane loved the long, hot soapy shower, scrubbing all the salt and sand from his body, never worrying that he would deplete the fresh water supply. Then fresh, clean white Turkish towels, crisp starched bed linens, and the air conditioner set on high. American television. The unblinking eye. *The Simpsons* and ice-cold Meyers's and Coke. Fucking paradise.

"How long do you think that they'll keep us here?" Britt asked.

"I don't know, babe. We are on island time, and on top of that, the bureaucracy here is agonizingly slow. Remember last trip? It took two days to get a fucking fishing permit, for Christ's sake. We bought our house in Tampa with less paperwork."

"Maybe we should call Lynwood. Didn't he say that he was going to call you back yesterday?"

"Yeah, but I turned off the Iridium for a while. I tried to reach him on the sail to Little Harbor, but no one answered. Probably too early. I'll try again." Coltrane retrieved the handset from their gear, and dialed Lynwood's number in Tampa.

"Lynwood here," he answered the phone abruptly.

"Lynwood, this is Coltrane. What did you find out about the patients on my list?"

"Doctor Coltrane, I tried to contact you yesterday, but I couldn't get through. I have interesting news," Lynwood sounded excited, and genuinely friendly. "Every single one of the patients you listed is on the HMO plan, and every one is a Medicare or Medicaid patient as well. In fact, Tallahassee tells me that a high proportion of these patients have been flagged for internal audit by the regional HCFA office. It seems that the billing activity on these accounts is suspiciously high. The lead HCFA investigator wants the rest of your list as soon as possible. It looks like I may owe you an apology."

"Forget about the apology, just tear up my arrest warrant."

"Consider it done. When can you get back to Tampa, Doctor Coltrane? I would like to meet with you immediately."

"We have a little problem down here. Do you remember the couple that was killed on their sailboat? Well, on what was supposed to be our sailboat. We are being detained for questioning in the murders. I have MasterCard receipts placing us a hundred miles from the murder, but the police are holding us here until they are sure of our part in the tragedy." Coltrane paused. "We'll be on a plane as soon as they release us."

"Maybe I can speed up the process. Were the victims Americans?"

"I am pretty sure they were."

"Where are you at now? I will try to contact the Bahamian authorities, and the American consulate in Nassau. Maybe we can get you released on your own recognizance."

Coltrane gave Lynwood their room number and the phone number of the resort, and the names and phone numbers of the investigating officers. Lynwood promised to call back within the hour with an update. Coltrane thanked him, hung up and turned off the Iridium handset. He turned to Britt, beaming a broad grin.

"Lynwood can bail us out of here?" Britt asked hopefully.

"Maybe. But the best news is that he's convinced that the list is legit. God, is that a relief." A wave of relief washed over him, and he walked to the balcony where Britt stood, and put his arms around her gently, kissing her neck. They looked out over the beautiful crescent bay, with the brand new marina and rows of sparkling yachts and sportsfishermen all neatly secured between concrete and metal pilings.

"If you have to be detained, this is the place," Coltrane laughed as he thought of the irony. "May I buy you a drink, my dear?" he asked with a lecherous grin.

"Myers's and Coke, with a lime, please. And lots of ice. Big, huge hunks of sparkling, clear ice."

After being on the boat for two weeks, and without the basic conveniences of life they always took for granted, rock-hard ice and a hot shower were obscenely luxurious.

They sat on the balcony of the hotel room, enjoying the huge glasses of ice and the cold Coke, savoring the sweet flavor of the Jamaican rum. Time passed as the sun slipped into the sea behind the island's green scrub. The heat of the day receded, and the warmth of the rum effused their tired bodies, bathing in the sunset. The silence was comfortable.

The gentle buzzing of the hotel phone roused him from his reverie. He picked it up.

"Hello."

"Doctor Coltrane, this is Agent Lynwood."

"Any luck?" Coltrane asked.

"Yes. I convinced the Bahamian police that you were not directly involved with the murders. They have consented to allow you to leave at any time. However, there may be a connection between you and the killers, and I have personally guaranteed that you will cooperate with their investigation. You don't have a problem with that, do you?"

"Certainly not."

"Good. I have taken the liberty to book you on the morning flight out of Marsh Harbor, connecting through Miami. Your previous reservations were canceled when you missed today's flight. Is that OK?"

"Yeah, that's fine. You're not taking any chances, are you?"

"Nope. You're an important witness now. I can't afford to lose you," Lynwood laughed.

"Thanks. I'll see you in Tampa," Coltrane finished and hung up the phone.

He turned to Britt, smiling happily. "Let's go down to the grill for some conch. Conch salad, conch fritters, fried conch. They have the world's best fried conch here."

"July 4th. The perfect way to celebrate our freedom. Life is good," Britt beamed radiantly at her lover, and they touched glasses.

Chapter 87

Marsh Harbor
July 5
8:22AM

They jumped the morning flight from Abaco to Miami, and enjoyed the noisy, bumpy trip over the emerald waters. All the small island hopper flights ended in a crowded part of Miami International Airport, in a jammed corner of the tarmac. From there, the passengers were herded onto busses, breathing heavy diesel fumes as they were shuttled to the main Customs Port of Entry at MIA.

The Miami Customs port clears millions of international visitors yearly, and is a vast, complicated and extremely efficient operation. Incoming passengers are separated into lines by citizenship, and by visa type. Luggage is electronically scanned for weapons, contraband, drugs and explosives. Special dogs are used to find cocaine and marijuana. The entire process is constantly monitored with electronic surveillance and recording equipment, and data banks kept on visitors and citizens alike.

The Coltranes passed through the green line for US citizens with passports, and entered the cavernous luggage and clearing depot. They stood around the carousel, and picked up their gear bags and luggage off the moving platform. They loaded everything onto a metal cart, and headed for the exit and their connecting flight to Tampa. Coltrane watched with amazement and disgust as full grown adults pushed and cut in line, trying to save a minute or two.

When they arrived at the Customs desk, the inspector smiled and scanned Britt's passport, briefly questioned her about the nature of their visit, then waved her through. He was about to do the same for Coltrane when something on his computer screen caught his eye. He swiveled on his stool, made eye contact with Coltrane, and asked him the same questions. Before Coltrane could answer, two armed Customs agents appeared and moved very close to the couple, blocking their exit. The desk inspector handed Coltrane's passport to one of the agents, and instructed the startled couple to take their baggage and follow the uniformed officers.

No one noticed the tall hispanic male just outside Customs on the other side of the glass partition in the main terminal, watching the action with intense interest. He wore the dark blue coveralls of the airport maintenance crews, and a filthy Miami Dolphins cap. They didn't see him curse and turn away as they were led into the hallway to the detention area.

Before Coltrane could protest, they were hurried out of the passenger area, herded through a metal detector and into a maze of corridors with low ceilings and naked flickering fluorescent bulbs. It all happened so quickly that they were awestruck and intimidated, too bewildered to resist. They found themselves sitting in a small, spartan interview room with an obvious two-way mirror filling one entire wall. Their luggage had disappeared. They sat for twenty minutes before the Miami Customs Port Director Chacon arrived.

Port Director Roberto Chacon had been in his office when the yellow alarm had been called. He immediately scanned the bank of video monitors in his office, and saw that Station Five had intercepted a passenger wanted for questioning by the FBI. Automatically, the information from the entry inspector's desk was displayed on his command monitor.

William Thomas Coltrane, MD
Passport Number
15336599648224

Threat Level	**Low**
Flight Risk	**High**
Priors	**None**

Wanted for questioning in regard to murder/extortion.
Detain for questioning.
Contact Agent Scott Lynwood/Miami FBI

Years ago, the United States Customs Service adapted computer and scanner technology to develop a passport with an integrated barcode identification band. Each time an American citizen enters or exits the country, the Customs agent or the airline employee swipes the passport through a scanner, and the validity of the passport and the identity of the traveler are recorded. This data is instantly cross-checked against the federal government's alert list. The alert list covers many levels of threat to the United States, both internal and external. Wanted criminals, convicted felons, suspected drug smugglers or money launderers as well as political terrorists are high priority on the alert list. In the event that anyone on the alert list is picked up by the entry desk scanners, simultaneous messages are flashed to all desk inspectors, the supervisors and the heavily armed tactical response team. Passenger processing is halted until the situation is cleared.

Director Chacon watched on the monitors as his response team reacted to the desk inspector's silent alarm, and intercepted the man and his wife. He coordinated the operation via his command Motorola radio, linked to earpieces worn by all the Customs inspectors. The operation went without incident. As he viewed the couple sitting quietly in the interview room on one of the video monitors, he turned to the other man seated in the office. Chacon leveled his gaze at the man, wondering if this display of professionalism and technology would impress him. The Customs Service never got the respect or credit it deserved, he thought as he stared at the impassive FBI agent across his desk. And these FBI assholes are the worst.

"Nice job. I thought all you guys did was confiscate Cuban cigars. And destroy them by 'incineration'," Lynwood laughed sarcastically.

"What is that supposed to mean?" Chacon was angered by the comment. He knew it was an insult, disguised as a friendly joke. And this *pindeho* was no friend of his.

"Sorry, just a joke. I'd heard you guys have a weekly cigar party, that's all. No offense, Director," Lynwood backed up. He immediately regretted fucking with this hot blooded, humorless Latino.

"Follow me. We will interview your suspects. But you had better have something substantial to detain them. I am not putting my ass on the line for you, *amigo*," Chacon said with distaste. He rose, and led Lynwood down through the clearing depot, toward the cubicle where the Coltranes sat waiting.

Chapter 88

Miami International Airport
US Customs
July 5
1:44PM

Coltrane sat on the metal folding chair, his mind running wild. Why had Customs detained them? He had assumed that Lynwood would have an alert posted for him when he returned, but doubted that the FBI agent would have ordered them taken into custody. Had the Bahamian police found evidence on his dive knife? He knew that he had lunged at the Cuban with it, but missed. It had happened so fast... Had the island police called Calvin? Had Calvin told them about the two men looking for them? Had Cal's wife said something? Did Lynwood have satellite surveillance photos of the yacht? Or of Coltrane's little trips out into Exuma Sound? The possibilities were endless. What would he say? How to respond? His heart and mind were racing beyond control.

Just when it seemed that the tension was unbearable, that his head was about to explode, the metal door to the cubicle opened. Director Chacon entered, with a single armed guard. Chacon sat at the table, and the guard moved to a far corner behind him. As he did so, Coltrane noticed a rectangle of gray light appear in the mirror, and a silhouette pass into the adjoining room. He felt a wave of unease wash over him.

"Doctor Coltrane, I am Roberto Chacon, Port Director. I am sorry for the inconvenience, but we need to ask you some questions."

"There must be some mistake. Why are we being detained?" Coltrane asked politely.

"A routine spot check," Chacon lied. "Do you have anything to declare?"

"Nothing. We are seasoned travelers, and have been through this port of entry many times. No Cuban cigars, no booze, no plant material, no ivory. We are clean, and our luggage is clean. Our flight to Tampa leaves in an hour, and..." Coltrane abruptly stood up, and moved to the two-way mirror. He knew the source of the vague unease he had experienced earlier. His subconscious mind had recognized Lynwood's profile in the hallway light. "Perhaps you would like to join us, Agent Lynwood."

Coltrane turned to Chacon. "Director Chacon, this is no routine spot check. I am an American citizen, and will not be detained illegally. I want my wife released immediately, and I want immediate access to a phone to contact my attorney. Show me an arrest warrant. Where is Lynwood?" Coltrane turned to the mirror again, the veins in his neck bulging. "Come on out here, Lynwood. Show me a warrant."

Chacon stood up from the table, and without a word, left the room. He took the guard with him, and summoned Lynwood from the observation room into the hallway. Their discussion was animated.

"Do you have an arrest warrant for them, either of them?" Chacon asked irritably.

"Not yet," Lynwood muttered, avoiding eye contact with Chacon.

"Any hard evidence?"

"No. But I'm sure he knows more than he's telling. I just want to sweat him for awhile." Lynwood was bending the rules, and he knew it.

"Listen, you idiot. This doctor is no fool. His luggage was clean. He knows his rights, he's got money, and he will retain a lawyer to come down here and *fuck me up* if I violate procedure. Which I'm certainly not going to do for your dumb ass. Now produce a warrant and arrest them, or I release them immediately. If they miss their plane, it'll be your fault."

"Let me talk to them," Lynwood said, and turned to enter the interview room.

"Just a minute," Chacon said, and deftly reached into Lynwood's jacket, removing his 9mm Sig-Sauer. He handed it to the guard, smiling disdainfully at Lynwood. "I'd hate to have you get shot by your suspect, on Customs Service property." With that, he turned and headed back to his office. He could watch the FBI asshole on his video monitor.

Lynwood composed himself as he entered the cubicle. He had lost the upper hand, the moral righteousness, that he had held earlier. Perhaps Coltrane sensed that, perhaps not. It didn't matter. There was always Plan B.

"I am sorry that you were detained, Dr. Coltrane," Lynwood lied. "I would like to place you under protective custody. I have reason to believe that the people who killed Hendricks and Ochoa will attempt to kill you as well."

"Protective custody? Not a chance. I have a practice to get back to. I'm long overdue. Besides, once you have the disk, there is no reason to kill us. The evidence will be in your hands," Coltrane reasoned.

"You will still have to testify in the trial, and that trial may be years away. A dead witness is not very credible, Doc."

"I'll tape my testimony. Look, we have had a long trip, and a rough couple of weeks. I want to get my wife home, and we are going to miss our plane." Coltrane stood up and helped Britt up. "Arrest me or let me go."

"I am not going to arrest you, and you are free to go. But you've missed your flight by now. I'll be glad to fly you back to Tampa, at the government's expense."

"When?" Coltrane was skeptical.

"Right now. I flew down this morning on a chartered plane. We can be in the air in thirty minutes. All I want to do is talk, get some questions answered. No more tricks, you have my word," Lynwood seemed sincere. He held his hands up in mock surrender.

"Fine. Let's go," Coltrane agreed and stood up, despite the strong opposition of his wife.

They all left the interrogation room together, and headed toward the huge, crowded terminal and the private aviation wing of the airport. As they walked through the maze of terminal gates and corporate aviation terminals, Lynwood spoke urgently on his cellphone to the charter pilot. He arranged for the plane to be fueled and taxied to a government gate, but refused to give him a flight plan or a manifest of passengers. He was obviously very concerned about security.

The plane was a new twin turbo-prop, sleek and streamlined. The flight crew, two young men in blue uniforms, welcomed them politely aboard and pulled the curved metal doors shut before disappearing into the curtained cockpit. The cabin was well-appointed, and laid out with pairs of seats facing each other. The three passengers settled into the spacious cabin, and seated themselves. Within seconds, they were underway. Finally, as they lifted off, Lynwood began to relax.

"Crowd control and security is very difficult in airports. That's why I asked Customs to hold you up," he continued the charade. "You're in danger until the government can present evidence showing that Athena has defrauded Medicare. And the sooner I can prepare that evidence, the sooner you will be safe."

"You've already got all the evidence. Susan Kerr gave you the disc, didn't she?" Britt asked bluntly.

"Right. She gave me a disc with a long series of numbers on it. But that wasn't the original disc, right? She told me that it was a copy of a file that you E-mailed to her from the Bahamas. Is that right?" Lynwood asked.

"Right," Coltrane answered, and shot a quick glance to his wife. "The original CD-R is in my safety deposit box in Tampa. I'll deliver it to you, in the presence of witnesses, as soon as possible. And I want a receipt, as well as something in writing about the whistle-blower arrangement. Who does that?" Coltrane didn't trust Lynwood for a second.

"I'll arrange for my district lead agent to be present, as well as representatives from HCFA. I'm sure that their Tallahassee investigators will be very interested in the disc. We can do the entire thing before a federal judge, if you like. You can give your statement at that time. You'll need to testify before a grand jury in the very near future, as well."

"Ah ha, Lynwood. Covering your ass in case we get killed, right? Once the trail of evidence is established for the disc, you won't need us any more. Is that it?" Coltrane laughed.

"Sorry, Doc. Just doing my job. I did offer you protection, remember? But you're right, we have to show that the disc came from Ochoa, then went to you and then to us. And I have to make some conclusive link to Hendricks from the disc. I need a trail of evidence, especially with digital data." Lynwood lectured smugly.

"No, you don't," Britt fired back.

"What do you mean?" Lynwood asked abruptly.

"Look, it may help the case against Athena if you can connect Hendricks to the disc, but the real evidence of wrongdoing is not on the disc. The evidence is in the patient files and billing records at the hospital. The disc is irrelevant at this point. All you need is the patient list, and you have that. Susan Kerr gave you that," Britt related.

"I'm sorry. I don't follow you," Lynwood was confused.

"AthenaHMO has committed fraudulent billing, and there is clear, undeniable proof in their own records. All you have to do is compare the patients' medical records with their billing records. The obvious discrepancy between the actual and the billed ICD-9 codes will be proof of the fraud. It really doesn't matter how you got tipped off. You can't prosecute Hendricks anyway. He's dead. To state the *obvious*," Britt said.

Lynwood glared at Britt, irritated by being censured by a woman. Without answering her, he turned to Coltrane. "How did you break the encryption? How did you get a patient list from those numbers?" Lynwood asked.

"Ask Britt. She's the one who figured it out," Coltrane told him.

Surprised, Lynwood pushed back into his seat and waited for an explanation.

"I'd have to show it to you on a computer," she answered sweetly, "but it really is a simple code. You have to know what you're looking for. I've spent years billing for the practice, so I'm familiar with the format used by HCFA for provider charges. We only decoded the first twenty or so patients, but there may be tens of thousands on that disc. Hopefully, your lab in Washington can finish the job." Britt knew that the FBI mainframe computers could complete the job much more efficiently than she could.

"Damn." Lynwood leaned back in the high backed seat, looked at Britt and shook his head. "I underestimated you. You're smart. Really smart. I thought you were just a trophy wife."

"Jesus. Do you realize how insulting that is?" Britt asked, shaking her head in amazement.

"No, I don't mean it that way. Look, I want to make amends with the both of you. I've screwed you around a little during the course of this investigation, and I'm sorry. Some of it you deserved, because you lied to me about your whereabouts and your plans. But it is clear to me now that you did not kill Hendricks or Ochoa. Part of my job is to suspect everyone. Sometimes we pressure innocent people. Let's try and start with a clean slate, alright?"

"Fine," Britt responded, knowing that her husband would not be as magnanimous. Coltrane sat quietly and said nothing.

"What's next?" Coltrane broke the silence.

"Well, like I said, I'll need to take a formal statement from you and get that disc to Washington as soon as possible. Maybe I could pick up the disc this afternoon, if you can arrange it. Then we have to get search warrants for any Athena hospital facilities that may be involved in this billing scheme, and start examining their charts. This could be as big as the Columbia/HCA investigation. The process will take months, maybe years." Lynwood paused, suddenly becoming very somber. "There is something that I need to discuss with both of you. If I am correct, the same person or persons who killed Hendricks also killed Ochoa. Both murders appear to have been done by professionals; there were no fingerprints or footprints at the scenes, no witnesses, and no viable suspects. Hendricks' death even fooled the coroner. Whoever committed these murders is still at large, and most likely, you are their next target."

"We've considered that. But they aren't after us, they're after the disc. Once the disc is in the hands of the FBI, they'll have no interest in us. That's the endgame. Why do you think I E-mailed you the encrypted contents? I was hoping that you would get the HMO off our backs."

"You think that the killers were hired by the HMO?" Lynwood was incredulous.

"Maybe not the HMO board of directors or the CEO. More likely a rogue executive within the company, or a small group of corporate officers who would benefit financially from the fraud. Hendricks may have been involved himself. Stock options, incentives, and promotions are all tied to productivity. Have you seen the stock price of Athena over the last two years? It has more than doubled, and is ready to split again. I'm sure you will find plenty of people with opportunity and motive."

"Still, I would like to place you in protective custody, at least until the HMO is aware that we have the disc, or the killers have been caught. They are very dangerous."

"I can't just disappear; I have patients and an office to run. I have surgery that has been scheduled months ago. It's impossible."

"You are going back to work immediately?"

"Of course. You don't understand how medical practices work. I've been gone far too long. My colleagues have been covering for me, and I can't abuse my friends. I have to return to my practice."

"Even if it means risking your life? Do you know how easy a target you are? ER visits in the middle of the night. Empty parking garages. Crowded hospitals. You follow a very predictable and consistent routine. Office in the morning and afternoon. Same hospitals every day. You're an easy mark. I know. I was on a detail that provided security for a plastic surgeon who was receiving death threats because he was creating 'Aryan features' on 'non-Aryan' patients. I've protected gynecologists at abortion clinics in seven different states. It is almost impossible to protect doctors."

"I can't just leave my practice," Coltrane repeated softly.

"You know, if this whistle-blower thing comes through, you will never have to work again. Take a month off. I may be able to get you into a federal witness protection plan. Or maybe get you a position in the military; the Army has several outstanding medical facilities and would love to have an experienced trauma surgeon. Shit, who causes more trauma than the military?" Lynwood was sincere and animated.

"Maybe we can take a few weeks off, darling. We could stay at my parents' place in Bradenton. The security is great there, and they won't be down this year." Britt looked at Coltrane, and raised her eyebrows in question.

Coltrane gazed at his wife, and leaned back and stared out the window at the clouds drifting by. He was tired, and he knew she was tired and drained as well. His shoulder wound still burned constantly, and had drained more blood than he had told Britt. He would need X-rays and a wound culture before he even *thought* of operating. Maybe a week or two off wouldn't be a bad idea. He could always give his cases to Hernandez; his friend was as good a surgeon as anyone in the state. Maybe it was time to get a partner, anyway. And her parents' place in Bradenton's Isla Pacifica was very nice, a two bedroom condo overlooking the water with a little marina where he kept his sportfisherman. Maybe he could get some fishing in.

Lynwood broke his reverie. "What's the security like?"

"The building is a twelve story high-rise on the water, in a gated development. Within the development, there are roving security patrols, and the gate is manned twenty-four hours. Access to the high-rise itself is by the underground parking ramp or by the front atrium doors. In both cases, you have to be buzzed in by the security guard, and pass directly in front of their booth. It's a very secure building. Most of the tenants are gone the majority of the year, so they want to have peace of mind about their belongings." Coltrane was liking the idea more by the minute.

"I could provide an escort to and from your office, if you like. What kind of gun do you carry?" Lynwood smiled mischievously.

"What?" Coltrane was startled.

"I know all about you, Coltrane. I do my homework. I have a file three inches thick on you on my desk. Concealed weapons permit with three renewals. Your practical shooting score was 249 out of 250. Who told you to miss the last 10 circle?"

"The instructor. He said a perfect score would be a mistake. Some jury might expect me to shoot the gun out of my assailant's hand instead of killing him. So I pulled the last shot."

"That's funny. That's exactly what they tell us at the academy. Never get a perfect score in qualification. Anyway, what do you carry?" Lynwood was curious.

"I've got a Glock 23 and a Walther PPK. But I've never carried either in public. They're too heavy for a dress belt with the type of clothing I wear, and it's so damn hot here I never wear a jacket. Plus, it's illegal to carry in a hospital, and I'm in a hospital all day long. It just turned out to be one of those ideas that look better on paper than in execution."

"You might want to carry something for awhile, Doc. At least until we get a handle on who killed Hendricks and Ochoa. Which brings me to a question I need answered. Why aren't you in the least concerned any more about the two men who were after you in the Bahamas? First you call me and tell me he, or they, are trying to kill you. Then nothing. And you haven't mentioned them in days. Why?" Lynwood leaned forward, and looked directly at Coltrane, then at Britt, waiting for an answer.

"I don't know, Lynwood. I discussed that in detail with the Bahamian police, and they seem to think those two were involved in the murder of the young couple who sailed out of Marsh Harbor in what was supposed to be our yacht. Maybe they mistook them for us. Maybe they wanted to get out of the islands after they killed those people. Or maybe they really thought that they had killed us. Who knows?" Coltrane wanted to cloud the issue with as many theories as possible.

"It's doubtful that they left that boat thinking that they had killed the Coltranes. Why they simply gave up, after traveling so far, and killing two innocents, seems very odd to me. There's more to this story." Lynwood's eyes told more than he was saying.

As they sat in silence, the pilot's voice came over the intercom. They would be landing in fifteen minutes, and the weather in Tampa-St. Pete was warm and clear. Each passenger checked their seatbelt, and looked out the windows as the plane banked and descended to land.

Chapter 89

Tampa
July 5
7:17PM

The ride home was uneventful. Lynwood insisted on sweeping the house before the Coltranes entered, and neither argued. The house was clean and undisturbed, and they were glad to be home. Lynwood arranged for a black and white police cruiser to remain out front, and Coltrane acquiesced. After extracting a promise from Coltrane to deliver the disc in the morning, Lynwood departed.

Coltrane was exhausted beyond human endurance. He checked the doors, and activated the security system. Finally, he slumped into an armchair, dead tired. He watched the local news as Britt showered, and dressed for bed.

Wearily, he dragged himself out of his chair to shower. He stripped off his traveling clothes, damp from the tropical humidity and soiled from hours in filthy cabs and airports. His shoulder was bandaged with a single sterile adhesive bandage, and was soaked through. He winced as he peeled off the tape, and bits of flesh came off with the bandage. Using hydrogen peroxide and bottled water, he sat in the bathtub and gently cleansed his wound. It looked pretty good, he thought. Minimal discharge, minimal inflammation, and the swelling was going down. Relieved, he lay back in the tub, and let the tension drain from his body.

Bathed, showered and refreshed, he put on silk boxers and slipped into bed. Britt was already sound asleep, turned away from him. He reached over and stroked her hair, marveling at the perfect parallel patterns of hundreds of rows of soft strawberry blonde strands, delicate and fragrant. Her skin soft and inviting, the smell of her body scented and sweet. He kissed her neck and shoulder lightly so as not to wake her, and lay back. Within minutes, he drifted off into a deep sleep.

Chapter 90

Tampa
July 6
10:33AM

They both slept late, luxuriating in the clean linen sheets and soft familiar bed. Britt made a huge breakfast of eggs, corned beef hash, English muffins and potatoes O'Brien. Coltrane savored the meal, and they sipped their coffee in silence. They both knew that today would be a huge day.

Coltrane was showered and dressed first, as usual. While Britt put on her makeup, he opened his safe, and pulled out the Glock 23. Made in Austria of high tech polymers using a revolutionary design, the Glock was brutishly ugly. But it was incredibly durable, and extremely accurate in Coltrane's hands. The .40 caliber round had been designed to FBI and Secret Service specifications, and was the optimum blend of a high velocity cartridge and a large caliber projectile. If it was good enough for them, it was good enough for Coltrane. He loaded the clip with .40 caliber hollow point slugs, and inserted it into the pistol grip. He adjusted the pancake holster high on his right hip, and stood before the mirror to see if the bulge of the squat weapon was visible through his linen jacket. Satisfied with the concealed carry, he went downstairs to call Lynwood and wait for Britt. He had learned long ago that hovering over her was useless, and could be risky.

They packed clothes and gear for a two week stay at the condo on the coast. Coltrane just unpacked his clothes from the islands, and hung seven starched white dress shirts and several pairs of tropical weight wool slacks in his hanging bag. Some fresh cotton shirts and shorts, and he was ready to go. Britt took two hours selecting and coordinating her packing, but they were ready before noon.

Coltrane thanked the officers on watch outside, and they followed as he pulled the Expedition out of the driveway, and headed to his bank. Lynwood met them all at the bank, and quickly went to the secured vault area. Coltrane opened his safety deposit box, and right on the top of his deeds and personal papers, lay the CD-R in its plastic jewel case. He picked it up carefully, and handed it to Lynwood. Lynwood placed it in a manila envelope, and dated and signed a receipt for Coltrane. He seemed greatly relieved.

"You need an escort to work, Doc?" Lynwood asked.

"No, thanks. I've decided to take a few weeks off, after all. Life is too short, and we didn't get much rest in the Bahamas. You can reach me through my answering service any time, and I'll give you my cellphone number. When do you want to arrange my testimony?"

"Probably next week. I need to explain the unique nature of this investigation to the judge, and coordinate with the HCFA boys in Tallahassee. But I'll give you plenty of notice. What's the name of your condo?" Lynwood asked as they all headed out of the bank.

"We'll just keep that my little secret, if you don't mind. The fewer people who know, the better."

"You've seen too many movies, Doc. But that's fine with me. Just be careful, and I'd advise that you rent a car for awhile. The FBI will pick up the tab. That Eddie Bauer Expedition with the brush bars is a bit too conspicuous for my taste. Nice vehicle, though." Lynwood shook both their hands, and got into his sedan with the envelope. "I'll get back to you with the lab results on this as soon as I know. Good luck."

Coltrane drove them to his office, and parked the Expedition in his parking place in the underground garage. They quickly visited the office, and Coltrane picked up some papers and journals that he could peruse during the week. Britt called and arranged for a rental car to be delivered to the front of the medical office building, and chatted with Cindy for some time about all the events during their absence.

When the rental car came, Coltrane transferred their luggage from the Expedition, and they headed for the coast. Britt had requested a 4WD F-150 SuperCrew, in case Coltrane wanted to tow their boat south for some fishing. The hour trip to Bradenton was soothing, with vast expanses of the tranquil Gulf of Mexico to the west, and colorful inlets and estuaries sheltering small sailboats and jetskis to the east. Sunlight shimmered off the sparkling blue water, and Coltrane felt the pressure of the past months ease away.

Isla Pacifica was located at the northern tip of a long barrier island that jutted out into the shallow Gulf of Mexico. Access to the island was by a two lane bridge at the extreme southern tip of the sandy island, and all traffic passed through the manned security gate. Coltrane showed his resident permit, and the security officer recognized him and waved him through. Coltrane was a frequent visitor to the marina on the island. During the summers, Coltrane spent many weekends at the condo, fishing the clear waters offshore and escaping the pressures of his practice.

They drove down the manicured boulevard of the master planned community, north toward the condo. The grounds were meticulously maintained, huge rushes of bright red bougainvillea everywhere, and tall palms bending gracefully from the constant onshore breezes. The island was lush and tropical in vegetation, bright and Caribbean in flavor. Ahead, the condominium tower rose above the white sand.

Coltrane guided the truck through the entry gate, and ran his plastic entry card through the automated sensor. The metal gate rolled up, and a uniformed security guard looked out through a glass window at the arriving vehicle. Not recognizing the pickup, he motioned for them to stop. After walking up to the truck's window and seeing Coltrane, he waved them through. They parked and carried their luggage to the elevators, and ascended to the eleventh floor.

The condo faced northwest, with a spectacular view of the Gulf of Mexico and the city skyline. Britt's parents had been looking for a summer home in Tampa ever since she married Coltrane. When Isla Pacifica's developer filed for Chapter 11 and the RTC sold off fifteen of the condo units to clear sub-contractor liens, Coltrane attended the auction. The fifteen units went very quickly, and the cash only terms discouraged speculators. But the prices were incredibly low, and Coltrane decided that if his in-laws didn't like the unit, he would keep it for himself. But they were delighted with the views and amenities, as well as the nearness to their daughter. They stayed in the condo several weeks each year, when they visited Tampa and Britt. The rest of the time, Coltrane used it as an occasional retreat.

The two bedroom unit had a large living room and dining area with floor to ceiling glass, and absolutely spectacular views of the Gulf. Britt had furnished it with comfortable, beach-style furnishings. Overstuffed cotton duck sofas and chairs surrounded a big screen television, and a huge pine dining table filled the other half of the room. The bedrooms were simply furnished, with a California king in the master, and two sets of bunk beds in the second bedroom. Coltrane frequently used the condo for all night poker games, or weekend fishing excursions when he wanted his buddies to be able to drink heavily and not have to worry about driving home. Coltrane viewed heavy drinking as a highly effective form of therapy.

Britt went to the master bedroom, and unpacked their luggage as Coltrane threw his briefcase and cellular phone on the dining room table. He unpacked the laptop, and connected the modem line to the telephone wall jack. As the computer hummed and dialed his Internet access number, he went into the well-equipped kitchen and poured a Coke over a tall glass of ice and a capful of Myers's. By the time he got back to the table, the AOL home page was up. He went to Internet access, and pulled up the *Caduceus* home page. He typed in his password, and opened his mailbox. There were over one hundred fifty E-mails in his mailbox. He smiled, shrugged, sipped the cold Coke, and opened the first one.

Chapter 91

Federal District Court
Middle District of Florida
Sam M. Gibbons U.S. Courthouse
Tampa
July 12
9:27AM

Lynwood led Coltrane down a wide hallway, and into an area that faced large, oaken double doors. The door had a simple brass plate mounted upon it, reading: Federal Courtroom 3. Across from the doors were austere, hard wooden benches. They sat in one of the long benches, the somber mood of their surroundings enveloping them.

Lynwood went through his briefcase, and reviewed his papers. He mumbled softly to himself, reciting his delivery for the judge. Coltrane sat ramrod straight, looking forward into space.

People came and went through the doors to Courtroom 3, occasionally giving apprising glances at the two men seated on the bench. Coltrane wondered what was transpiring in the room, and how they would know when to enter. Lynwood continued his shuffling of court documents and his preparation. Coltrane waited.

Eventually, Lynwood leaned back and closed his leather attaché. He stood up, and motioned Coltrane to follow. They walked through the double door into a small, dignified courtroom paneled in oak with a massive, high judge's bench of polished mahogany. To Coltrane's surprise, the courtroom was completely empty. The eighteen chairs of the jury sat in austere and mute observation of their approach. The sound of street traffic could be heard over the faint music of a desktop radio in a distant office. Above them, a domed, hand plastered ceiling, gave testimony to skilled artisans of the past century. Behind them, rows of wooden pews sat empty.

Only upon careful observation could two doors be seen hidden in the paneling and wainscoting that led out of the courtroom into private chambers. They went past the wooden rail that separated spectators from the legal teams, and sat at the table on the right side of the courtroom. Set up in the area to their right was a video camera and lighting and sound recording equipment.

Several minutes later, a young woman carrying camera equipment entered the courtroom through the double doors, and approached Lynwood.

He conferred with her briefly, and she took her position behind the videocamera, and adjusted her equipment.

At this time, a uniformed bailiff entered from one of the side doors. "All rise. Federal District Court is in session. The Honorable Judge Jefferson presiding."

Federal Judge Corrine Anne Jefferson, a stern black woman in her sixties, entered through a concealed door in the mahogany paneled courtroom, and strode to her bench, seating herself without once looking up at the courtroom.

The proceedings went rapidly. As Lynwood was in court to obtain search warrants and establish Coltrane's testimony, the protocol normally required for legal matters was truncated. Lynwood stood before the judge and recited the probable cause he had for searching the records of Athena facilities. He delineated the evidence trail of the disc, and detailed the forensic evidence pertinent to the murders of Hendricks and Ochoa. He described the manner in which Athena was fraudulently billing Medicare, and how he had come to believe that the scheme was, in fact, a conspiracy to systematically defraud the Health Care Financing Administration. Finally, he summarized and asked for statewide search warrants for all Athena facilities, and for the convening of a grand jury to pursue indictments on multiple charges of fraud and conspiracy.

Judge Jefferson looked down on them from her bench, peering over gold rimmed spectacles. Her face wore a frown. She summoned Lynwood to the bench and, placing her hand over the metal microphone, spoke to him in low tones. Coltrane couldn't make out the words, but it was clear that she was admonishing Lynwood in no uncertain terms. He was calmly nodding his head in assent. After several minutes of intense discussion, he returned to the table, and called Coltrane to the witness stand.

Coltrane was duly sworn in by the bailiff. After identifying himself to the judge, videotechnician and court reporter, he was prepared to give testimony. Lynwood rose from the table, and approached the witness stand. Before he could begin to question Coltrane, Judge Jefferson halted the proceedings, and turned to Coltrane.

"Dr. Coltrane, I know you only by reputation. You are the president of the Bay Area Medical Society, am I right?" Judge Jefferson scowled down at him.

"Yes, your honor."

"In addition, are you not involved in civil litigation with regard to this HMO's alleged negligence in a local boy's death recently?"

"Yes."

"You will address me as 'Your Honor'."

"Yes, Your honor."

"I believe that the so-called 'medical conference' you held was merely a thinly disguised labor action, and find the entire affair reprehensible. I can tell you that if you are coming before me today to attempt another manipulative stunt like that conference, you will be very sorry. I will hold you in contempt, and you *will* do jail time. I have discussed this with Mr. Lynwood, and he understands. The question is, do you understand?" She leaned forward, awaiting an answer.

"Yes, Your Honor." Coltrane was taken aback by the vehemence of her accusations.

"Very well. Continue."

Lynwood slowly and carefully walked Coltrane, step by step, through the events that brought him into possession of the CD-R, and how they had decoded the sequence of numbers. He elicited a narrative of the phone call to Athena, and how Coltrane had deduced that the hospital was using ICD-9 diagnoses of cancer to falsely increase bills submitted to Medicare. The judge listened attentively, occasionally turning to write notes on her legal pad. At length, Lynwood concluded. The judge sat for several minutes reviewing her notes, and arranging her thoughts before making her decision.

"I am granting your request for a search warrant for three Athena facilities in the Bay area. I will limit your investigation to the Tampa-St. Petersburg area for the time being, however. Come back to this court when you have conclusive evidence of fraud or conspiracy. I further acknowledge and record the whistle-blower claim of Dr. William Coltrane in regards to this alleged fraud against the United States Government." She leveled a hard stare at Lynwood, then at Coltrane. She hit her gavel, and ended the hearing. She rose quickly, and left the courtroom.

"Shit. I was hoping to search Miami and Orlando as well. Now they have time to destroy evidence, and shift personnel around to cover their tracks. Ah well, you can't win all the time." Lynwood gathered his papers, and took the videotape handed him by the technician.

"What are you crying about? She wanted to put my ass in jail."

"You weren't prepared for the hostility, were you?" Lynwood laughed.

"I'm glad you enjoyed it. Now what's next?"

"I've got lots of work to do, preparing for the search, organizing teams to collect and review documents, and so on. Nothing for you to do at this point. I'll keep in touch." With that, Lynwood turned and headed down the hallway toward the wing of the Federal Building that housed the FBI offices. Coltrane turned and exited to the street, somewhat depressed.

Chapter 92

Federal Building
Saint Petersburg
July 14
10:00AM

Davis Clark sat in the waiting room of the FBI office in the Federal Building in downtown St. Petersburg, anxiously awaiting his appointment with Scott Lynwood. His hands were sweating profusely, despite the fact that the air-conditioning was chilling his face. He was constantly rubbing his palms on the cloth of his trousers, an action that the receptionist had noticed with mild revulsion. His heart beat loudly and irregularly, and his stomach churned. God, God, God, what a fool I've been, he thought to himself. When the disinterested secretary told him to go in, he stood on weak knees, and entered Agent Scott Lynwood's office.

"Thank you for coming so promptly, Mr. Clark," Lynwood said, remaining seated behind his desk. He motioned Clark to a chair in the center of the office, facing him. To Clark's surprise and shock, seated in a corner of the office, was Dr. William Coltrane.

"Coltrane!" Clark turned to Lynwood. "What's he doing here?" he demanded.

"Dr. Coltrane is cooperating with my investigation, just as you are, Mr. Clark. Please be seated," Lynwood pointed to the chair again. Clark reluctantly sat. He turned this head awkwardly behind him, nervously aware of Coltrane in his peripheral vision. Coltrane sat in a black leather chair, impeccably dressed in cuffed gray wool trousers, navy blazer and Italian deerskin loafers. Coltrane calmly turned his wedding band on his ring finger, and smiled icily at Clark.

"I am conducting a capital murder investigation into the deaths of Dr. Stephen Hendricks and Carlos Ochoa," Lynwood said aloud, purposefully dictating into a large cassette recorder prominently positioned on his desk. "It is July 14, 10:05AM, and present are Dr. William Coltrane and Mr. Davis Clark." Lynwood paused, and looked straight at Clark. "Both men are voluntarily present at this interview, and consent to the proceedings being recorded. Is that correct?" Lynwood asked.

Both men consented aloud.

"Mr. Clark, please describe to me how you came to be in possession of a microcassette of Dr. Coltrane's conversation with Dr. Hendricks."

"Coltrane asked me to meet him after hours one evening," Clark squirmed in his chair, looking off to the side and behind him to where Coltrane sat. "He had a tape of a conversation with Hendricks, and had a wild scheme to blackmail Strahan's attorney with it. He wanted to get himself off the defendant list in the lawsuit, or something. And he wanted a percentage of the judgment, if Strahan won. The whole scheme was loony, and illegal. I didn't know what to do."

"Did Dr. Coltrane act oddly or inappropriately?" Lynwood asked.

"He was angry about the lawsuit, but that was all."

"But you took the tape?" Lynwood asked benignly.

"Yeah."

"Did Dr. Coltrane play the tape for you?" Lynwood continued.

"No, he just handed it to me and I put it in an envelope."

"He put it directly into your hands?"

"Yes."

"Were you wearing gloves at that time?"

"No."

"Was Coltrane wearing gloves?"

"I don't remember," Clark felt a constricting band tighten around his chest, knowing he was being slowly drawn into a spider's web from which there was no escape.

"I asked you if Coltrane was acting oddly. Wouldn't wearing gloves, indoors, in a social situation be considered very odd?"

"I guess."

"Well, was he wearing gloves or not?"

"No."

"Surgical gloves, leather gloves, any kind of gloves?"

"No." Clark hesitated, confused.

"You saw the microcassette at that time. Did it look unusual?"

"No. Just a cassette. Why?"

"I'll ask the questions, if you don't mind. If the tape implicated Coltrane, why do you think that he would want you to keep it? Wouldn't it make more sense to destroy the tape?"

Clark began to shift uneasily in his chair, looking over his shoulder at Coltrane. He hadn't prepared for the many different avenues down which the interrogation could lead, and half-realized that he was burying himself in lies. Too far gone to extricate himself, he was doomed to continue.

"I don't know. I didn't know what was on the tape. But when I had a chance to listen to it, it was obvious that Coltrane was responsible for the boy's death. So I felt obliged, as an officer of the court, to deliver it to John Alistair, who is Strahan's lawyer."

"Why? Didn't that violate the attorney-client relationship?" Lynwood asked gently.

"No. Coltrane was never my client. He just asked me to put the cassette in the hospital safe. He thought someone was trying to steal it. He was never my client."

"Even so, why did you give it to Strahan's attorney? You have no obligation to Strahan." Lynwood continued to direct Clark toward the answer he wanted.

Clark was silent.

"Are you aware that the microcassette recording had been altered, electronically edited?" Lynwood took another tack.

"No."

"The tape that you gave to Strahan's legal team, was that the original tape? The same tape that Coltrane gave you?"

"As far as I know," Clark slowly responded. He was getting lost, and afraid.

"The FBI lab in Washington examined the tape. It has been altered, and Dr. Coltrane's conversation changed. It's a very good forgery, but as with all analog magnetic tapes, there are unique characteristics of each individual recording. These distinguishing electronic features were obviously altered. In addition, yours were the only fingerprints on the tape cassette. I find that odd."

Lynwood paused in the questioning, and let the silence sit heavily on the room. Clark shifted uneasily in his chair.

"I still don't understand why you gave the tape to Strahan's lawyers. What's your obligation to Strahan?" Lynwood asked again.

Clark shrugged his shoulders, and looked nervously behind him to see Coltrane.

"Isn't it true that you are a member of the Strahan legal team? When did you become involved with that case?" Lynwood demanded.

"Around the time of the tape."

"Before or after you supplied them with the tape?"

"Before."

"Before or after you met with Dr. Coltrane?"

"I think before." Clark glanced over his shoulder at Coltrane, nervously.

"How much before?" Lynwood pressed the questions, even though he already knew all the answers.

"I don't have to listen to this," Clark complained, rising from his chair.

"Read this," Lynwood pushed a folded document across his desk, as he rose from his desk, towering over Clark. It was a signed federal arrest warrant for Davis Clark, citing multiple counts of perjury, falsification of evidence and obstruction of justice. "Cooperate, or I will arrest you right now."

Clark slumped into the chair, and held his head in his hands. He was very close to crying, his breathing fast and shallow. After several moments of silence, he slowly sat up.

"What do you want?" Clark begged.

"The whole truth. Exactly to whom you gave the tape, and why. All your contacts. If you help us, I can help you."

"I have to keep my license," Clark pleaded.

"Your license is long gone, Clark. You'll never practice law again. We're talking about your freedom here. Do you want to go to federal prison?"

"No, no. I have a family. I made a mistake. I got greedy. I gave the tape to an executive at Athena's home office in Atlanta. I knew him from law school, and our fraternity in college. I don't know what he did with it. At first, we were just going to destroy it. Coltrane said that it was the only copy. Then Avery..."

"Avery?" Lynwood interrupted.

"Marc Avery. He's the executive in Atlanta. Then he decided to alter the conversation to get Athena off the hook, and to implicate Coltrane. How he altered it, I don't know. But he returned it to me, and I gave it to Alistair. That's all I know. I did nothing criminal. I didn't alter the tape. I'm just a messenger," Clark pleaded.

"You are much more than just a messenger, Clark. You're an officer of the court and you presented falsified evidence. Furthermore, you destroyed crucial evidence that would have cleared Dr. Coltrane. I have personally begun proceedings to have you disbarred. If it was up to me, you would do time as well," Lynwood growled. He stared contemptuously at the man, and slid a yellow legal pad across the desk to him.

"Give me a handwritten statement, detailing all your contacts with Dr. Coltrane and exactly what went on in his office. Then detail all your phone calls and personal contacts pertaining to the tape from that time to present. You leave one thing out, and you will be in jail by nightfall. My secretary will show you to a conference room," Lynwood rose and led the broken man out of his office, and walked him to his secretary's desk.

Lynwood found Coltrane brooding when he returned to his office. Even from across the room, he could see the arteries in the doctor's temples pulsing hotly. This guy's had a rough month, he thought.

"That slimy asshole," Coltrane spat. "I stitched up his kid in the middle of the night and never asked him for a dime. I agreed to his fees to represent me, he would have made whatever he wanted on that case. And he goes and fucks me anyway. Jesus, some people are such pieces of shit. Strahan is the same thing. He calls me in the middle of the night, begging for my help. I stay up all night calling Miami and trying to help his kid out, never thought of charging him a dime, and he tries to fuck me *too*. Goddamn asshole sues me. Maybe I'm getting old. Maybe I expect too much from people. Now I've got a fucking headache." Coltrane stood up, massaging his temples. "I wanted to choke that prick so bad. What's going to happen to him?"

"That depends on what we get from Marc Avery. I suspect that his story is genuine, and he just delivered the tape to Avery. We'll get a search warrant for Avery's office and see what shakes out. These white collar criminals are quick to deal. They don't want to lose their families, or their comfortable lifestyle. And they're scared shitless of going to prison and getting raped. In all probability, Avery will tell us something."

"Good luck," Coltrane shook Lynwood's hand, and started to leave the office. "By the way, how did you know the tape was a forgery?"

"Do you have an antique wristwatch?" Lynwood asked with a smile.

"No. I don't usually wear a watch. Taking one on and off for surgery gets old. Why?"

"Our technicians picked up a regular, one second interval ticking on the tape. Usually this would be caused by a watch on the wrist of someone holding the phone receiver. That doesn't apply to quartz watches, obviously. When the tape was analyzed, the frequency of the ticking changed at several critical junctures during the conversation. That indicates the sequences that were dubbed. Maybe Hendricks had an old watch."

"No, it was my desk clock. Britt gave me a brass mariner's clock for my birthday one year, and it makes a barely audible ticking. Incredible. Have you found anything on the disc yet?"

"Oh, yeah, I forgot to tell you about that. The lab pulled a couple of good prints off that disc, a thumb of Hendricks and partial index of Ochoa. And the data was transcribed using the same program that Athena uses on all their computers. The HMO, of course, is claiming that they know nothing about any of this. I suspect that they will take the position that the fraudulent billing was the independent criminal act of their rogue employees, and that they bear no responsibility for those acts," Lynwood explained as the two men walked out of his office.

"Will that work?" Coltrane wondered aloud.

"Not in court. But it'll get heavy play in the media, and help avoid a public relations nightmare. Finding a scapegoat is as old as sin itself. By the time this goes to trial, the public will have forgotten the entire mess. My guess is that Athena will pay as much for PR as for their legal defense."

"What next?" Coltrane asked as he headed out.

"I have hundreds of boxes of seized Athena documents to look through and process. If I need you, I'll call. Watch your back, Doc." Lynwood smiled, and turned to return to his office.

Coltrane left the suite of FBI offices, wandered down the wide Federal Building hallways, and down the marble steps into the brilliant Florida sunshine. The heat baked his face, and he felt it warming his skin through his clothes. Sensing the end of this ordeal, he smiled and headed for his F-150.

Chapter 93

AthenaHMO Corporate Offices
Atlanta
July 18
11:45AM

The office on the twenty-sixth floor was expansive, and furnished with impeccable taste. Oriental carpets graced the hardwood floors, and the walls were paneled and wainscoted in solid mahogany. One wall was solid glass floor to ceiling, and commanded a spectacular view of the city skyline. But the fat man seated at the massive desk was not enjoying the view. He was running his hands rapidly and frantically through his thinning hair, as if pounding on his forehead would bring an end to his anguish. Finally, he reached for his phone.

He dialed a three digit extension. The line picked up after one ring.

"I need to talk to you. Right now!" he whispered.

"Of course, sir," the voice responded, "but let's meet for lunch. I'll meet you at Doyle's in an hour."

"Fine," the man sighed, and slowly hung up the phone.

Again he hammered his own forehead, blinding himself with pain and rage. His carefully manipulated world was not responding obediently any more. Over the past few months, Marc Avery's life had gone from a dream to a nightmare. Events, and people, were no longer responding to his omniscient guidance. Anger had slipped into frustration, and frustration had slipped into fear. Now he was fully, completely within the grasp of sheer terror.

His scheme had been brilliant. He had thought it was foolproof. For years, he had planned, designed, deliberated. For years, he spent every spare hour examining his strategy. He looked at the scheme from the inside, and from the outside; he tried to find a flaw, a weakness, an Achilles' heel. A way he could be discovered. Or beaten at his own scheme. In the end, he concluded it was perfect. Then he implemented it.

It had begun when he realized that the Athena board of directors was considering using an outside agency for Medicare and Medicaid billing. It had become simply too expensive to maintain an in-house staff dedicated to Medicare/Medicaid billing, due to the complex and intricate nature of the federal and state governments' constantly changing regulations. Many insurance entities were increasingly relying upon independent contractors to process Medicare/Medicaid claims. And these independent contractors only charged a small percentage of accounts receivable. Of the three agencies bidding, the highest charge was 2.67% of fees received. Less than three cents on the dollar. It was a huge savings to Athena in terms of staffing, personnel, paperwork, employee benefits and pension costs that could not be ignored.

Avery quickly realized that he could profit from this arrangement. Initially, he simply used his insider information to invest modestly in the three front runners in the bidding war for the Athena contract. He set up a small LLC, a limited liability corporation, to shield his identity. Federal law demands full disclosure of all significant investments by board members of a publicly held company, and disclosure of stock option packages, and selling and buying of stock by board members, corporate officers and directors. All this stock market information is available on EDGAR, the US government's website. Avery had a very substantial corporate salary, and he was not willing to lose that as a result of some housewife stockholder doing her due diligence, sitting at home by the computer in a pair of fuzzy slippers. Everything had to be concealed.

When the winner of the billing contract was announced, he invested further. The billing agency was small, only thirty employees, and had made a solid reputation by servicing physicians and outpatient facilities. But it was going to need to expand in order to handle the volume from Athena. Expansion meant money. Avery invested heavily, but he only had so much. He met with the owners, a pair of retired nurses, and advised them well. Through his contacts in the financial sector, he helped them organize a small private stock offering in return for future stock options. Avery purchased stock in the offering as well. Slowly, quietly, he became a major shareholder in the company.

The contract with Athena was complex, and very one sided. Initially, the agency had a two year agreement that could be extended, at the sole discretion of Athena, if so desired. Incentives were in place that benefited both entities. Of specific interest to Avery was the sliding scale provision for the agency's fee. In order to give incentive to the agency to aggressively pursue collections, there were built-in rewards for high collection rates. If the agency was capturing greater than average return, based on quarterly averages, they were given bonuses. The formula was very intricate, but, simply put, the more money for Athena, the more money for the agency.

Initially, Avery was content with the hundreds of thousands of dollars that his scheme was pouring into his LLC. He could not easily spend it without raising suspicions. His marriage was unsteady, and he had no desire to share his ill-gotten gains with his wife and her boyfriend. But greed is a very powerful thing. He realized that if he could boost the billable dollar amount, he could boost the return in two ways. First, any increase in the billable fee would directly increase the return, and therefore the agency's charge. Secondly, if the returns were high enough, the percentage charged could be increased as well. The returns would be boosted exponentially. He sat down with a calculator, and projected his monthly return. When billable fees are in the tens of millions of dollars per day, the income generated was astronomical. He had rubbed his fat little hands with glee.

But now all this was crashing down around him. Everything was happening too fast. The events of the past month had become increasingly chaotic. As he had taken every step, that step had seemed logical, and necessary. It had seemed, each time, that step would solve the complication; end the confusion and extract him from the quagmire. But each time he sank deeper. Like quicksand. Like the tar pit, deeper and deeper into the depths he sank. From insider trading to stock fraud to murder. Now multiple murders were on his bloody hands. He was not equipped to handle this kind of intensity, this kind of gravity. He didn't have the inner strength, the constitution.

He was disintegrating.

An hour later, he entered Doyle's, a trendy downtown pub frequented by a business clientele. In a booth at the far end of the bar sat the head of security for Athena. In recent years, the executive had gradually become involved in increasingly more dangerous and illegal acts using the willing security man as his agent. With each step, he had become more deeply entangled in the web of lies and deceit, but the thrill of danger and the vast wealth he had stolen from the corporation and the government had made the game grow sweeter. The security man seemed to be involved only for the pleasure of the kill.

"I've got big problems," he said breathlessly as he sat opposite the other man.

"The wife again?" The man laughed as he motioned the executive to sit and then placed his index finger to his pursed lips to silence him. He pointed to his ear, and then to the open room, indicating that their conversation may be heard. As he continued with small talk, he reached into his suit pocket and retrieved a small palm held computer. He typed a message on the PDA's LCD screen, and slid it in front of the executive.

Write on this

The message glowed in green letters on the little computer's screen.

The upset executive slowly responded.

Clark has fingered us for the altered tape

Us?

Me

so what. He has no proof. I sanitized the tape case, and no one could trace it to you

they will subpoena me

lawyer up and deny deny deny

what do I say?

That he never gave you any tape, he never gave you anything, you are just old frat buddies

I am scared shitless

that is normal it will pass

I want you to kill clark

no. we already killed hendricks and ochoa. The cops are investigating both jobs and the contract is still out on coltrane. More is insane. Someone will get caught.

Then cancel the contract on coltrane, just kill clark

The head of security read the message and slowly raised his gaze to meet the other man's. The executive sat on the wooden bench, squirming on the hard surface and visibly sweating. His right eye was twitching rapidly, and he was twisting the starched cotton napkin into a crumpled ball. His eyes pleaded. The security man looked at him for a long time.

You don't just cancel the contract, like returning a sweater. You still have to pay him. And I haven't heard from him in weeks he's probably laying low stalking coltrane

I don't care what it costs, work it out with him, just get it done

Fine, but I want twice what you were going to pay my cuban associate for the doctor.

Sure. Of course. But you have to act fast.

When can you have the money?

Tonight. The usual arrangement??

Yes. The usual arrangement.

The executive pushed the little computer back to his companion with a sweaty hand, and leaned back in the booth, sighing heavily. They ordered and ate in silence.

Chapter 94

Isla Pacifica
July 19
10:05AM

The cellphone on the dining room table chirped, and Coltrane answered on the third ring.

"Coltrane, this is Lynwood. I have bad news. Marc Avery has been found dead at his hunting cabin. They think that it was suicide."

"How is that bad news?" Coltrane smiled grimly.

"I don't think it was suicide. I think that the killers are still out there, trying to eliminate all the witnesses against Athena. And you are the linchpin of our entire case. We can make the case against AthenaHMO without your testimony, but having you present to tie Hendricks to Strahan and then to the fraud evidence is very powerful theatre. And trial law is ninety percent theatre. You make a very credible and respected witness. It will be better for Athena if you were absent. I'm afraid you and your wife are in grave danger."

"Now, you think that I'm respectable? A dramatic change from last month, when I was a murder suspect, eh?" Coltrane laughed outloud.

"Just doing my job, Doc. By the way, I should bring you up to date on Ochoa's murder investigation. He was probably killed while you were still in Tampa, on or around June 21. But when his girlfriend came down off her speedballs, she remembered Ochoa getting into a car with a tall, skinny, white male, in front of her apartment late one night. From her vague description of the car, it may match tire tread imprints left near the murder scene. Probably a mid-size rental car. We are canvassing the hundreds of rental facilities in the area, but it will be difficult to find that car. We checked, you haven't rented a car in the past year. And the fingerprint analysis of your office is consistent with a burglary by Ochoa, not a social encounter. So, for the time being, you are not a suspect." Now it was Lynwood's turn to laugh.

"Thanks."

"I would like to arrange a security detail for you and Britt, ASAP."

"I'm really touched by your concern, Lynwood. But we're fine here. Very safe. And you have my testimony on videotape, anyway, right? Even if I'm killed, you can still make the case, right?"

"Sure. Actually, we don't really need your testimony. Your wife was right. All we need is the medical records, and HCFA has the bills Athena submitted. But, the thing is, there may be a killer out there who doesn't know that. He may still try to kill you and your wife. And I've never gotten a satisfactory answer from you or the Bahamian Police about the two men who were looking for you down there. Or how that ties into the murder of the two kids on your boat."

"I am so sorry about them. Innocents." Coltrane was immediately subdued by remembrance of the gruesome murders.

"It appears that those men hired two boats during the time you were in the Exumas, and one boat disappeared without a trace. Along with both men. And the second boat was found abandoned and beached in the area you were cruising. Strange, isn't it?"

"Lotta strange things happen down there, Lynwood. That's in the Bermuda triangle, right? The devil's triangle. Cocaine smuggling. Refugees. Piracy. Bad mojo. Certainly you don't think I had something to do with any of that?"

"You were cleared by the Bahamian authorities with regard to the young couple's murder. You were placed on another island miles away, by several yachtsmen and locals. The mysterious two men who vanished are most likely criminals, who want to stay lost. The Bahamian Police are gradually putting together their movements, but given the number of tourists coming to the Bahamas from all over the world, it will take time. I find it fascinating that the only consistent common thread in the investigation is William Coltrane, MD. What I don't understand is if those two men killed Hendricks and Ochoa, why aren't you even the least bit concerned about them wanting to kill you? Or your lovely wife? Explain to me why they would kill Ochoa when he had nothing to give them; he had no tape, no CD-R. You, on the other hand, have a tape and the CD-R. Yet you seem totally indifferent to the prospect of imminent death. It's the only thing that doesn't make sense in this entire, bizarre story."

"You told me the answer yourself, just minutes ago. You have the evidence you need already, you don't need our testimony. If you recall, I was trying to get that CD-R to you from the beginning. Now, there is no necessity to kill us, we can't do any further harm to Athena at this point. Why risk it?"

"You're still a target, Doc, even if you refuse to admit it. I can't force you to accept protection. But I am going to have the US Marshall Service keep an eye on you both. From a distance. Try not to shoot at them."

"Fine. I am grateful for your concern." Coltrane thanked him, and hung up.

In his office in the Federal Building, Lynwood leaned back in his chair and reflected. The doctor was not telling him everything, there was no question about that. Maybe an examination of the satellite passes for the past few weeks would make for interesting viewing. Even if the US Customs or the French Space Agency photo stills were unproductive, he had other options. There were hundreds of surveillance satellites up there; checking for illegal water resource usage, keeping track of real estate development, monitoring logging and mining operations, and cross-checking tax and permit rolls. Someday, he would have to look into that.

Chapter 95

Gulf of Mexico

Three hundred meters offshore, a small aluminum rental boat was tossed by the swells. The fisherman cursed, as the tide and current ran against the wind, creating an irregular chop, just at the perfect amplitude to unbalance the twelve foot craft. He constantly struggled to keep the bow into the waves, while he peered through his salt encrusted binoculars at the shore. The sea spray, seeping through the fractures in the gasket seals of the cheap lenses, made seeing through the instrument nearly impossible.

The man in the grimy Miami Dolphins cap could barely make out the high rise complex in the distance. Each three foot wave sent his field of view five stories up, then five stories down. He was getting seasick, from the binoculars and the action of the seas. Somewhere in that building, he knew his quarry lay. But where?

The condominium tower was twelve stories high. Perhaps the architect had been a superstitious man. Only five apartments on each floor faced the water on the west side of the building. He had spent six days watching the east, north and south faces of the tower, to no avail. But this kind of work is so much easier on land, he thought. Now, there were still sixty more units to watch. Somehow, somewhere, he would find the doctor that his brother wanted to kill. Lying on the wet bottom of the skiff was a worn lever action Model 94 Winchester. The constant pitching of the boat kept the rifle skittering along the metal, rattling the bargain scope he had hastily attached.

Fear and caution had kept him far offshore. But he could not see into the illuminated windows from that distance, and he was getting tired. His back and hands hurt from the exertion and weather. It was getting colder, and a front was moving in. In anger and frustration, he edged closer to the beach. Soon he was able to make out the residents of the brilliantly lit condos.

Only three units were occupied. One was an obviously older woman, heavy-set, in a billowy house dress. In the second unit, several young children were playing. He knew that the doctor didn't have children. That left the third unit. He motored even closer.

He watched as a man walked from the dining room into a darkened or curtained room, and then back minutes later. The man was talking on a cordless or cellular phone. The conversation seemed animated, and the man was writing on a pad of paper as he spoke.

The man in the boat wanted this guy to be his target. There was an easy way to find out. Fumbling in his jacket, the man found his cell phone. He dialed a number from memory.

"Doctor Coltrane's service," a woman's pleasant voice answered on the second ring.

"Can I speak with the doctor?" the man asked politely.

"Are you a patient?" the operator asked.

"Yes. He saw me in the Emergency Room last month."

"Your name, please?"

"Roberto Huertes." He lied.

"One moment, Mr. Huertes."

As the operator put him on hold, he shifted his gaze to the man in the window. Through the fogged binoculars, he saw the man remove the phone from his ear, and push the keypad twice. Instantly, he heard the connection go through.

"Dr. Coltrane."

"Yeah, hi, Doc. You sewed up my arm last month, and I missed all my appointments. Can I take my stitches out myself?" He watched intently as he spoke into the small phone.

"Does the incision look good?" Coltrane asked.

"Yeah, fine."

"Just come to the office next week. I should take out the stitches. Call the office."

"Okay, thanks." The man in the boat hung up.

As he watched, the man in the condo again lowered the phone, and punched the keypad twice. He continued the conversation that had been interrupted.

This was his guy, the man in the boat thought. If not, he would know tomorrow anyway. He pulled the Winchester onto his lap, and turned the boat closer to the high-rise tower. He hadn't had the time or the knowledge to sight in the scope. But he knew if he was close enough, it would not matter. As he aimed the bow directly at the lit windows, the first raindrops began to fall.

The sky, unseen in the darkness, had become swollen and gray. The tropical moisture, moving up from the Caribbean and the Gulf of Mexico, needed to return to the earth. Through the thick air came raindrops, first small, then larger, until they slammed into the waves with a crescendo of sound. The cold raindrops hit the water with such force that they threw little geysers upward upon impact. The deluge stung his face and hands and eyes. Within seconds, he was drenched to the bone; cold and wet. The storm rapidly obscured his riflescope, and lowered a curtain of water between the boat and the tower.

Screaming curses into the unrelenting storm, the man whipped the boat around, flung the rifle down, and headed back to the rental marina.

There was always tomorrow.

Glossary

Aft	at or toward the rear of the boat
AMBU	a handheld device to pump air into a patient's lungs
Article 553	a law that requires all physicians be notified of a lawsuit
Attending	a practicing physician who has completed all training
BDF	Bahamas Defense Force, fulfills military and police duty
COBRA	Federal legislation governing health insurance issues
Code Blue	Hospital alarm indicating life threatening condition
CPT	Coding system that delineates procedures
CVA	Cerebrovascular Accident, stroke
Discovery	Stage of a trial when facts are presented
DRG	Diagnosis Related Groups, coding by diagnosis
ED	Emergency Department
EDGAR	Electronic Data Gathering, SEC watchdog system
EMT	Emergency Medical Technician
ENT	Ear, Nose and Throat, a surgical specialty
ER	Emergency Room
Fore	at or toward the front of the boat
Forepeak	Triangular storage area in fore of boat
Furling	A method of rolling or storing a sail

GPS	Global Positioning System using satellites
Gunnel	Gunwale, upper edge of boat's side surfaces
H&E	Hematoxylin and Eosin, a stain technique for tissue
HCFA	Health Care Financing Administration, a federal agency
Halyard	a line used to raise sails, booms, flags
Hemodynamics	Pertaining to blood flow and perfusion
HMO	Health Maintenance Organization
ICD-9	Medical diagnosis codes
Intern	Physician, in his or her first year after medical school
IPA	Independent Physicians' Association, HMO variant
Jib	foresail of sailboat, the prime mover of boat
Leeward	Direction the wind is going, sheltered from the wind
Level I Trauma	Designation of the highest level of trauma and care
Main	Sail in the center of a sloop rigged sailboat
Maxillofacial	Surgical specialty treating the face and facial structures
McGuyver	Fictional heroic character known for miraculous feats
MI	Myocardial Infarction, heart attack
MVA	Motor Vehicle Accident
Port	Pertaining to the left side of the boat
PPO	Preferred Provider Organization, a HMO variant
RBRVS	Relative Value System, published by McGraw Hill

Resident	Physician in training, post internship
Rode	a rope used to attach, i.e. the anchor rode
Roller furling	a roller mechanism of retracting a sail on a winding shaft
Rule Out	Medical evaluation to determine if a condition exists
Scut	Dirty, thankless hospital ward work
Sheet	Line on a sailboat, usually attached to a sail
Shoals	Shallow water, or sand bar
Shroud	Metal high tension wires supporting the mast
Starboard	Pertaining to the right side of the boat
STAT	Hospital term meaning extremely urgent
Swami	A surgeons' mocking term for an internist
Telltale	a piece of bright yarn, tied to a shroud, to see wind
Third Party Payer	Insurance companies, government agency payers
Triage	Categorizing and treating injuries by their severity
Universal Fee	Fee payment that covers all aspects of the treatment
Weathervane	Motion a sailboat makes under wind, like a weathervane
Winch	Mechanical device to crank in lines, sheets, halyards
Windlass	Powerful electric winch for raising the anchor
Windward	Direction from which the wind is coming, into the wind
Zodiac	A manufacturer, model of high quality inflatable boats

About the Author

Adrian Philips, MD, is a Board Certified surgeon with the knowledge, perspective and insight into modern medicine only attained through decades of private practice. He writes with the wisdom of an insider, and his work, though fiction, is a naked, brutal prophecy of the impending doom in American healthcare.

Dr. Philips received his Medical Degree from the University of California, then completed General Surgery Residency and a Fellowship in Hand Surgery. He has served on medical insurance review boards, on physician credentialing committees, on medical ethics committees, as chief of his division of surgery, and as an academic teaching professor of surgery. He is an avid outdoorsman and hunter, a certified scuba diver and an accomplished blue water sailor.

www.ingramcontent.com/pod-product-compliance
Ingram Content Group UK Ltd.
Pitfield, Milton Keynes, MK11 3LW, UK
UKHW041431210726
13854UKWH00010B/1873